I0786090

KETOGENIC DIET CROCKPOT COOKBOOK

360

EASY RECIPES

FOR KETOSIS LIFESTYLE

Keto Guide for

Beginners

Oliver Cooper

Text Copyright © Oliver Cooper

All rights reserved. No part of this guide may be reproduced in any form without permission in writing from the publisher except in the case of brief quotations embodied in critical articles or reviews.

Legal & Disclaimer

The information contained in this book and its contents is not designed to replace or take the place of any form of medical or professional advice; and is not meant to replace the need for independent medical, financial, legal or other professional advice or services, as may be required. The content and information in this book has been provided for educational and entertainment purposes only.

The content and information contained in this book has been compiled from sources deemed reliable, and it is accurate to the best of the Author's knowledge, information and belief. However, the Author cannot guarantee its accuracy and validity and cannot be held liable for any errors and/or omissions. Further, changes are periodically made to this book as and when needed. Where appropriate and/or necessary, you must consult a professional (including but not limited to your doctor, attorney, financial advisor or such other professional advisor) before using any of the suggested remedies, techniques, or information in this book.

Upon using the contents and information contained in this book, you agree to hold harmless the Author from and against any damages, costs, and expenses, including any legal fees potentially resulting from the application of any of the information provided by this book. This disclaimer applies to any loss, damages or injury caused by the use and application, whether directly or indirectly, of any advice or information presented, whether for breach of contract, tort, negligence, personal injury, criminal intent, or under any other cause of action.

You agree to accept all risks of using the information presented inside this book.

You agree that by continuing to read this book, where appropriate and/or necessary, you shall consult a professional (including but not limited to your doctor, attorney, or financial advisor or such other advisor as needed) before using any of the suggested remedies, techniques, or information in this book.

Introduction

Greetings! It's great that you have finally found time to join us here!

Nowadays the most part of the people in our society is on the go. The majority of us is busy all the workweek and even on the weekends. This makes us dependent on such things as fast food. Having such a great helper as the Crock Pot is a half of a deal! It saves your time greatly and helps you to be in tempo, you don't need to spend all your time on cooking. But to be the owner of the Crock Pot is a half of a deal, to bring it into production is a must! If you have decided to keep the Ketogenic diet you have made a great challenge. But what if I tell you that the Crock Pot that is standing on the table in your kitchen is a magic wand you have forgot about? Are you looking for some ideas that must correspond your ketogenic diet but don't know how? In this case, you have chosen the right book and moreover, I'm sure you'll find your favorite delicious recipes right here!

If you are a great food lover, the owner of the Crock Pot and you follow the ketogenic diet, you can find here a plenty of necessary information basing on the last achievements of the technic such as the Crock Pot and the benefits of the ketogenic diet. The ketogenic diet includes lots of «complicated» rules, but it will be easier to keep it using this book and recipes in it. The recipes of the Keto Crock Pot Cook Book are rather simple, accessible, adaptable to understand and to perform in the Crock Pot that is in your kitchen already! You can enjoy your favorite products bought at the nearest market or shop. The recipes are divided in the cookbook into easy chapters. So, let's cook together and have fun!

Table of Contents

CHAPTER 1

What is the ketogenic diet?

A keto or another called a ketogenic diet is a widely known diet in the modern world sometimes also called as a low-carb diet that allows the individual's organism to run out rather small fuel molecules that are named "ketones" and are mostly used as a considerable source of the energy. It is used mostly when the blood sugar, another called glucose, is in a short supply. The glucose is actually the easiest molecule in the individual's organism and is exploited as a prime mover. If a person eats food high in carbs, the organism begins to produce both insulin and, of course, glucose. Insulin is generated by the body to remake the glucose in a bloodstream taking it around your body. There is no need for the fats in the organism since the glucose is in an action. In this case, fats are stored in the organism. During a higher carb diet, peoples' organism exploits glucose – it is the main prime mover. By the lower consumption of carbohydrates, the organism is induced into ketosis. The ketones are generated by the organism if an individual eats a low quantity of carbs that are destroyed into the blood sugar quickly, and perform a plenty of protein. The small fuel molecules are generated in the liver from fat then the organism uses as fuel including our important organ - the brain. The last one is «hungry» to consume a lot of energy during all day long and in fact, it can't go along fat directly, but only on ketones or glucose. The main aim of a ketogenic diet is to compel the organism into the metabolic state. The human's body is uncreditable adaptable to everything an individual puts into it – as soon as a person overloads the body with fat taking away all carbohydrates, it begins quickly to burn the ketones. The optimal keto level is a source of person's health and of course, weight loss that is so important for women, it has also both mental and physical benefits. This book could help you in keeping a keto diet based on simple recipes from real foods.

What you can eat during the ketogenic diet

If an individual is not fully sure what is allowed during a keto diet and what must be strictly avoided, this part of our book will be of terrifically use for you! Keeping any diet isn't an easy thing, I think the most part of women know what I'm talking about. It gets more complicated when you have no idea what you should consume today. It may become a real challenge to keep a keto diet if it is new for you. But the quick food list of well complicated keto-friendly foods that an individual can find here is a great helper to make a right choice. Remember the main rule - following this diet you have to be focused on eating real food, but not food low in carbs. A short list of allowed products and of that, you must avoid is introduced to you below. An easy visual guide of the expendable products that correspond to the ketogenic diet is amazing for the beginners who would like to make a right decision on what exactly they are consuming and of course, shopping for.

- *Oils and fats*

Fats make the base of the calorie consume through a day. Here you take the option, what you prefer and what you don't like. Basic lovely dressings, sauces, toppings could be added to your precious chicken or beef, combine them as you wish! Fats are significant for the organism, but a plenty of them could bring you harm. The ketogenic diet allows the next fats and also fats conjunctions: saturated (like ghee, butter, green bacon, coconut oil); as well as monounsaturated fats (nut, avocado, olive oil). Be attentive with polyunsaturated fats (eat fatty fish and animal protein, but strictly avoid margarine spreads). Trans-fats – escape it entirely! This fat is inflected by chemical means they lead to the heart diseases. Keep a counterpoise between the level of omega 6's and omega 3's, consume of tuna, wild salmon, trout will help you to keep this sufficient counterpoise necessary for your health. Pay attention to the general consume for spunk founded foods you know that there is a perfect number of inflammatory omega 6's. Almonds, pine nuts, walnuts, corn oil are of this type of spunk based foods. The food that could be ideal for you keto diet is – animal fat, fatty fish, lard, avocado, ghee, butter, mayo, macadamia/avocado/olive/coconut oil, cocoa and coconut butter, vitellus, tallow. Among the wild savage springs and grass-fed meat are such as lamb, beef or lamb, seafood and wild-caught fish, pastured pork, grass-fed and namely heart, liver or kidneys as well as the organ meats.

- *Protein*

Chose the dark meat it means poultry because it includes more fat than the white meat like chicken. If you prefer to eat red meat it is not so much to elude here, eat a ribeye, ground beef. What according to the sausages you have to elude buying those with added sugar. Don't consume too much protein, because it can cause the low level of ketone production, as a result, it will cause in the heightened production of non-wished glucose. Some examples of allowed products you will find right here: fish (flounder, cod, mackerel, halibut etc.); shellfish (lobster, mussels, clams, oysters); beef (steak, stew meat, roasts etc.); eggs; pork, liver, kidney, heart etc.; poultry; goat; lamb; turkey; sausages and bacon (control the labels of sausages!); nut butter (unsweetened and natural nuts, eat the fattier versions of it).

- *Fruit and veggies*

The best random among the vegetables for this diet is green and leafy, they are grown above the ground. What according to veggies that grow below the ground, consume them in moderation. Actually try to eat your favorite vegetables in moderation or for a flavor. The vegetables that allowed to eaten are: spinach, lettuce, chives, radicchio, endive, etc.; radishes, kale, kale turnip, asparagus, summer squash, cucumber, bamboo shoots. Eating berries strictly control the level of carb in them.

- *Dairy (milk)products*

Milk products are usually consumed by an individual within a keto diet in a complex with other variety of products. The better part of an individual's consumed foods must be based on veggies, added fats. Favored are organic, raw products, chose full fat products. For those individuals who are lactose sensitive, consume indefinitely long-term storage and some hard dairy. The patterns of the dairy products are: mozzarella, blue, brie, Monterey Jack, Greek yogurt, spreadable, hard cheese (Swiss or etc.), mayo, mascarpone, sour crème etc.

- *Spunks and nuts*

You may take spunks and nuts, especially when they are parched, using them as appetizers or as flavorings to the main dish. If it is conceivable exclude peanuts, as these nuts are legumes. I think, you know, the nuts are a perfect spring of fat, that's why be attentive consuming them in keeping your level of protein. Next time around, you open the wrapping of nuts, remember what you are allowed to: Brazil and macadamia nuts, pecans, almonds, walnuts, pine nuts, peanuts, hazelnuts also.

- *Spices and cooking*

Sauces and seasoning are intricate part of the keto diet, but an individual still continue to use his/her preferable ones. There is no reason to roll all the allowed and avoided species, as there are a great number of them at the market stores. Some of them are amazing to use the others – have high glycemic index. The sea salt is preferable than table salt. The spices and habitual herbs that are allowed to this type of diet are: cinnamon, chili powder, cayenne pepper, Greek oregano, cumin, cilantro, basil, rosemary, parsley, thyme. Be sure, you can consume pepper and salt without worrying.

- *Sauces and condiments*

The groutings, sauces as well as other condiments are at the twilight zone on keto diet. Principally, if you try to keep strictly the keto diet, you should avoid the most part of all beforehand prepared sauces as they could have commonly obtained sugars and sweeteners as aren't appropriable on the diet. The sauces or some gravies that you select to cook must be based on xanthan gum or guar. They are low carb than the others. Also, it depends on a brand mark some of sauces could include sugar some of them are without that's why you have to read the ingredients on the label attentively! The allowed are: mustard, Dijon mustard, ketchup, hot sauce, mayo, sauerkraut (without sugar or low), relish, Worcestershire Sauce, salad dressings (the fattier ones), flavored syrups (with permitted sweeteners).

- *Sweeteners*

It will be not so easy to keep this keto diet for those individuals who are real sweet-tooth. But running all from something sugary is also possible by two means – by keeping a floor stage of them or by using the substitutes. If you still wish to consume sweeteners, chose the fluid versions. You may also identify that tastes better for you as it is a great number of diverse sorts and new altered substitutions of them. The most popular are: Stevia (preferred in liquid form), sucralose (rather sweet substitution), monk fruit, erythritol etc.

- *Beverages*

Among the preferred beverages during a keto diet are coffee with coconut milk or cream, water, black or herbal tea.

What you can't eat during the ketogenic diet

And now, after you have already a clear agenda of products you might consume during a ketogenic diet, it is the right time to complete the roll of forbidden products. If you still have a thought you are not sure about the products that aren't keto appropriated, the enquire schedule will definitely help you:

- Sugar – it could be found almost in soda, mostly all juice, the plurality of sports drinks, sweet candies (even if these are your favorite ones!), chocolate, ice cream.
- Grains - the wheat products (these include also bread and buns), gruels, pasta, cakes, paddy and corn, beer must be escaped too. Here we include also whole grains like rye, wheat, buckwheat, barleycorn and quinoa.
- Starch – during the keto diet an individual has to escape some vegetables (like potatoes, yams) oats, etc. Only some of the edible vegetables are well in moderation.
- Trans-fats – paste like alternate butter like margarine and other variations of it should be escaped as they maintain hydrogenated fats. These are also bad for our health.
- Fruit – a person who is keeping the low-starches diet must escape consuming large fruits like apples, bananas, oranges, because of the reason they include an extremely high rate of sugar. Consume the berries in moderation, check the labels if you buy them at the store markets.
- Low-fat foods – these products admit as usual much higher in carbs and sugar than other full-fat versions. Be sure you read the package at the store to escape mistakes.
- Factory-farmed pork and fish - are almost high in inflammatory omega 6 fatty acids, farmed fish could include PCBs, escaping fish high in mercury.

- Milk isn't recommended because of some reasons (what according to full-fat milk it is allowed). First of all, it is rather complication to digest, it lacks the "good" bacteria and even maintain hormones. Then it is high in starches (it is about 5 grams of starches per about 100 ml). As for coffee and tea, if you prefer to drink them with milk, substitute milk with cream, but in this way follow the reasonable amounts.

-    Sweet and alcoholic drinks (sweet wine, beer, all the mixed drinks, etc.).

- Pistachios and cashews - consumed rarely as they're very high in starches (for example, two fulfils of cashews is almost a clear day's allowance of starches).

Benefits of the ketogenic diet

Despite the variety of the diets that have come and still take someplace at people's life with more or less success level, the ketogenic or the keto diet has been started to practice not so long ago. This type of diet is fully based on the knowing theoretically and understanding of nutrition science and human's physiology. When an individual relies upon counting the consumed calories, sorting the portions, avoiding fats strictly, the keto diet works in a full difference through changing a «fuel spring» that an individual uses to keep energy and be fit all day long 7/24. But the ketogenic diet hasn't met an agreement among the professors and food/health professionals at once. Since 2002 more than 15 studies were based on the rules and principals of the ketogenic diet. Almost everyone has proved that this diet was at the top three of the other diets. Below you could find the reasonably benefits of a keto diet, they are 1 – the ketogenic diet kills the appetite: hunger was always the adverse reaction to any diet you have already practiced. This is the main reason why individuals refuse and terminate the diets. Consuming fats and low-carb products reduces the appetite. 2 – Keeping the keto diet allows you to lose more weight than during other diets: the main reason of this point is that fact, the low-carbs tend to get rid of overage liquid from the human's organism. People, who keep this keto diet, could lose weight two times quicker. The keto-diets seem to be effective for up to 5 months, after this time an individual's body begins to creep back, it occurs usually when individuals give up and begin to eat the old products. 3 – The fat loose of the abdominal cavity. The bodies of the individuals differ from each other. People have two fat storages – in the abdominal cavity, it means the visceral fat, and, subcutaneous fat, it means under the skin. The keto diet reduces the visceral fat of the organism that could lead to insulin stamina, distraction, and is the mainspring of metabolic indigestion. 4 – The fat moieties called triglycerides tend to go to zero. 5 – The level of the high-density lipoprotein (HDL) that is also called as the «good» cholesterol could be increased thanks to the keto diet. The higher is the level of the individual's HDL, the lower is the risk to suffer from the heart disease. Eating fat is the best way to increase your HDL level. 6 – The ketogenic diet reduces the insulin level and the level of sugar in blood through escaping the consuming of the carbs that are dragged down into glucose in the gastrointestinal tract. 7 – The ketogenic diet reduces the high blood tension and as a result, the risk of saccharine disease gets lower. 8 – It is a good method against the metabolic syndrome. The last one is the medical condition that is also combined with heart problems risk and diabetes. 9 – The keto diet is good for brain disorders because of therapeutic effect. A part of an individual's brain can incinerate the glucose only. But the other one can also burn ketones that are mostly formed, for example during starvation. The method of the keto diet was applied earlier for treating epilepsy by kids. Nowadays this diet is being searched for Parkinson's and Alzheimer's disease.

Keto for beginners

Now you know the most information about the ketogenic diet, what to eat and what products are not allowed. I hope you have already understood how healthy is this type of the diet and you are going to keep it right with me. Sure, every beginning is rather complicated, but if you have a Crock Pot in the kitchen it solves the majority of problems that could arise. In order to decrease the difficultness of the keto beginning, try to consume keto food slowly, week after week. Remember that the keto diet could change the mineral and water balance at the organism, that's why you may add some extra salt to the consumed food. It is essential to eat until fullness, escaping restricting calories too much. A short list of frequently asked questions according to the keto diet using the Crock Pot will definitely help you at the starting stage:

- Is it dangerous for health to refuse eating carbs fully? – No, after some months (2-3) you might eat them occasionally, but then return to the keto diet cooking your meals at the Crock Pot.
- I have heard ketosis is dangerous. Is it true? – Don't modificate the ketoacidos with ketosis. Ketoacidosis occurs in uncontrolled diabetes. By the way, using your Crock Pot by cooking is already healthier than usual cooking and roasting without it.
- Must I count my calories? – Be attentive of them, read the labels at the markets and escape fat-trans and sweeteners.
- May I prepare the dishes late at the evening to eat them in the morning for breakfast? – Sure, cook at your great helper and then turn on WARM, in the morning you will have the warm breakfast at table.
- How much protein should I eat? – Don't eat it too much, the high level of eat could increase of the insulin level at the organism. Consume not more than 30-40% of general calorie intake.
- Is it possible to combine the keeping of keto diet with the high rhythm of my life as I work all day long 7/24? – Sure! This keto Crock Pot cookbook is definitely for you! Save time, eat well and keep the diet!

Moreover, the keto diet using the crock pot is great for diabetics, people who are overweight, busy men and women, moms and dads.

CHAPTER 2

Crock Pot. What is it?

I think every person has already heard this combination of words «the Crock Pot» in his/her life. It is appeared in 1970, marketed as only a bean cooker. But as it was modified it was almost used to heat the food and dishes for a long period of time. With time humans began to use it mostly for cooking delicious dishes. It is a small perfect kitchen appliance contains a glass lid, a porcelain or a ceramic pot (it is inside of the heating unit) and, of course, a heating element. The modern Crock Pots could be of oval or round form and of various sizes, from small ones to bigger. All the Crock Pots have two regulations: LOW (it corresponds to the temperature of 200°F mostly) and HIGH (up to the temperature 300°F). The WARMing option that is among the options of the majority of the Crock Pot nowadays allows keeping the prepared dish warm for a long period of time. Some of the Crock Pot models have a timer that allows you to control cooking time if you are busy.

What are the benefits of using the Crock Pot?

What is the most difficult for you in the kitchen? You spend too much time in the kitchen when you might go to the cinema with friends? You spend too much money for products and your fantasy of what to prepare today is running down? I know the solution to all your problems… It is the Crock Pot!

Firstly, it is possible to prepare meals when you are not at home. If the mornings of your family are the crazy beginning, just put all the ingredients following the recipe, switch the machine and go work.

Second, you don't prefer washing the dishes? Me too! Just clean the Crock Pot and the plates after delicious meals. That's all! Crock Pot means fewer dishes to wash.

Third, the Crock Pot cooks the delicious meals and save your money!

These meals taste even better than usual you may eat it the next day or even keep the dish in the refrigerator. How perfect are the species at the dishes if you eat them right after cooking! You might taste the cayenne pepper, cumin, ginger and other favorite species of yours. Buy simple products and follow the cookbook. It is easy!

Fourth, the Crock Pot is the best way to keep your meal tender and always warm.

Fifth, the Crock Pot reduces calories and fat. No oil (just olive or avocado oil), no frying is necessary.

Six, step by step preparation.

Step by step preparation facilitates the everyday cooking especially for those who are not the great lover of this process. In the most recipes, all the ingredients are added at one time to the Crock Pot.

Seven, it is energy saving. It needs less electricity in comparison with the usual oven.

The flexibility of the Crock Pot. You can take it to the trip, put it on the kitchen table or somewhere else. It doesn't need too many places.

And finally - large quantities of final foods. The most of the recipes make large quantities of the end products, so you may feed all the family and even freeze for tomorrow, make easy and quick lunches or suppers.

So, are you already looking for some recipes to get started? Check my great keto Crock Pot cookbook and you'll find the best and delicious dishes there! Cooking keto recipes in the Crock Pot will help you to manage day schedule and be healthy. After a long working day, you'll back home and delicious meal will wait for you.

CHAPTER 3

28-Day Ketogenic Diet Plan

Everybody is looking for the diets that are easy to follow. The keto diet with the list of the recipes prepared in the Crock Pot and meal plan for each week is everything you are looking for. When it comes to starting the keto diet, you must have a plan.

Firstly, you must make sure of what you are eating and what you actually need to be fully satiated. Moreover, you must be sure you're satisfied with what you're eating. I'm sure, if someone has to force himself/herself to eat something, it will never work out in the end. This is just a short guideline on how a person can eat following a ketogenic diet. So, you are welcome to change your lifestyle and a kind of foods you eat every day! What's more, it's of great importance to make sure your ketogenic diet is well-planned when you are eating keto-style products, because these products you can choose from are limited. I advise you to check your most recent bloodwork levels for the things such as vitamin D, cholesterol and other indicators of health because these can be changed while you are following the keto diet.

I tried to make the best meal plan for you, but I'd ask you to look a few days ahead in the meal plan, as you have to know what you are going to eat, the list of the products you need to buy, etc. If you have already cooked some recipes during the first week, you are also welcome to reuse them again. I also advise you to freeze some things if you have too many leftovers, as these products could be also re-used later on! Make sure that you are drinking a lot of water and eating enough amount of salt. Keeping the water and salt intake high enough is of great importance, allowing the body to re-supply and re-hydrate the electrolytes. If you are worried about consuming salt and high blood pressure, don't be! The recent studies have shown that the blood pressure and sodium intake are not as correlated as people so once believed.

Further, I suggest you buying some special items prior to need them for cooking. Usually, the most part of these items could be easily found in the stores or online if you wish, and by the time you need them, you will actually have them. Make a short list of what you order firstly and have it by the time you need it.

1st week of the ketogenic diet

Breakfast

During the first week, some people have a drastic cut of carbohydrates that leave them really hungry. The thoughts, they have to count carbs, what is allowed to eat and what is actually forbidden attacks the brain and as a result, a person gets fully dissatisfaction with the keto diet. Be sure, the appetizers you may cook in the Crock Pot and eat early in the morning or before breakfast could help to prevent your crazy hunger feelings during the first week. Eat more greenery and vegetables. The main goal during the first week is to stay rather simple at first. I think simplicity is a key for somebody that is just starting out on a keto diet. I'm sure, nobody wants to keep a difficult diet, because it could be boring and lasting during the first week (and second week also). For breakfast, you want to get something tasty, quick and easy. I suggest starting the first week from cooking light and easy recipes in the Crock Pot. The first week must be rather simple for you. Nobody wants to cook breakfast before going to work! You can use leftover meat from previous nights or use easy accessible canned fish or chicken. Using canned fishy or meats, don't forget to read the labels at the stores and get that one that corresponds to the keto diet!

Dinner

Dinner is usually a combination of soups or stews with some essential dishes of fish or meat. I highly recommend you to use leafy greens (usually, cauliflower, broccoli or spinach) with some meat. You are going high on the fat and moderate on the protein. Keep in mind that every person has different needs. So do you. You will also have to adjust the keto plan as you lose weight since your needs will change. Some people are rather busy during a day. Staying all day long in the office they don't have a chance to have a normal dinner, to eat soups or stews and moreover to cook them in the Crock Pot. This time, I recommend you to have an essential meal for dinner (even if it happens rather late) but remember – do not overeat. I don't recommend you to consume at the end of the day all you have in your fridge.

Supper

It's a pity, but **No** dessert for supper time for the first 2 weeks… Yes! But I'm sure, following my recommendations it is rather simple to keep the keto rules and don't eat desserts at all. Only first two weeks.

So, here you have a diet plan that includes breakfast, dinner, and supper with different variations of dishes depending on the products you prefer to eat. Dinner includes soups (stews) as well as an essential meal of meat dishes. The vegetarians and those who prefer eating the seafood can find the correspondent dish plans here also. Breakfast and supper include two recipes you must choose depending on your preference.

Monday (the first week)

Breakfast:　　Scrambled eggs with smoked salmon

(alternative) Broccoli and Cheese Stuffed Squash

Dinner:　　Ginger and turmeric keto dip

(alternative) Crock Pot veal stew /

For those who prefer seafood: Crock Pot Tuna Mornay /

For the vegetarians: Crock Pot keto aubergines

Supper:　　Crock Pot keto Pesto chicken

(alternative) Keto cheese pancetta cauliflower

Tuesday:

Breakfast:　　Garlic-Parmesan Asparagus Crock Pot

(alternative) Crock Pot benedict casserole

Dinner:　　Crock Pot Moroccan lamb stew

(alternative) Crock Pot creamy salsa chicken /

For those who prefer seafood: Crock Pot Indian fish curry /

For the vegetarians: Italian vegetable keto bake

Supper: Crock Pot Sausage and Fennel

(alternative) Keto easy cheesy zucchini gratin

Wednesday:
Breakfast: Keto broccoli and bacon Alfredo /

(alternative) Persian omelet Crock Pot

Dinner: Keto garlic butter chicken

(alternative) Keto Crock Pot pizza soup /

For those who prefer seafood: Crock Pot keto sea bass /

For the vegetarians: Crock Pot pumpkin chili recipe

Supper: Lemon Herb veal Crock Pot

(alternative) Zucchini noodles in a creamy tomato sauce

Thursday:
Breakfast: Keto seafood dip Crock Pot

(alternative) Keto crock pot gingerbread with Crock Pot cauliflower hummus recipe

Dinner: Crock Pot chicken Thai soup

(alternative) For those who prefer seafood: Keto shrimp Crock Pot /

For the vegetarians: Keto Vindaloo vegetables /

Supper: Crock Pot White Chicken Chili

(alternative) Squeak and Bubble Crock Pot

Friday:
Breakfast: Garlic butter Keto spinach

(alternative) Keto Crock Pot chili recipe

Dinner: Crock Pot Zuppa Toscana soup

(alternative) Keto meaty paleo chili /

For those who prefer seafood: Jamaican salmon Crock Pot recipe /

For the vegetarians: Crock Pot vegetable soup

Supper: Crock Pot Scrambled Eggs with Green Herbs

(alternative) Cheddar cauliflower bacon bites Crock Pot

Saturday:
Breakfast: Keto Crock Pot tasty onions

	(alternative) Keto pumpkin spice pie
Dinner:	Hearty Crock Pot Fish Stew
	(alternative) Crock Pot sweet garlic chicken /
	For the vegetarians: Crock Pot easy keto soup /
Supper:	Italian sausage and egg bake
	(alternative) Crock Pot Keto Cheesy zucchini

Sunday:

Breakfast:	Keto sweet kielbasa /
	(alternative) Bacon, Egg and Cheese Bread Boxes
Dinner:	Keto Crock Pot Chicken Soup
	(alternative) Crock-Pot Beef Tips Recipe /
	For those who prefer seafood: Broiled Sea Bass with Chili Basil Glaze /
	For the vegetarians: Crock Pot Broccoli Tofu soup
Supper:	Crock Pot Yorkshire Pudding /
	(alternative) Rosemary garlic cauliflower Crock Pot

Here I have prepared the list of the products you need for cooking during the first week. Of course, it may vary depending on the dishes you choose, preparing a seafood or meat, or keeping the vegetarian eating plan.

Food list for the first week:

Cauliflower	3-5 heads
Broccoli	0,5 lb
Aubergines	0,5 lb
Pesto sauce	1 package
fat cream cheese	5 ounces
unsalted butter	2 tablespoons
garlic	20 cloves
fresh rosemary	1 bunch
shrimp	2 - 3lbs
Worcestershire sauce	1 bottle
BBQ sauce	1 can

yellow onion	5 -10 pcs
hot green chilies	2-5 small
fresh ginger	2-3 pcs
ground cumin	1 package
ground coriander	1 package
brown mustard seeds	1 package
ground turmeric	1 package
tomatoes	1 lb
sweetener	1 package
Kosher salt	
fish fillets (such as tilapia, cod or halibut)	3-5 lb
tuna	1 lb
sea bass	1 lb
chicken breasts	2 -4 pounds
olive oil	1 can
Splenda	1 package
ground beef	1-2 pounds
chunks of beef	1 pound
green pepperoncini	2 pcs
bell pepper	1 package
tomatoes	1 can
chili powder	1 package
bone broth	1 can
almond flour	1 package
garam masala	1 package
curry powder	1 package
chicken thighs	3 lb(s)
cashews	1 package
jalapeno pepper	1 pcs
tomato paste	1 can

Greek yogurt	1 package
salsa	1 package
taco seasoning	2 ounces
cream of celery soup	2 ounces
dried oregano	1 package
avocado	2-3 pcs
Italian sausage	1 pound
kale	1 head
coconut milk	2 cans
chicken stock	2 can
fish sauce	1 can
peanut butter	1 package
mozzarella cheese	0,5 lb
Parmesan cheese	0,5 lb
Cheese cheddar	1 lb
Cheese American	0,5 lb
Lobster	1 large
Shrimps	0,5 lb
Crabmeat	0,5 lb
Bay leaf (optional)	1 package
Gouda cheese	0,5 lb
Eggs	10 pcs
Bacon	0,5 lb
Pumpkin	2 pcs
Lemon	1 pcs
Spinach	0,3 lb
Green herbs	1 package
Kielbasa	0,5 lb
Tofu cheese	0,5 lb
Zucchini	4-5 pcs

Fennel   3-4 pcs

2nd week of the ketogenic diet

So, the first week is over. I'm sure if you follow my instructions you must still do well on the ketogenic diet and realize simply it is so easy breezy to keep on track with everything!

Breakfast

The next week (week two) you are going to keep it simple for breakfast again. Don't forget about fats! Eating fat leads to greater amounts of energy, efficient energy usage during a whole day and more effective weight loss (don't forget about his option!). I think, you have already understood - it's the main component of the keto diet. I don't think the rules of this diet are rather difficult for you, but make your diet easier - feel free to add various sweeteners and spices to this if you're not the biggest fan of the taste. Vanilla extract, cinnamon, stevia, hot chili... Whatever you like, it will get your dish great taste. You may even switch up the taste every day so you don't get bored! If you have long periods of breakfast and dinner, you are busy at work, so just incorporate more meat or fish to the breakfast. Green vegetables and high-fat dressings are the key points. Make sure to balance out the fats with the amounts of protein that is very important.

Dinner

We are going to eat meats, vegetables, soups and stews, high-fat dressings that are the center of the keto diet. Don't over think things during the first two weeks; remember, simple is a success.

Supper

You may vary from both dishes listed below or from the general list you would like something else. Don't take the meal right before going to bed. This way your keto diet will not work absolutely. Balance the meat (fish) consuming with essential amount of vegetables prepared in the Crock Pot. No desserts for this week either, wait a little bit for the next one!

Monday (the second week):

Breakfast: Cauliflower with celery puree and garlicky greens

                (alternative) Crock Pot Scrambled Eggs with Green Herbs /

Dinner: Keto Beef Stroganoff Soup Crock Pot

                (alternative) Keto chicken curry Crock Pot /

                Seafood: Sea bass with fennel and tomatoes in Crock Pot /

                Vegetarian: Crock Pot cauliflower Bolognese with zucchini noodles

Supper: Creamy Greek Zucchini Crock Pot

                (alternative) Keto bacon and Goat cheese cauliflower

Tuesday:

Breakfast: Twice baked spaghetti squash Crock Pot

                (alternative) Bacon, Egg and Cheese Bread Boxes

Dinner: Crock Pot vegetable and lamb soup

(alternative) Chicken sliders with an Indian twist /

Seafood: Crock Pot cod with red curry /

Vegetarian: Easy Vegetarian Roasted Chestnut Soup

Supper: Crock Pot French onion-zucchini

(alternative) Mashed Cauliflower with Chives and Parmesan cheese

Wednesday:

Breakfast: Keto Crock Pot cheesy smoky

(alternative) Keto Crock Pot zucchini bread

Dinner: Southern keto soup recipe

(alternative) Crock-Pot Homemade Italian Beef Recipe /

Seafood: Pepper lemon tilapia with asparagus

Vegetarian: Crock Pot keto ratatouille

Supper: Keto collard with cherry tomatoes

(alternative) Cauliflower with mustard butter

Thursday:

Breakfast: Brussels Sprouts with Lemon and Pine Nuts

(alternative) Broccoli Gratin with Parmesan and Swiss cheese

Dinner: Keto Crock Pot BBQ chicken soup

(alternative) Crock Pot Strawberry-Habanero Pulled Chicken /

Seafood: Crock Pot Seabass in Coconut Cream Sauce /

Vegetarian: Crock Pot cauliflower Bolognese with zucchini noodles

Supper: Cauliflower with celery puree and garlicky greens

(alternative) Asiago zucchini and sun-dried tomato bread

Friday:

Breakfast: Crock-Pot keto artichoke, spinach recipe

(alternative) Keto bacon cheeseburger pie Crock Pot

Dinner: Keto pumpkin and coconut soup Crock Pot

(alternative) Seafood: Crock Pot Vietnamese Braised Catfish /

Vegetarian: Creamy Roasted Red Pepper Soup /

Supper:	Cauliflower casserole with tomato and Goat cheese /
	(alternative) Crock Pot veal meatballs with tomato sauce

Saturday:

Breakfast:	Crock Pot cream cheese French toast
	(alternative) Garlicky zucchini noodles with Buratta and tomatoes
Dinner:	Keto pumpkin and coconut soup Crock Pot
	(alternative) Crock Pot Pulled Pork with Fried Shallots and Chiles /
	Seafood: Crock Pot creamy garlic king prawns /
	Vegetarian: Crock Pot Mediterranean eggplant salad
Supper:	Cauliflower casserole with tomato and Goat cheese
	(alternative) Crock Pot chicken with 40 garlic cloves

Sunday:

Breakfast:	Keto small meatballs the Mediterranean
	(alternative) Keto Crock Pot turkey stuffed peppers /
Dinner:	Crock Pot Andouille sausage cabbage soup
	(alternative) Crock Pot keto whole chicken in a hot sauce /
	Seafood: Crock Pot spicy barbecue shrimp recipe /
	Vegetarian: Crock Pot flavor Brussels sprouts
Supper:	Low Carb Spinach & Artichoke Dip Cauliflower Casserole
	(alternative) Crock Pot Pulled Pork with Fried Shallots and Chiles

Food list for the second week:

onion	5-8 pcs
garlic	10 cloves
ginger root	2 thumb-size pieces
garam masala	1 package
cumin	1 package
turmeric	1 package
cayenne pepper	1 package
coconut milk	3 cans

tomato paste	1 can
chicken thighs	3 lb
whipping cream	2 cans
beef roast	3 pounds
Italian dressing dry mix	1 package
pepperoncini peppers	16 ounces (1 jar)
beef broth	3-4 cans
strawberry purée	1 can
Sweetener	1 package
vinegar	1 bottle
liquid smoke	1 bottle
chicken breasts	1 pound
avocado	1 pcs
pork shoulder	3 lb(s)
barbecue sauce	1 bottle
sweetener	1 package
chili powder	1 package
scallions	3 pcs
Vegetable oil	1 bottle
Eggs	10 pcs
almond flour	1 package
Fresno chilies	4 pcs
caraway	1 package
whole chicken	1 pcs 4- to 5-lb
Ketchup	1 package
andouille sausage	12 ounces
cabbage	1 medium head
chicken broth	1-2 cans
beef rump steaks	2 large pcs
Dijon mustard	1 package

lemon	1 pcs
Cauliflower	2 small heads
Parmesan cheese	1 lb
coconut flour	1 package
baking soda	1 package
xanthan gum	1 package
eggs	10 pcs
zucchini	2- pcs
walnuts or pecans	1 package
squash	2-3 pcs
fennel	2-3 pcs
asparagus	1 lb
collard	1 pcs
artichoke	1 lb
spinach	0,5 lb
pumpkin	2-3 pcs
bacon	1 lb
Goat cheese	0,5 lb
Green Herbs	1 package
Lamb	3 lb
Cod	1 pcs
Tilapia	2 lb
Veal	3 lb
Prawns	1 lb
Shrimp	1 lb

3rd week of the ketogenic diet

The third week I'm going to inform you that you are going to get full of fats in the morning during breakfast and all the way until dinner time. It's also easy for your both cooking and eating schedule.

Breakfast

I recommend eating the breakfast at 7 am and then having dinner and supper in 4-5 hours. No lunch! Don't worry – the fats from the breakfast will keep you feeling energized and full all the time till afternoon. This will help put your body into a fasted state, at this time the body of a person can break down the extra fat that is stored mostly for the energy it needs. Breakfast should come to quite a lot of calories and keep you definitely full all the time to dinner. Remember to continue drinking water to be sure you are staying hydrated. When you don't get the success of the food you eat or the process of keeping keto diet, don't to worry about it try to cook more delicious using the Crock Pot!

Dinner

Dinner is staying the same as previous week. Fish, a variety of meats, stews and soups, cooked vegetables, and fats are almost always going to be the dinnertime norm.

Supper

After a hard working day or even during weekends it is highly recommended to eat some vegetable side dishes and fish or meat for a supper. Use hot and spicy dressings to make the dishes tastier. And… this week you may finally eat desserts! Don't be skeptical – desserts prepared in the Crock Pot and sugar-free will not damage your ketogenic diet!

Monday (the third week):

Breakfast: Crustless Crock Pot Spinach Quiche with Savory keto bread Crock Pot

Dinner: Crock Pot Authentic Scotch broth

(alternative) Crock Pot keto whole chicken in a hot sauce /

Seafood: Crock Pot spicy barbecue shrimp recipe /

Vegetarian: Crock Pot vegetarian stew keto recipe

Supper: Brussels Sprouts with Lemon and Pine Nuts

Desserts: Chewy ginger cake Crock Pot

Tuesday:

Breakfast: Crock Pot Brussels sprouts casserole

Dinner: Keto Crock Pot Chicken Cordon Bleu soup

(alternative) Crock Pot Pulled Pork with Fried Shallots and Chiles /

Seafood: Crock Pot spicy barbecue shrimp recipe /

Vegetarian: Crock Pot vegetarian stew keto recipe

Supper: Keto Pork Meatballs in Marinara Sauce

(alternative) Roasted Summer Squash with Lemon, Mint, and Feta

Desserts:	White Chocolate Green Tea Mug Keto Cake

Wednesday:
Breakfast:	Keto Crock Pot meatloaf breakfast

Dinner:	Crock Pot Andouille sausage cabbage soup

(alternative) Keto Veal With Cabbage Crock Pot /

Seafood: Crock Pot Vietnamese Braised Catfish /

Vegetarian: Crock Pot Mediterranean eggplant salad

Supper:	Crock Pot caramelized onion beef stew

Desserts:	Keto lemon coconut cake with cream cheese icing

Thursday:
Breakfast:	Cauliflower casserole with tomato and Goat cheese

Dinner:	Old-fashioned Crock Pot veal stew

(alternative) Keto pork roast with creamy gravy /

Seafood: Mediterranean octopus casserole /

Vegetarian: Red Thai veggie curry

Supper:	Asiago zucchini and sun-dried tomato bread

(alternative) Crock Pot Butternut Dhal

Dessert:	Crock Pot Pumpkin Pecan Bread Pudding

Friday:
Breakfast:	Crock Pot keto «English muffin»

Dinner:	Crock Pot keto Hungarian beef stew

(alternative) Crock Pot chicken and broccoli /

Seafood: Crock Pot sole in onion sauce /

Vegetarian Korma Crock Pot keto

Supper:	Keto ginger pork with broccoli

Desserts:	Crock Pot raspberry-vanilla pudding cake

Saturday:
Breakfast:	Keto Crock Pot Mediterranean frittata

Dinner:	Crock Pot spicy chicken stew

(alternative) Seafood: Crock Pot crab and shrimp bisque /

Vegetarian: Crock Pot tomato soup recipe /

Supper: Jalapeno popper cauliflower casserole

Desserts: Chocolate-Cinnamon Latte Cake Recipe

Sunday:

Breakfast: Greek eggs breakfast casserole

Dinner: Keto Crock Pot buffalo chicken soup

(alternative) Crock Pot chicken gizzard recipe /

Seafood: Crock Pot Soy-Ginger Braised Squid /

Vegetarian: Crock Pot flavor Brussels sprouts

Supper: Low Carb Spinach & Artichoke Dip Cauliflower Casserole

(alternative) Crock Pot Chicken Korma

Desserts: Crock Pot giant chocolate pie recipe

Food list for the third week:

Eggs	10 pcs
Almond milk	1 package
dried oregano	1 package
baby arugula	1 package
red peppers	2-3 pcs
red onion	1 pcs
Goat cheese	1 lb
Spinach	0,3 lb
Brussels sprouts	6-10 pcs
Lemon	2 pcs
Shallots	10 pcs
Squash	2-3 pcs
Mint	1 bunch
Cabbage	1 pcs head
Zucchini	2-3 pcs
Broccoli	10 pcs

Ginger	1 pcs
Tomatoes	5-8 pcs
Jalapenos	5-7 pcs
Artichoke	4-6 pcs
Cauliflower	0,5 lb
Hot sauce	1 package
Pine nuts	1 package
Marinara sauce	1 package
Feta cheese	0,5 lb
Almond flour	1 package
Shrimp	2 lb
Pork	2-3 lb
Veal	2-3 lb
Catfish	1 lb
Octopus	0,5 lb
Chicken	3-4 lb
Bay leaf	1 package
Sweetener	1 package
almond flour	1 package
coconut flour	1 package
ground ginger	1 package
ground cinnamon	1 package
unsalted butter	1 can
powdered erythritol	1 package
eggs	1 large
liquid stevia	1 package
coconut oil	1 bottle
vanilla extract	1 package
matcha powder	1 package
baking powder	1 package

| xanthan gum | 1 package |
| frozen sugar-free white chocolate chips | 1 package |

4th week of the ketogenic diet

During the fourth week, we are getting stricter with keeping the keto diet. Remember all the time, water is your best friend! Keep drinking to make sure you are not thinking about the stomach.

Breakfast

We are still going on! Though ketogenic diet takes some time for the body to get used to, I recommend putting your best efforts into the last week. Not because only the health benefits are fantastic, but the self-control that you gain from keeping it is really a great thing. If you get bored, try to experiment more with tastes and dressings. Make sure you keep yourself hydrated.

Dinner

A plenty of recipes will cover your needs. Dinner is a fantastic time for a person who keeps the keto-diet, normally you need two essential balanced meals to get the macros.

Supper

Supper is just the same as the previous week. Vegetables, fish, and meat are your base for this week. Don't forget about the desserts!

Monday (the fourth week):

Breakfast: Crock Pot Turkish breakfast eggs

Dinner: Crock Pot tomato basil Parmesan soup

(alternative) Keto Mississippi roast beef /

Seafood: Crock Pot keto mackerel /

Vegetarian: Crock Pot salmon curry

Supper: Keto collard with cherry tomatoes

Desserts: Crock Pot keto coffee cake

Tuesday:

Breakfast: Keto pumpkin spice pie

Dinner: Spring Soup with a poached egg

(alternative) Keto spicy beef curry /

Seafood: Crock Pot lemon dill halibut /

Vegetarian: Crock Pot keto aubergines

Supper: Mashed cauliflower with rosemary

Desserts: Crock Pot Mocha Pudding Cake

Wednesday:
Breakfast: Crock Pot broccoli omelet

Dinner: Keto butternut squash soup

               (alternative) Crock Pot Burgundy beef /

               Seafood: Crock Pot Cilantro-Lime Fish Tacos /

               Vegetarian: Crock Pot flavor Brussels sprouts

Supper: Indian spiced cauliflower rice

               (alternative) Crock Pot Sunday gravy

Desserts: Keto Crock Pot pumpkin custard

Thursday:
Breakfast: Keto Crock Pot pizza chicken

Dinner: Bacon-cabbage chuck beef stew

               (alternative) Crock Pot simple corned beef /

               Seafood: Crock Pot Ginger Steamed Pompano /

               Vegetarian: Red Thai veggie curry

Supper: Crock Pot crack chicken

Desserts: Keto pumpkin cake Crock Pot

Friday:
Breakfast: Keto Crock Pot meatloaf breakfast

Dinner: Crock Pot Cuban seafood stew

               (alternative) Keto Crock Pot Chicken Parmesan /

               Seafood: Crock Pot Miso-Poached Salmon /

               Vegetarian: Crock Pot cabbage soup

Supper: Keto chicken and sausage mix

Desserts: Crock Pot milk cake low-carb

Saturday:
Breakfast: Crock Pot sausage with bok choy

Dinner: Crock Pot vegetable beef stew recipe

               (alternative) Whole Tuscan chicken Crock Pot /

Seafood: Crock Pot seafood cioppino /

Vegetarian: Keto creamy cauliflower soup

Supper: Crock Pot Chicken Cacciatore

Desserts: Berry cobbler Crock Pot recipe

Sunday:

Breakfast: Keto breakfast lemon cake

Dinner: Keto Crock Pot Korean Beef Stew

(alternative) Crock Pot herb chicken and veggies /

Seafood: Crock Pot Indian-style fish curry /

Vegetarian: Spicy Maple Meatballs

Supper: Crock Pot keto butter chicken

Desserts: Keto brownies Crock Pot

Food list for the fourth week:

coconut oil	1 bottle
onion	8-9 pcs
ground pork	2-3 lbs
eggs	10 pcs
almond flour	1 package
maple syrup	1 bottle
garlic powder	1 package
fennel seeds	1 package
dried oregano	1 package
red pepper flakes	1 package
ground sage	1 package
dried thyme	1 package
black pepper	1 package
paprika	1 package
fat milk	1 bottle
chili powder	1 package

cooking spray	1 package
garlic	3-5 cloves
broccoli florets	5-8 florets
Parmesan cheese	0,5 lb
Cheddar cheese	0,5 lb
tomato	5 pcs
raw pecans	1 package
Swerve Sweetener	1 package
coconut flour	1/3 cup
protein powder	1 package
baking powder	2 teaspoon
ground cinnamon	1 package
ground ginger	1 package
pumpkin puree	1 can
vanilla extract	1 package
Chicken parts	1 clear chicken
Tomato sauce	1 can
Laurel leaf	1 package
Italian seasoning	1 package
Mozzarella	0,5 lb
xanthan gum	1 package
butter	1 package
whipping cream	1 can
lemon	1 pcs
Pure	1 can
Basil	1 bunch
Collard	1 pcs
Pumpkin	2-3 pcs
Aubergines	3-5 pcs
Cauliflower	1 head

Rosemary	1 bunch
Dill	1 bunch
Broccoli	3-4 heads
Squash cabbage	2-3 pcs
Bok choy	1 bunch
Shallot	7-8 pcs
Lime	1 pcs
Beef	2-3 lb
Mackerel	1 lb
Salmon	1 lb
Halibut	1 lb
Ground beef	2-3 lb
Sausage	1 lb
Maple syrup	1 bottle

Top products for the ketogenic diet:

Almond (coconut) flour

Olive (avocado) oil

Cooking spray

Butter

Veggies (tomatoes, cauliflower, broccoli, onion, garlic, pumpkin, celery, zucchini, artichoke, kale, shallot)

Meat (veal, chicken, beef, pork, lamb, sausage, ground beef, ground pork)

Fish (salmon, prawns, shrimp, sea bass, cod, etc.)

Baking soda

Xanthan gum

Sweetener

Eggs

Parmesan, Cheddar, mozzarella, Swiss, American cheese

Whipping cream

Salt

Pepper

Lemon

Sauces and species

APPETIZERS

1.Keto squash cake Crock Pot

This keto squash cake or pie (as you like) is a great appetizer and simply easy and low-cost dish. It doesn't need to much time but the variations of eating it are great – you may add mayo, different sauces, both hot and sweet, cheese cream.

Ingredients (9 servings):

Summer squash	1 pound
salt	1 teaspoon
eggs	2 large
scallions	1 1/2 ounce
lemon pepper	1 1/2 teaspoon
baking soda	1/2 teaspoon
almond flour	1/2 cup
coconut flour	1/4 cup
grated Parmesan cheese	1/4 cup

oil for frying

Directions:

1. Wash the squash, dry it with a paper towel.
2. Grate the squash in a food processor. Put the grated squash into a large bowl and sprinkle with salt.
3. Stir the squash gently to spread the salt and let the mixture sit for about 10 minutes.
4. Squeeze the zucchini with hands after this put into a mixing bowl.
5. Add the eggs to the mixture and toss everything.
6. Peel the scallions and chop finely. Mix together with the grated squash.
7. Take a small bowl, stir together lemon pepper, baking soda, almond and coconut flour. Add the mixture to the squash and mix finely altogether.
8. Spray the bottom and the sides of the Crock Pot with cooking spray or oil, pour the mixture into the Crock Pot. Cover and set on LOW for 2 hours.
9. Once the cooking time is over, check the readiness with the toothpick.
10. Remove the squash cake from the Crock Pot on a plate and dress with grated Parmesan cheese.
11. Eat warm.
12. Bon Appetite!

2.Broccoli and Cheese Stuffed Squash

I can't forget the taste of the broccoli and cheese squash as I tasted it for the first time. I like this dish because of many reasons – this recipe is low in carbohydrates, is cooked rather quickly, tastes delicious, is healthy and simple to prepare. I think everyone who tries it will definitely like it!

Ingredients (7 servings):

squash	1 pcs
broccoli florets	2 cups
garlic	3 pcs
red pepper flakes	1 tsp
Italian season	1 tsp
mozzarella cheese	1/2 cup
Parmesan cheese	1/3 cup
cooking spray	
salt and pepper at will	

Directions:

1. Wash and dry with a paper towel the squash. Cut in two halves. Take off the seeds. Set aside.
2. Wash broccoli thoroughly and cut into florets.
3. Peel garlic and mince it.
4. Spread the spray over the bottom and the sides of the Crock Pot. Put the halves in the Crock Pot.
5. Add a little bit water of room temperature to the bottom of the Crock Pot.
6. Cover the Crock Pot and put on LOW for about 2 hours, until squash is mild. Check the readiness once the time is over.
7. Take off the squash and let it cool for about 15 minutes.
8. Take a medium skillet, add pepper flakes and a little bit oil and cook for 20 seconds, stir it constantly.
9. Add broccoli, minced garlic to the skillet, continue to stir thoroughly, until the broccoli is tender.
10. Take the squash (previously cooled) and using a fork, take off the flesh of the squash. Add it to the medium bowl and conjoin with the broccoli mixture.
11. Shred carefully the Parmesan cheese, join salt and pepper at will, add seasoning to the mixture. Mix everything well and fill the squash.
12. Put the filled squash again in the Crock Pot, dress with mozzarella cheese each squash half.
13. Add a little bit water if needed to the bottom of the Crock Pot.
14. Cover and cook on LOW for about 1 hour.
15. Remove the dish and enjoy!
16. Bon Appetite!

3.Roasted Spaghetti Squash and Browned Butter

I know a lot of people who like spaghetti squash like their favorite pasta with tomato sauce. Today I advise you to create spaghetti squash keto-friendly dish that means to conjoin delicious species, butter, and tender squash. All these ingredients on one plate! The butter gets a new taste in this dish.

Ingredients (9 servings):

spaghetti squash	2 pcs
olive oil extra-virgin	1-2 tablespoons
salt	1 tsp.
black pepper	1 tsp.
butter	4 tablespoons
hazelnuts	1/4 cup
sage leaves	2 tablespoons
red pepper flakes	1/4 tsp.
ground cinnamon	1/4 tsp.

Directions:

1. Wash and dry squash with a paper towel. Cut in two halves. Take off all seeds and set aside.
2. Lightly sprinkle the flesh with oil, add salt at will and pepper.
3. Put the halves into the Crock Pot, cover the lid and set on LOW for 2 hours, squash must be tender.
4. Take off the squash once the time is over and let it cool.
5. Flip the halves carefully. Use a fork, scrape the flesh, try to keep the sides as they are. Set aside.
6. Take a saucepan, put the butter and melt.
7. Cook the butter, whisk carefully all the time until it foams and turns brown and about 2 minutes.
8. Add finely chopped hazelnuts, sage leaves, pepper flakes, cinnamon and continue cooking for about 30 seconds more.
9. Top the butter over the squash.
10. Serve warm.
11. Bon Appetite!

4.Twice baked spaghetti squash Crock Pot

This is the best full spaghetti squash that is so creamy and rich. You need to use your Crock Pot twice during the preparation of this recipe, but be sure it is not so difficult as you think. Try to cook it for the first time and you'll cook it always.

Ingredients (5 servings):

cooked spaghetti squash	2 cups

egg whites	2 pcs
Herbes de Provence	1 Tsp
Light Swiss Cheese	6 wedges
pinch of salt	
mozzarella cheese	1 cup

Directions:

1. Wash and dry with a paper towel squash.
2. Cut squash in half (lengthwise), remove the seeds.
3. Pour a little bit water into the Crock Pot, put the squash, cover and cook on HIGH for 1 hour. Check the readiness with a fork. Let it cool.
4. Remove the squash, make spaghetti squash. Put them on a plate and add olive oil.
5. Put the cooked spaghetti squash into the bottom of the Crock Pot.
6. Take a bowl, mix egg whites, shredded cheese, seasoning, salt. Blend everything together.
7. Pour the mixture over the spaghetti squash.
8. Season with the rest of cheese.
9. Cover the Crock Pot and set on LOW for 1 hour.
10. Serve warm.
11. Bon Appetite!

5.Keto broccoli and bacon Alfredo

This appetizer is easy to cook and it is the favorite dish of whole my family. Creamy Alfredo sauce gets the dish special taste and tender. It is almost impossible to change the sauce with another creamy one. Try to follow all the instructions strictly.

Ingredients (10 servings):

broccoli florets	8 cups
avocado oil	1/4 cup
salt	1 tsp
pepper	1/2 tsp
butter	2 tbsp
garlic	2 cloves
heavy cream	1 cup
pepper	1/8 tsp
Parmesan cheese	1/2 cup
bacon slices	6 slices
salt	

Directions:

1. Wash the broccoli and cut into florets.
2. Peel the garlic and mince.
3. Spray the bottom of the Crock Pot with cooking spray.
4. Take a medium bowl, combine broccoli florets with oil, pepper, and salt.
5. Spread the mixture of broccoli over the bottom of the Crock Pot.
6. Cover and cook on LOW for 1 hour.
7. While the broccoli is cooking, take a large saucepan, place it over medium heat, melt butter.
8. Add garlic and roast it until tender. It may take you about half a minute.
9. Reduce heat, add cream, pepper, salt and let it simmer.
10. Shred the cheese, add it to a pan and continue to cooking until thickened.
11. Add the mixture to the broccoli and slice the bacon.
12. Serve warm.
13. Enjoy!

6.Garlic-Parmesan Asparagus Crock Pot

What kind of appetizer could be so flavor as the garlic-Parmesan asparagus? Do you know?! Yes, it is simple but delicious appetizer every beginner could prepare. Everything you need here is just to buy garlic, asparagus, Parmesan and organic fresh eggs. Nothing more!

Ingredients (6 servings):

olive oil extra virgin	2 tablespoons
minced garlic	2 teaspoons
egg	1 pcs fresh
garlic salt	1/2 teaspoon
fresh asparagus	12 ounces
Parmesan cheese	1/3 cup

Pepper at will

Directions:

1. Peel the garlic and mince it.
2. Wash the asparagus. Shred the Parmesan cheese.
3. Take a medium-sized bowl combine oil, garlic, cracked egg, and salt together. Whisk everything well.
4. Cover the green beans and coat them well.
5. Spread the cooking spray over the bottom of the Crock Pot, put the coated asparagus, season with the shredded cheese. Toss everything finely.
6. Cover and cook on HIGH for 1 hour.
7. Once the time is over you may also season with the rest of the cheese.
8. Bon Appetite!

7.Keto asparagus with soy sauce

This recipe is quite well for a keto diet. Asparagus is tender, delicious and low in carbs. Don't forget to read the ingredients on a bottle of the soy sauce or just use the coconut aminos. Add this recipe to your private collection of the keto appetizer Crock Pot recipes.

Ingredients (5 servings):

Asparagus	1 lb.
peanut oil	1 Tbsp + 1 tsp.
soy sauce (sugar-free, keto-friendly)	1 T
toasted sesame oil	1 tsp.
sesame seeds	2 tsp.

Directions:

1. Wash the asparagus.
2. Spray the cooking spray over the bottom of the Crock Pot.
3. Put asparagus on a bottom and sprinkle with oil, turn asparagus in a way it could be coated on all sides.
4. Whisk together the 1 tsp. oil, soy sauce, sesame oil.
5. Cover the Crock Pot and put on HIGH for 1 hour.
6. Once the half an hour is over, open the Crock Pot and sprinkle with the soy mix. Cover again and do the same every 10 minutes.
7. Take off the asparagus from the Crock Pot and dress with toasted sesame seeds.
8. Serve warm.

8.Bok Choy with butter and soy sauce

This recipe of the appetizer is really healthy and amazing. Taste the oyster sauce and sugar-free version of the soy sauce. It's perfectly well. I think almost all the things of this recipe are already in your refrigerator and wait until you combine them in a delicious dish.

Ingredients (8 servings):

Water	2 Tbsp
soy sauce (sugar-free)	2 tsp.
sesame oil	1 tsp.
oyster sauce	1 Tbsp
vegetable oil	1 Tbsp
head bok choy	2 heads
salt (optional)	1/2 tsp
butter	1 Tbsp
sesame seeds for dressing	

Directions:

1. Wash the bok choy, remove the ends, chop crosswise into strips.
2. Take a medium bowl, combine water, soy sauce, sesame oil, oyster sauce. Mix everything well and set aside.
3. Spray the cooking spray over the bottom of the Crock Pot.
4. Add bok choy on the bottom of the Crock Pot, add salt, a little bit water, cover and cook on LOW for 1 hour.
5. Once the time is over, add soy sauce mixture and butter and cover the Crock Pot once more. Put on WARM until bok choy is tender.
6. Serve hot.
7. Sprinkled with sesame seeds at will.
8. Bon Appetite!

9.Garlic butter Keto spinach

I was always sure that the easiest and delicious recipes are cooked from rather simple ingredients. This appetizer is a great proof of my words. Garlic butter spinach is full of vitamins like C and A, iron, is keto-friendly and tender one!

Ingredients (4 servings):

salted butter	2 tablespoons
garlic, minced	4 cloves
baby spinach	8 oz
Pinch of salt	
lemon juice	1 teaspoon

Directions:

1. Wash the spinach.
2. Peel the garlic cloves and mince finely.
3. Heat up a little skillet, add the butter, melt.
4. Sautee the garlic until a little bit tender.
5. Spray the cooking spray over the bottom of the Crock Pot.
6. Put the spinach into the Crock Pot, season with salt and lemon juice, tender garlic, butter.
7. Cover the Crock pot and put on LOW for 1 hour.
8. Once the time is over, garnish with fresh lemon wedges.
9. Serve hot.

10.Keto warm cheese dip Crock Pot

I began to think about this tasty cheese dip and wished to prepare this amazing one already. I remember as I ate it for the first time. How wonderful was the taste! It's light, easy and corresponds to your ketogenic diet. It is my version of cheese dip, but you might also use your favorite type of cream cheese, also Swiss or Parmesan as an example. Here you are!

Ingredients (6 servings):

Can of chili	1 (15 ounces) pcs

Salsa	1 cup
Cream cheese (room temperature)	1 (8 ounces) pkg.
Cheese (cheddar)	1 cup
Garlic	1 teaspoon minced
Onion	1 clove
Sea salt at will	

Directions:

1. Take your Crock Pot and spray with a non-stick cooking spray that you have at home.
2. Peel the onion and garlic, press the garlic and mince the onion carefully.
3. Open the can of chili and a package of cream cheese (your favorite one), shred the cheddar. Leave a little bit cheddar for serving.
4. Put all the ingredients in the Crock Pot on the bottom and mix well thoroughly with a long spoon.
5. Switch on the Crock Pot and cook on LOW for about 4 hours. Another saying, until the Crock Pot completely heated. Stir occasionally during cooking. I made it 2-3 times.
6. Stir carefully before serving once more, right before time ends.
7. Top your cheese dip with green onions at will and the rest of cheddar.
8. You may also eat with veggies.
9. Bon Appetite!

11.Keto seafood dip Crock Pot

It is a warm/hot seafood dip of tasty lobster, delicious shrimps, and crabmeat. I have used cheddar and American cheese but you may involve your favorite one. Creamy celery soup makes it perfect and it is rather easy to prepare! If you like, you may use only crabmeat or shrimps. As you like. As a result, you will get about 6 cups of seafood dip.

Ingredients (9 servings):

Celery soup condensed cream	2 cans (10 3/4 oz each)
Cheese cheddar	1 cup
Cheese American	1 cup
Lobster	1/2 to 1 cup
Shrimps	1/2 cup
Crabmeat	1 cup
Paprika at will	
Nutmeg at will	
cayenne pepper (optional)	
salt to taste	

Directions:
1. Prepare at hand all the ingredients – the cooked and diced lobster; cooked shrimps and crabmeat that is also chopped.
2. Butter a little the bottom of the Crock Pot, also the sides of it.
3. Shred the cheese.
4. Put creamy celery soup, both kind of cheese American and cheddar, cooked and chopped lobster, shrimps and crabmeat to the bottom of the Crock Pot and combine them well with a spoon.
5. Add a little bit cayenne pepper (optional), paprika and nutmeg, salt.
6. Cover the Crock Pot and switch on for 2-3 hours. Cheese must be melted at the end of the time.
7. Keep the Crock Pot on LOW for further serving.
8. Bon Appetite!

12. Kale, Spinach, Artichoke dip Crock Pot

Oh dear, don't you know the easiest and the most delicious dip prepared in the Crock Pot? Haven't you tried it yet? Traditional artichoke, as well as spinach in a mixture of kale and other ingredients, could make a perfect addition to your keto diet! If you don't like kale or spinach, you may prepare it without these ingredients. This dip is very scrummy pasta sauce eating with keto bread. It is highly recommended here to use the Parmesan cheese of high quality! You'll taste the difference

Ingredients (11 servings):

Garlic	2 cloves
Onion	½ cup
Artichoke	28 oz canned
spinach	10 oz
kale	10 oz
Parmesan cheese	1 cup
Mozzarella	1 cup
Greek yogurt	1 cup
sour cream	3/4 cup
mayonnaise	1/4 cup

Salt and pepper to taste

Directions:
1. Peel the onion, garlic and chop everything into pieces.
2. Put garlic, onion, and artichokes in the food processor and mix together.
3. Wash spinach and chop it. Chop the kale, grate Parmesan cheese, cut the mozzarella cheese.
4. Add the mixture of garlic, onion, and artichokes in the Crock Pot and stir together.
5. Add cheese, mozzarella, mayo, sour cream, Greek yogurt, kale, spinach to the mixture in the Crock Pot.

6. Cover the Crock Pot and cook for 4 hours on HIGH.
7. Season the ready dish with salt and pepper at will.
8. Bon Appetite!

13.Keto Crock Pot tasty onions

This recipe is for those who really like the onion. Yes, the onion! Have you never tried to eat the onion as a simple dish? The onion could be stored in the refrigerator for weeks, so you can prepare this dish at all time. Just to chat with a friend in the kitchen and eat the tasty onions like chips. But don't forget about limit! You are still keeping the keto diet. It is a cheap dish, I must say. Quick and perfect one!

Ingredients (4 servings):

Onions   4 (or 5) large pcs

Butter or coconut oil   4 tablespoon

coconut aminos   1/4 cup

Splenda (optional)

Salt and pepper at will

Directions:

1. Peel the onion. Wash it and dry with paper towel.
2. Slice the onions into ¼ thickness. Slice them into circles.
3. Place the onion slices into the Crock Pot.
4. Top the onion slices with coconut aminos and butter, you might add Splenda at will.
5. Cover the Crock Pot and cook it on LOW during 6-7 hours.
6. Serve over the grilled vegetables or eat it directly without anything!

14.Keto Crock Pot ranch chicken dip

Do you prefer eggs but don't know how to cook them in a new way because all the old dishes are too boring? Do you have some hash browns like Trader Joe's or another one at the refrigerator? Some cheddar cheese, green onion, and few bacon strips? This time you have a new tasty dish! Try to cook it in the Crock Pot.

Ingredients (6 servings):

white meat chicken   2 (12.5 fl oz) cans

Cheddar cheese   1 cup

Greek yogurt   1 cup

taco sauce   1/4 cup

taco seasoning mix   1 (1.25 ounce) package

ranch dressing mix   1/2 (1 ounce) package

Directions:

1. Shred the cheddar cheese.
2. Cut the cooked white chicken.
3. Take a large tureen, mix here shredded cheddar cheese, taco sauce, Greek yogurt, ranch dressing, seasoning mix.
4. Add there cut cooked chicken.
5. Cook everything on LOW 2 hours in the Crock Pot.
6. Spread the rest cheddar cheese at the end of the cooking time, add salt and pepper at will.
7. Bon Appetite!

15. Keto Crock Pot sweet pepper and sausage hash

If you prefer to eat chicken sausages you can prepare this tasty, easy and healthy dish, mixing vegetables and chicken sausages at one plate! Sweet peppers of various colors are like a rainbow on your plate! This recipe is great for the keto diet using your Crock Pot! Vitamins are always essential for human's organism.

Ingredients (11 servings):

chicken sausage (sugar-free)	12-ounce package
olive oil	1 slop-feeder
green onion	1 ½ cup
cauliflowers	1 ½ cup
fresh thyme	2 slop-feeder
ground, black pepper	½ slop-feeder
chicken broth	¼ cup
green, red, and/or yellow sweet peppers	1 ½ cup
Swiss cheese (2 ounces) (optional)	½ cup
fresh parsley	2 slop-feeder
salt	

Directions:

1. You may prepare the dish without prior cooking of the sausages or if you wish, take a large skillet and cook the sausages over medium heat, it takes you 5 minutes approximately. Wait until they are browned. Remove them from the skillet.
2. Peel the onion and cut it. Wash cauliflowers. Shred the cheese and crush the thyme. Slice the green onion.
3. Wash and dry with the paper towel the peppers. Clean them with corns and cut.
4. Use the readymade broth.
5. Spread the bottom of the Crock Pot with oil. Combine here the onion, sausage, cauliflowers, black pepper and thyme. Pour the broth over the mixture in Crock Pot. Add salt.
6. Cook on LOW for 5 hours or on HIGH 2-3 hours.
7. When the time is over, open the lid, add cheese, parsley, peppers, black pepper, green onion. Cover for half an hour or put on WARM.

8. Bon Appetite!

16.Keto crock pot Asian slides

Prepare the keto Asian slides as usual appetizers or for a next party. This dish is a tasty combination of pork prepared in the Crock Pot, keto bread homemade seasoned with juicy slaws. I'm sure it is better than all previous slides or sandwiches you have eaten!

Ingredients (15 servings):

For the Asian Pork

Pork (Ribeye)	3 pounds
Xylitol	2/3 cup
Garlic	1 - 2 cloves
hot sauce	1 tablespoon
sesame oil	1 tablespoon toasted
Chinese five spice powder	1 teaspoon
black pepper	1 teaspoon
water	1 cup
sesame seeds optional	2 tablespoons
salt	

For The Asian Slaw

broccoli slaw	12 ounces
sesame oil	1 slop-feeder
seasoned rice vinegar	1/4 cup
garlic minced	1 clove

For The Sliders

Keto (coconut) bread or homemade 1 package

Directions:

Preparing the pork:

1. Peel the garlic and mince it or press as you wish.
2. Take a medium bowl and mix here Xylitol, pressed or minced garlic, hot sauce, powder of Chinese five spice, a little bit black pepper. Mix thoroughly all the ingredients until it gets a wet paste.
3. Prepare the pork ribeye at the table.
4. Add a cup of water to the Crock Pot.

5. Put the pork ribeye in the Crock Pot, add the wet paste you have already prepared on the top, spread it along the sides of the pork.
6. Cover and cook on HIGH for 5 hours or on LOW for 9 hours.
7. After the time is over, remove the pork from the Crock Pot and put it on the plate. Let it cool a little.
8. Slice the readymade pork and put it again into the Crock Pot, add sesame seeds (optional) and mix with the remaining juice of pork.

For The Slaw

1. Prepare the broccoli slaws. Peel the garlic and press it or slice as you wish.
2. Take a small bowl, toss the broccoli slaw with sesame oil, rice vinegar, pressed garlic.
3. Cover the bowl, let it cool at the refrigerator for some minutes.

For The Sliders

1. Slice the keto bread and place the readily prepared pork and add the slaw on a top also.

17. Keto Crock Pot Garlic Chicken Wings

Prepare these tasty chicken wings as an appetizer or as part of the main dish. Only 5 simple ingredients for this serving! The wings will taste delicious when you use your favorite sauce, it may be chili sauce or another hot one. Either way, they will be perfect!

Ingredients (5 servings):

chicken wings	3 pounds
your preferred hot sauce	1/2 cup
vegetable oil	2 slop-feeder
garlic	2 cloves
salt	

Directions:

1. Wash the chicken wings, dry them with the paper towel.
2. Peel garlic, press it or mince.
3. Take a bowl, add preferred sauce there, oil and already pressed garlic and shake up to combine.
4. Put the wings into the crock pot add the sauce over the wings.
5. Toss with a long spoon the chicken wings in the sauce. All the wings must be covered.
6. Coat and cook in the Crock Pot on LOW for 7 hours.
7. If you would like to have keto garlic chicken wings in the morning you may switch the Crock Pot late in the evening and you'll get it ready.
8. Bon Appetite!

18.Keto Crock Pot cheesy smoky

How will you find a mixture of smoky sausages and cheese? Gouda cheese tastes best for this dish but you also may choose the other one. I definitely recommend you to use here the hot sauce, it is toothsome with the smoky. To let the cheese melt and be sticky, switch the Crock Pot on WARM.

Ingredients (4 servings):

Smoky Sausages   (sugar-free)   28 ounces

Gouda cheese   2 pounds

hot sauce   24 ounces

pepper at will

cooking spray or olive oil for spraying

Directions:

1. Spray a cooking sauce over the bottom of the Crock Pot.
2. Grate the Gouda cheese to a little bowl.
3. Place the sausages into the Crock Pot. Cover the sausages with cheese.
4. Pour the hot sauce over the sausages, add black pepper at will.
5. Cover and cook on LOW 2 hours.
6. Stir the ingredients in the Crock Pot every 25 minutes to be sure they aren't burnt, the cheese must be melted.
7. As soon as the cheese is melted the sausages are ready to serve.
8. To keep the cheese melted and nice, turn your Crock Pot on WARM.
9. Bon Appetite!

19.Keto crock pot glazed walnuts

If you are a great lover of short but tasty and healthy snakes or appetizer this will surely be among your favorites. It is simple to prepare just some buttons on the Crock Pot, a little number of ingredients - only walnuts, butter, maple syrup and vanilla extract - and a keto glazed maple walnuts on your table!

Ingredients (4 servings):

Walnuts   16 ounces

Butter   ½ cup

Maple syrup   (unsweetened)   ½ cup

Vanilla extract   1 slop-feeder

Directions:

1. Put the walnuts, butter, maple syrup and vanilla extract into the Crock Pot.
2. Turn the Crock Pot on LOW and cook for 2 hours.
3. Stir every 25 minutes to be sure, all the walnuts are covered and not burned.
4. After the time is over, take the walnuts off and cool on a parchment paper.

5. Eat as appetizer or store in a Ziploc bag.

20.Keto sweet kielbasa

For this recipe, you need just 5 servings and you'll get this easy sweet kielbasa. The unsweetened sauce that could be found at any store market near your house adds the sweetness to the dish, but garlic and Dijon mustard put a touch of savory.

Ingredients (5 servings):

kielbasa sausage	2 pounds
unsweetened sauce low carb	1 cup
Sukrin Gold	3/4 cup
Dijon mustard	2 tablespoons
garlic	2 cloves

Directions:

1. Peel the garlic and press it or mince as you wish.
2. Cut the kielbasa sausage into slices.
3. Mix in the Crock Pot the kielbasa sausage with sauce, Sukrin Gold, Dijon mustard, add garlic.
4. Cover and cook on LOW for 5 hours.
5. After the time is over, stir everything once more and put on WARM.
6. Bon Appetite!

21.Keto small meatballs the Mediterranean

If you or your family members prefer to take some essential food for an appetizer, the easy/cooking and keto-friendly Mediterranean meatballs are the right choices among the other recipes. Here you could add parsley to fell the taste deeper than usual or add some other seasonings.

Ingredients (9 servings):

Ground Beef	2 ½ lbs.
Keto (coconut) bread	1 slice
Parsley (optional)	½ cup
Onion	1 pcs
Eggs	2 pcs
Coconut flour	¼ cup
Vinegar	1 slop-feeder
Water	¼ cup
Salt and black pepper at will	

Directions:

1. Combine the bread with water and after this cut it into small pieces.
2. Peel and cut the onion, cut the parsley, mince the meat.
3. Take a medium bowl, mix here bread with meat and eggs, add the onion, parsley (optional), pepper and salt.
4. Knead the mixture using clean hands.
5. Make the small meatball from the mixture.
6. Roll each of the meatballs in flour.
7. Place the water into the Crock Pot, put the meatballs here also.
8. Cover and cook on LOW for 5 hours.
9. Serve hot and add fresh parsley.
10. Bon Appetite!

22.Appetizer spare ribs in a Crock Pot

Mouth-watering ribs don't let anyone be apathetic! Only water, garlic powder, the onion powder, a little bit avocado oil and you have a tasty dish! Amazing!

Ingredients (6 servings):

Spare ribs	2 lbs
Water	2 cups
Garlic powder	1 slop-feeder
Avocado oil	1 cup
Onion powder	½ slop-feeder

Salt and pepper to taste

Directions:

1. Wash the ribs and make them dry with the paper towel.
2. Season the ribs with garlic powder to taste.
3. Pour water into the Crock Pot. Lay the ribs, add onion and garlic powder. Cover the lid and cook almost for 7 hours on LOW.
4. After the time is over, remove the ribs from the Crock Pot and serve hot, seasoning with pepper and salt
5. Bon Appetite!

23.Keto pepperoni dip recipe

Could you imagine it is possible to create a perfect appetizer combining just three simple ingredients! The luscious recipe for famous pepperoni dip is amazing. Be hurry to cook this for your family breakfast! Dip the favorite vegetables in amazingly simple and tasty dish!

Ingredients (3 servings):

cream cheese	8 ounces
cream of celery soup	10.5 ounces

| pepperoni | 7 ounces |

Pepper and salt to taste

Directions:

1. Wash and cut pepperoni into slices.
2. Mix cream cheese, sliced pepperoni and canned cream of celery soup in a Crock Pot (you may use the small version). Dress with pepper and salt.
3. Cover and cook on LOW at least 1 hour. After first 15-20 minutes, stir the mixture carefully. Then after the second quarter – do the same once more time.
4. After the time is over, keep the dip on WARM or serve at once.
5. Bon Appetite!

BREAKFASTS

24.Crock Pot keto «English muffin»

I think the majority of us have heard this word combination - «English muffin». Don't be surprised that we cook it today in the Crock Pot and as a result, we get one, a large muffin that we could cut with a knife and eat like small muffins from the usual oven Cooking in the Crock Pot doesn't need too much time as in the oven. Try to cook this following my easy instructions!

Ingredients (6 servings):

Almond flour   3 tbsp

Coconut flour   1/2 tbsp

Butter (or coconut oil) 1 tbsp

Egg   1 large

Sea salt   1 pinch

baking soda   1/2 tsp

salt at will

Directions:

1. Take a medium-sized skillet, melt the butter. It takes usually 20-30 seconds.
2. Take to the skillet with melted butter coconut and almond flour, egg, salt and stir everything well.
3. Take from the heat and add baking soda.
4. Open the Crock Pot, spray the bottom of the Crock Pot with cooking spray. Pour the mixture.
5. Cover the lid and put on LOW for 2 hours. Check the readiness with a fork.
6. Remove the baked «muffin» from the Crock Pot and eat with bacon slices, cheese or other ingredients.
7. Bon Appetite!

25.Crock Pot benedict casserole

Benedict casserole is a variation to prepare keto eggs benedict using the Crock Pot. You have to be patient to get this tasty dish that I recommend to prepare late in the evening to enjoy it in the morning. Try to surprise your family!

Ingredients (7 servings):

For the Casserole

English muffin   1 large (cut into portions)

canadian bacon   1 lb thick cut

eggs   10 large

milk	1 cup
salt and pepper	
chives at will for garnish	

For the Sauce

egg	6 yolks
lemon juice	1 1/2 TBSP
unsalted butter, melted	1 1/2 sticks (3/4 cup)
salt	
pinch of cayenne	

Directions:

1. Cook the English keto muffing in my recipe:
   (using a medium-sized skillet, melt the butter. Add coconut and almond flour, egg, salt and stir everything well. Add baking soda. Open the Crock Pot, spray the bottom of the Crock Pot with cooking spray. Pour the mixture, put on LOW for 2 hours. Remove once the time is over).
2. Spray the bottom of the Crock Pot with cooking spray (the second time), cut the muffin into equal pieces, put on the bottom
3. Slice the bacon, sprinkle half of it over top of muffin (pieces).
4. Take a large bowl, whisk together milk, eggs, season with salt and black pepper at will.
5. Pour the egg mixture evenly over the muffin pieces and top with the rest of the bacon.
6. Press down on the muffins to be sure that they are all coated with the egg mixture.
7. Cover the lid of the Crock Pot, put on LOW for 2 hours.
8. Remove the dish from the Crock Pot once the time is over and keep the muffins covered before ready serving.
9. Prepare the sauce while the main dish is cooked in the Crock Pot: Set up a double boiler, put the egg yolks and squeezed lemon juice in the bowl and whisk thoroughly until it begins to thicken (it must also double in size). Be patient! It could take some time.
10. Put your bowl over the double boiler, continue whisking carefully, the bowl mustn't get too hot.
11. Drizzle in the melted butter while continuing to whisk.
12. Season with salt and pepper at will. You may also add a little bit more lemon juice or cayenne at will.
13. Enjoy the sauce together with keto Crock Pot «muffin».

26.Crustless Crock Pot Spinach Quiche

This crustless spinach quiche is perfectly well for the breakfast both for adults and kids. It is easy, keto-friendly, cheep and quickly. It doesn't take you too much time to prepare this quiche. Add your favorite species once the dish is ready.

Ingredients (11 servings):

frozen spinach	10 oz package
butter or ghee	1 Tbsp
red bell pepper	1 medium
Cheddar cheese	1 1/2 cups
eggs	8 pcs
homemade sour cream	1 cup
fresh chives	2 tablespoons
sea salt	1/2 teaspoon
ground black pepper	1/4 teaspoon
ground almond flour	1/2 cup
baking soda	1/4 tsp

Directions:

1. Let the frozen spinach thaw and drain it well. Chop finely.
2. Wash the pepper and slice it. Take off the seeds.
3. Shred the cheddar cheese and set aside.
4. Chop finely the fresh chives.
5. Open the Crock Pot and spray the bottom and sides with cooking spray.
6. Take a little skillet, heat the butter over high heat, sautee pepper until tender, about 6 minutes.
7. In a large bowl combine together eggs, sour cream, salt, pepper.
8. Add grated cheese and chives and continue to mix.
9. In another medium-sized bowl, mix together almond flour with baking soda. Pour into the egg mixture, add peppers in the eggs mixture, pour gently into the Crock Pot.
10. Cover the lid and set on high for 2 hours.
11. Bon Appetite!

27.Crock Pot Brussels sprouts casserole

This easy and flavor Brussels sprouts casserole is quick, healthy and tender. An amazing combination of cheese and Brussels sprouts are great and keto-friendly. You may also add the shredded cheese.

Ingredients (9 servings):

Brussels sprouts	32 oz bag frozen
ground turkey sausage	1 pound
eggs	6 large
heavy cream	2 tablespoons
dried thyme	½ teaspoon

garlic powder	½ teaspoon
salt	¼ teaspoon
pepper	⅛ teaspoon
Colby jack cheese	1 cup shredded

Directions:

1. Open the Crock Pot and spray the bottom and sides with cooking spray.
2. Shred the cheese. Set aside.
3. Add about ⅔ of the bag of Brussels sprouts on the bottom of the Crock Pot.
4. In a medium-sized bowl whisk together eggs, heavy cream, thyme, garlic powder, salt pepper.
5. Pour over the Brussels sprouts in the Crock Pot.
6. Take a medium-sized skillet, put over high heat, brown a little bit sausage.
7. Add cooked sausage on top of eggs and Brussels sprouts.
8. Top it all off with remained Brussels sprouts, add shredded cheese.
9. Cover the lid and cook on high for 2 hours.
10. Bon Appetite!

28.Crock Pot Turkish breakfast eggs

Turkish-style breakfast is low-calories, keto-friendly, full of vitamin C and tasty dish for early morning. Begin your daily routine with full energy, smile, green veggies, hot species and a good mood. Let's enjoy this recipe together!

Ingredients (9 servings):

olive oil	1 tbsp
onions	2 pcs
red pepper	1 pcs
red chili	1 small
cherry tomatoes	8 pcs
keto bread	1 slice
eggs	4 pcs
milk	2 tbsp
small bunch of parsley	
natural yogurt at will	4 tbsp
pepper at will	

Directions:

1. Peel the onions and chop finely.
2. Wash parsley and chop finely. Wash the cherry tomatoes and dry with a paper towel.
3. Wash the pepper and chili, take off the seeds from the bell pepper and slice.

4. Cube the keto bread.
5. Spray the inside of the Crock Pot with oil or cooking spray.
6. In a large skillet, heat the oil, add the onions, pepper, and chili. Stir everything together.
7. Cook until the veggies begin to soften.
8. Put them in the Crock Pot and add the cherry tomatoes and bread, stir everything well.
9. Cover and cook on LOW for 4 hours.
10. Season with fresh parsley and yogurt.
11. Bon Appetite!

29.Crock Pot sausage with bok choy

Keto sausage with bok choy is ideal for serving making breakfast or serving for a big company. The right proportion of eggs and milk, finely browned sausage, healthy bok choy and tender spinach –is a perfect beginning for the whole day!

Ingredients (11 servings):

pork breakfast sausage	1 pound
yellow onion	1 small pcs
dried oregano	1 1/2 teaspoons
baby spinach (about 4-5 packed cups)	5 ounces
bok choy	2 cups
shredded Swiss cheese	1 1/4 cups
grated Parmesan cheese	1/4 cup
eggs	8 large
whole or 2% milk	2 cups
Dijon mustard	2 teaspoons
kosher salt	1 1/2 teaspoons
ground black pepper	1/4 teaspoon
hot sauce for serving	
Cooking spray	

Directions:

1. Peel and dice the onion.
2. Wash and chop bok choy.
3. Shred the Swiss cheese. Grate the Parmesan cheese and set aside.
4. Take a large skillet over medium heat, add sausages, onion, add oregano.
5. Toss everything well and cook until sausages are browned. It takes usually 7 minutes.
6. Add the spinach and stir well.
7. Spray the inside of the Crock Pot with oil or cooking spray.

8. Put the sausage and spinach mixture into the Crock Pot. Add bok choy, half of the Swiss cheese, and half of the Parmesan cheese. Combine well everything.
9. Take a large bowl and combine freshly cracked eggs, milk, mustard, salt, pepper. Whisk everything until smooth.
10. Pour the egg mixture into the Crock Pot.
11. Cover and set on the LOW for 5hours.
12. Remove the dish from the Crock Pot and sprinkle with the remained amount of cheese.
13. Cover the lid and wait until the cheese melts fully or put on WARM for 1 hour.
14. Serve hot!
15. Bon Appetite!

30.Scrambled eggs with smoked salmon

This is a tasty, flavor, easy and delicious recipe of the tender smoked salmon and fresh organic eggs. What could be easier for breakfast? I don't recommend to use another kind of fish in this keto recipe.

Ingredients (6 servings):

smoked salmon	¼ lb(s)
eggs	12 pcs
heavy cream	½ cup
almond flour	¼ cup
Salt and black pepper at will	
Butter	2 Tbsp
fresh chives at will	

Directions:

1. Cut the slices of salmon. Set aside for garnish.
2. Chop the rest of salmon into small pieces.
3. Take a medium bowl, whisk the eggs and cream together.
4. Add a half of the chopped chives, season eggs with salt and pepper. Add flour.
5. Melt the butter over medium heat and pour into the mixture
6. Spray the inside of the Crock Pot with oil or cooking spray.
7. Add salmon pieces to the mixture, pour everything into the Crock Pot.
8. Cover the lid and put on LOW for 2 hours.
9. Garnish the dish with remaining salmon, chives.
10. Serve warm and enjoy!

31.Bacon, Egg and Cheese Bread Boxes

The egg, bacon and cheese boxes are cooked usually in my family not only for each morning but for parties and crowds. This dish is easy to cook and to serve, comfortable to consume and flavor. Add any cheese Swiss, Parmesan or Cheddar if you want.

Ingredients (6 servings):

Keto bread	1 loaf
unsalted butter	6 Tbsp
American cheese	8 slices
Bacon	8 slices
whole milk	⅓ cup
eggs	12 large

Hot sauce for dressing

Directions:

1. Slice bacon into 1/2-inch pieces. Set aside.
2. Shred the cheese.
3. Remove about 1/4 inch of the crust from the ends of the keto loaf, cut the keto loaf crosswise into 4 pieces.
4. Using a fork make a box from each piece of keto bread. Leave about 1/2-inch of bread around the bottom and walls.
5. Take a little skillet, melt the butter about 1 minute. Brush the bread boxes inside and out with the melted butter, add salt.
6. Put small cheese slices at the bottom of keto bread box.
7. Open the Crock Pot and spread the cooking spray over the bottom and sides.
8. Place the boxes on the bottom of the Crock Pot.
9. Meanwhile, take a large bowl, whisk eggs and milk adding salt and pepper.
10. Add the mixture to the keto bread boxes, put the bacon slices over the top of the boxes.
11. Spread the shredded cheese.
12. Cover the lid and put on LOW for 3 hours.
13. Serve hot with hot sauce and additional salt and pepper.
14. Bon Appetite!

32. Persian omelet Crock Pot

This vegetarian recipe is full of fresh sunny herbs, green onions, organic eggs and pine nuts. This recipe is cooked until golden brown. I usually top it with the Greek yogurt but you may also add the sour cream.

Ingredients (14 servings):

olive oil	2 Tbsp
butter	1 Tbsp
red onion	1 large
green onions	4 pcs
garlic	2 cloves
spinach	2 oz

fresh chives	¼ cup
cilantro leaves	¼ cup
parsley leaves	¼ cup
fresh dill	2 Tbsp
Kosher salt and black pepper at will	
pine nuts	¼ cup
eggs	9 large
whole milk	¼ cup
Greek yogurt at will	1 cup

Directions:
1. Peel the onion cut thinly.
2. Chop carefully green onions. Chop chives.
3. Wash spinach after this carefully chops it.
4. Peel garlic and mince.
5. Finely cut cilantro and parsley, dill.
6. Take a saucepan melt the butter. Add red onion, stirring occasionally, it takes about 8-9 min.
7. Add green onions, garlic, continue cooking for 4 minutes.
8. Put the spinach, chives, parsley, cilantro, add salt and pepper at will. Remove the skillet, add the pine nuts.
9. Take a bowl, crack the eggs, add milk and a little pepper and whisk.
10. Mix the eggs with veggie mixture.
11. Open the Crock Pot and spread the cooking spray over the bottom and sides. Pour the mix into the Crock Pot.
12. Cover the lid and put on LOW for 3 hours. Serve with Greek yogurt.
13. Bon Appetite!

33.Crock Pot cream cheese French toast

Keto cream-cheese French toasts are great at the beginning of the day. Light keto bread slices, covered with cream mixture in a combination with almonds are delicious and amazing! I usually dress these toasts with maple syrup.

Ingredients (9 servings):

cream cheese	1 (8-oz) package
slivered almonds	¼ cup
keto bread	1 loaf
eggs	4 pcs
almond extract	1 tsp
sweetener	1 Tbsp

milk	1 cup
butter	2 Tbs
Cheddar cheese	½ cup

Maple syrup, at will, for dressing

Directions:

1. Take a large bowl, mix together cream cheese with almonds.
2. Slice the keto bread into 2-inch slices. Try to make a 1/2-inch slit (horizontal) in the bottom of every slice to make a pocket.
3. Fill all the slices with cream mixture. Set aside.
4. In a little bowl mix eggs, extract the sweetener in milk. Coat the keto slices into the mix.
5. Open the Crock Pot and spread the cooking spray over the bottom and sides.
6. Put the coated keto slices on the bottom of the Crock Pot. Put on the top of each separate slice additional shredded cheese.
7. Cover the lid and put on LOW for 2 hours.
8. Serve hot.
9. Bon Appetite!

34.Keto Crock Pot meatloaf breakfast

Would you like to eat meat for breakfast? Do you like to consume bread for breakfast also? But what is the meatloaf? It is made of pork, but you may also use another meat. The breakfast meatloaf has no chances of falling apart or to be not tasty! By no mean!

Ingredients (15 servings):

coconut oil or avocado oil	1 slop-feeder
onion	2 cups
ground pork	2 lbs
eggs	2 pcs
almond flour	½ cup
maple syrup	2 slop-feeder
garlic powder	1 slop-feeder
fennel seeds	2 slop-feeder
dried oregano	2 slop-feeder
red pepper flakes appetizer	2 slop-feeder
ground sage	2 slop-feeder
dried thyme	2 slop-feeder
black pepper	1 slop-feeder
paprika	1 slop-feeder

| sea salt | 1 slop-feeder |

Directions:

1. Peel the onion. Chop it carefully.
2. Take a medium bowl, add eggs, chopped onion, almond flour, maple syrup, garlic powder, fennel seeds, dried oregano, red pepper, sage, thyme, black pepper and sea salt.
3. Prepare the pork at the table. Add the pork to the mixture at the bowl. Using your clean hands combine all the ingredients once more.
4. Make with using your hand a loaf, put it into the Crock Pot that must be covered a little with avocado or coconut oil previously (both bottom and sides).
5. Put your loaf in such a way the will be a half inch gap between the sides of the loaf and the wall of the Crock Pot.
6. Cook on LOW about 3-4 hours.
7. Remove the meatloaf at once the time is over, let it cool a little bit and place in the refrigerator for a night.
8. Take the meatloaf in the morning and slice it for breakfast.
9. Bon Appetite!

35.Crock Pot broccoli omelet

Do you prefer to have some eggs for a breakfast? The broccoli omelet could be a great addition to your morning herbal tea or coffee that doesn't need to much time and a lot of ingredients. I think you have all the ingredients in your refrigerator.

Ingredients (14 servings):

Eggs	6 large
fat milk	1/2 cup
Salt	1/4 slop-feeder
Pepper	1/2 slop-feeder
garlic powder	1/4 slop-feeder
chili powder	1/4 slop-feeder
shortening or non-stick cooking spray (for greasing the crockpot)	
yellow onion	1 pcs small
garlic	3 cloves
fresh broccoli florets	1 cup
parmesan cheese	1 tablespoon
cheddar cheese	1 - 2 cups
tomato chopped	1 pcs medium
green onions	1/4 cup

Directions:

1. Peel the yellow onion and cut it. Peel the garlic and press, shred the cheese and wash the medium red tomato, dry with paper towel and cut also. Chop the green onions.
2. Take a cooking spray and spread it over the bottom and all the sides of your Crock Pot, just to prevent sticking.
3. Crack the eggs into a large bowl, add the cup of milk mix well, add all the species and mix it once more carefully.
4. Add the onions to the mixture, then garlic, Parmesan cheese, and broccoli florets. Continue whisking it thoroughly.
5. Put your mixture into the Crock Pot, cover and cook on HIGH for 2 hours.
6. As soon as the time is over, with using the long keen knife cut along the edge of the Crock Pot into quarters.
7. Take your omelet to the plate and serve with remaining cheddar and green chopped onions.
8. Bon Appetite!

36.Keto pumpkin spice pie

This keto Crock Pot pumpkin pie recipe is great! I can't quite decide if it's pie or if it's bread. It is well in both situations, depending on how you treat this after it is ready. Eat it in the morning and you'll get a wonderful full breakfast meal. In another way, it is delicious at any time.

Ingredients:

raw pecans	1 1/2 cups
Swerve Sweetener	3/4 cup
coconut flour	1/3 cup
unflavoured whey protein powder	1/4 cup
baking powder	2 teaspoon
ground cinnamon	1 1/2 teaspoon
ground ginger	1 teaspoon
ground cloves	1/4 teaspoon
salt	1/4 teaspoon
pumpkin puree	1 cup
eggs	4 large
butter melted	1/4 cup
vanilla extract	1 teaspoon

Directions:

1. Spread the bottom of the Crock Pot with cooking spray.
2. Grind the pecans in the food processor until the coarse meal, but don't let turn them into the butter.

3. Transfer pecans to the bowl and whisk together, add coconut flour, sweetener, baking powder, whey protein powder, ginger, cinnamon, salt garlic and whisk once more.
4. Mix in another bowl pumpkin puree, cracked eggs, vanilla, butter until well mixed.
5. Join everything together, add this mixture to the Crock Pot and set on LOW for 3 hours.
6. As soon as the top of the pie is barely firm to the touch the pumpkin spice pie is ready.
7. Bon Appetite!

37.Keto Crock Pot pizza chicken

The latest achievements of the technic like a Crock Pot give us a variety of possibilities to use the preferred products in different combinations to get the best meals and loved one. Combine the chicken breast with flavored tomato sauce, garlic, and laurel leaf and you'll get a Crock Pot chicken pizza!

Ingredients (7 servings):

Chicken parts	1 clear chicken
Tomato sauce	8 one can
Garlic	2 cloves
Laurel leaf	2 leaves
Italian seasoning	1 slop-feeder
pepper at will	
Mozzarella	½ cup

Directions:
1. Wash the chicken thoroughly and make it dry with paper towel. Cut into parts.
2. Place the chicken parts into the Crock Pot.
3. Peel the garlic and mince it or press. Shred the cheese.
4. Add tomato sauce and all the species into the Crock Pot right over the chicken. Combine everything carefully with clean hands.
5. Cover and cook on LOW for 4 hours.
6. Serve with rubbed cheese on top.
7. Bon Appetite!

38.Keto Crock Pot zucchini bread

Bread is the base of the breakfast for many people. But what about the delicious keto zucchini bread basing on the almond, coconut flour that corresponds to the rules of a keto diet and is prepared at the Crock Pot? Try it and you'll find it is no worse than usual one at the shop shelf.

Ingredients (13 servings):

almond flour	1 cup
coconut flour	1/3 cup
cinnamon	2 slop-feeder

baking powder	1 1/2 slop-feeder
baking soda	1/2 slop-feeder
salt	1/2 slop-feeder
xanthan gum optional	1/2 slop-feeder
eggs	3 pcs
coconut oil or butter	1/3 cup
sweetener	1 cup
vanilla	2 slop-feeder
zucchini	2 cups
walnuts or pecans	1/2 cup

Directions:

1. Take a medium bowl mix here coconut and almond flour, baking powder with baking soda, xanthan gum. Set this aside.
2. Take another little bowl, combine here cracked eggs, sweetener, butter or coconut oil and whisk all together thoroughly.
3. Add the dried ingredients from the first bowl to the second one and combine everything once more.
4. Wash zucchini, shred it and crush the nuts.
5. Spread the oil or butter into the bottom of the Crock-Pot, place your mixture into it.
6. Cover and cook on HIGH for 3 hours.
7. After the time is over, cool it completely and enjoy!
8. Bon Appetite!

39. Keto crock pot gingerbread

Among my preferred bread recipes is also a gingerbread, but it almost for those who like it. This recipe includes a variety of species for those who are great lovers.

Ingredients (13 servings):

almond flour	2 1/4 cups
Swerve Sweetener	3/4 cup
coconut flour	2 tablespoon
ground ginger	1 1/2 tablespoon
ground cinnamon	1/2 tablespoon
baking powder	2 teaspoon
ground cloves	1/2 teaspoon

salt	1/4 teaspoon
butter melted	1/2 cup
eggs	4 pcs
milk	2/3 cup
freshly squeezed lemon juice	1 tablespoon
vanilla extract	1 teaspoon

Directions:
1. Spread the bottom and the sides of the Crock Pot with the butter or cooking spray.
2. Shred the ginger, peel the cloves and press.
3. Take a large bowl, add the almond flour, sweetener, shredded ginger, coconut flour, cinnamon, salt and baking powder, pressed cloves.
4. Mix in another little bowl melted butter, milk, cracked eggs, lemon juice and vanilla extract.
5. Combine everything together from the first and second bowls.
6. Put everything into the Crock Pot, cook on LOW for 3 hours.
7. Let it cool a little!
8. Bon Appetite!

40. Keto Crock Pot chili recipe

An easy keto recipe of chili with the ingredients that strictly correspond to the ketogenic diet. The common ingredients are rather cheap and could be found at any store market or even your kitchen! You may choose another species if you like.

Ingredients (13 servings):

Ground beef	2 1/2 lb
Onion (chopped)	1/2 large
Garlic (minced)	8 cloves
Diced tomatoes (with liquid)	2 15-oz can
Tomato paste	1 6-oz can
Green chiles (with liquid)	1 4-oz can
Worcestershire sauce	2 slop-feeder
Chili powder	1/4 cup
Cumin	2 slop-feeder
Dried oregano	1 slop-feeder
Sea salt	2 slop-feeder
Black pepper	1 slop-feeder
Bay leaf (optional)	1 leaf medium

Directions:
1. Peel the onion and garlic and cut them carefully, or press the onion.
2. Take a large bowl, mix the ground beef with onion, pressed or cut garlic, diced tomatoes as well as tomato paste, green chiles, chili powder, cumin, salt, pepper, Worcestershire sauce and mix everything carefully with hand or loaf.
3. Transfer the mixture to the Crock Pot, cover and cook on LOW for 4 hours.
4. Add bay leaf at the end of the time.
5. Remove the dish to the plate and eat warm.
6. Bon Appetite!

41.Keto Crock Pot Mediterranean frittata

What kind of dish looks like super tasty and doesn't need too much time for breakfast? Yah, it is the keto Crock Pot Mediterranean frittata! You just put all the vegetables into the Crock Pot, pour the eggs mixture and make your business. In the morning you have a great breakfast at the table!

Ingredients (8 servings):

Eggs	8 pcs
Almond milk	⅓ cup
dried oregano	1 teaspoon
Salt and freshly ground black pepper at will	
baby arugula	4 cups
red peppers	1¼ cups
red onion	½ cup
goat cheese	¾ cup

Directions:
1. Peel the onion and slice it thinly.
2. Crumble the goat cheese.
3. Take a medium bowl, crack the eggs into it, add milk, oregano and combine. Add pepper and salt at will.
4. Put the roasted red pepper, baby arugula, goat cheese and onion into the Crock Pot. Pour the eggs mixture over vegetables.
5. Cover and cook on LOW for 3 hours.
6. Serve the dish immediately.
7. Bon Appetite!

42.Keto breakfast lemon cake

Have you already tried a keto Crock Pot cake for early breakfast? The recipe for the lemon keto cake was conformed especially for the Crock Pot that doesn't demand too many movements with it. Dress in whipped cream at the end or with strawberries!

Ingredients (14 servings):

For cake:

almond flour	1 1/2 cup
coconut flour	1/2 cup
Pyure	3 soup spoon
yeast powder	1/2 slop-feeder
xanthan gum	1/2 slop-feeder
butter	1/2 cup
whipping cream	1/2 cup
Juice of lemon	4 soup spoon
Lemon peel	1/2 slop-feeder
Eggs	2 pcs

Topping:

Pure	3 soup spoon
water	1/2 cup
butter	2 soup spoon
juice of lemon	2 soup spoon

Directions:

Baking cake:

1. Take a medium bowl and conjoin coconut flour, almond flour, sweetener, xanthan gum, yeast powder carefully.
2. In another little bowl mix the cracked eggs, cream, fused butter, lemon juice, peel of lemon.
3. Add the dry mixture to the wet one and combine it well.
4. Cover the bottom and the sides of the Crock Pot with cooking spray or drawn butter.
5. Place the mixture into the Crock Pot, cover and cook on LOW 4 hours.

Topping:

1. Mix all the ingredients for topping in a little bowl – Pyure, drawn butter, boiled water, lemon juice.
2. Take the bun off and pour the garnish on the cap of the cake.
3. Serve warm with whipping cream.
4. Bon Appetite!

43.Keto breakfast casserole

The keto breakfast casserole containing the almond milk, riced cauliflower, sweet bell pepper, and a combination of the fragrant species, cheddar cheese, and bacon, pouring with eggs' mixture make your breakfast unforgettable! You may use also your favorite cheese (Swiss or Parmesan) instead of the cheddar.

Ingredients (11 servings):

Eggs	8 large
unsweetened almond milk	1/4 cup
dry mustard	1/4 teaspoon
Himalayan salt	1 teaspoon
Pepper	1/2 teaspoon
Cauliflower	1 head
onion	1 pcs
bell pepper	1 pcs
additional salt and pepper to season the layers	
turkey bacon	8 slices
cheddar cheese	2 cups

Directions:

1. Wash and dry with paper towel cauliflower, peel the onion. Shred cauliflower or rice it in the food processor. Cut the onion and shred the cheese. Cut the sweet pepper.
2. Spray the Crock Pot with the cooking spray or the coconut oil as you wish.
3. Take a large bowl, crack the eggs, mix them accurately with almond milk, dry mustard, salt, and pepper.
4. Put a third of the riced/shredded cauliflower in the bottom of the Crock Pot, top it with also a third of the bell pepper and chopped onion.
5. Sprinkle everything with pepper and salt, top once more with a third of bacon slices and the same part (about a third) of shredded cheese.
6. Repeat such layers three or four times.
7. Pour everything into the egg mixture and cook on LOW for 5-6 hours.
8. The eggs on the top must be browned, it means – your dish is ready!
9. Bon Appetite!

44. Keto Crock Pot turkey stuffed peppers

The delectable keto Crock Pot turkey stuffed peppers is a great healthy recipe, matching for family breakfast on weekend, as well as during the day. If you have too little time to cook it right now in the Crock Pot, you can freeze the peppers and prepare them in the Crock Pot later. Instead of ground turkey, you may use the ground beef if you wish.

Ingredients (7 servings):

olive oil	1 tablespoon
ground turkey	1 lb
onion	1 pcs

garlic	1 clove
green bell peppers	4 pcs
tomato sauce/pasta sauce (low carb)	24 oz jar
water	1/2 cup

Directions:

1. Peel and cut the small onion, peel the garlic and press or mince it.
2. Wash the bell peppers, cut off the tops and clean them accurately.
3. Take a medium bowl, put there ground turkey, cut onion, pressed or minced garlic and add pasta sauce.
4. Separate the compound into four equal parts, place the compounds into the prepared cleaned peppers.
5. Spread the olive oil over the Crock Pot bottom and sides put the peppers to the Crock Pot and top them with sauce.
6. Add a little water into the Crock Pot too, cover and cook on LOW for 6-7 hours.
7. Serve with remaining sauce and enjoy!
8. Bon Appetite!

45.Crock-Pot keto artichoke, spinach recipe

An easy keto recipe with artichoke hearts and frozen spinach is light and hearty. It updates your usual boring morning breakfast with balmy relish. You may serve it with vegetables or keto bread.

Ingredients (6 servings):

jarred artichoke hearts	14 - 15 ounces
spinach (frozen)	10 ounces
cream cheese	8 ounces
Parmesan cheese	1 cup
Garlic	3 cloves

Sea salt and pepper at will

Directions:

1. Peel the garlic, mince it.
2. Grate the cheese.
3. Prepare the frozen spinach, don't defrost them.
4. Drain half of the liquid from the jarred artichokes.
5. Conjoin all the components – artichoke, spinach, cream cheese, Parmesan, minced garlic in the Crock Pot. Savour sea salt and pepper at will.
6. Cap and cook on LOW for two hours. The cheese must be melted.
7. Stir from time to time.
8. Serve with keto bread or vegetables.

46.Keto Jalapeño popper Crock Pot

If you prefer jalapeño poppers, a combination of hot peppers with cheese, you are going the right way! I'm sure you'll love this hot recipe that is great for a lot number of family members. If you have a big family, prepare this tasty one with the same ingredients but double the portions and cook this recipe in a large Crock Pot if you have. Serve with your favorite veggies!

Ingredients (7 servings):

cream cheese	16 ounces
mayonnaise	1 cup
green chilies	4 ounces canned
jalapeño chilies	4 ounces canned
Mexican cheese	1/2 cup
mozzarella cheese	1/2 cup
Parmesan cheese	1/4 cup

Directions:

1. Prepare the cream cheese softened and cubed.
2. Drain the green chilies and chop them carefully.
3. Drain the jalapeno chilies and slice them also.
4. Blend the Mexican cheese.
5. Rub the Parmesan and cut mozzarella into cubes.
6. Combine all the ingredients in the bowl, add mayonnaise and stir it thoroughly.
7. Put the mixture into the Crock Pot, cover and cook on LOW 1 hour.
8. Stir the mixture 2-3 times during an hour.
9. Serve warm.
10. Bon Appetite!

47.Keto asiago spinach dip

Keto asiago spinach dip is a great mixture of simple 5 ingredients for cooking in the Crock Pot! If you haven't tried the asiago cheese yet, it would be perfect finding for you. So easy and full of flavor.

Ingredients (5 servings):

neufchâtel cheese or cream cheese	1 pound
asiago cheese	1 pound
fresh baby spinach	6 ounces
garlic powder	1 teaspoon
Italian seasoning	1/2 teaspoon
Seal salt and pepper to taste	

Directions:

1. Shred the asiago cheese, chop the washed fresh baby spinach leaves roughly.
2. Combine in the large bowl the asiago cheese, Neufchâtel cheese, garlic powder, spinach with Italian seasoning and stir carefully.
3. Smooth this to the Crock-Pot, cover and cook on LOW for 2 hours.
4. The spinach must wilt and the asiago cheese must be melted.
5. Stir every 15-20 minutes, to be sure your dish doesn't burn or stick.
6. After 2 hours set the Crock Pot on WARM and serve it!
7. Bon Appetite!

48.Crock-Pot all in hot dip recipe

This recipe needs to use the previously cooked ground beef as well as sausages that could be made previously in the same Crock Pot. Recipes made with American cheese taste especially great! Balmy dip must be served warm! Enjoy great melted cheese in a combination of ground pork and cream celery soup.

Ingredients (6 servings):

Cooked ground beef	1 pound
Cooked sausages	1 pound
cream of chicken soup	10.75 ounces canned
cream of celery soup	10.75 ounces canned
jarred salsa	24 ounces
American cheese	1 pound

Salt and pepper at will

Directions:

1. Shred the American cheese, prepare at hand all the ingredients.
2. Mix in the Crock Pot the ground beef, sausages, cream of chicken soup, cream of celery, shredded American cheese, jarred salsa, salt and pepper at will.
3. Cover and cook everything on HIGH for 2 hours. Stir from time to time.
4. Turn the Crock Pot on WARM to keep it warm and tasty while serving.
5. Bon Appetite!

49.Keto venison tenderloin

If you are from a hunting family or just a fan of venison, don't hesitate to prepare keto venison in the Crock Pot for breakfast! The flavor of venison doesn't leave you indifferent. But you may also prepare this dish of beef tenderloin. Use the dressing mix or do-it-yourself. My mouth has already started to water...

Ingredients (5 servings):

venison tenderloin	2 pounds
cheese cream	10.5 ounces can

cream of chicken soup	10.5 ounces can
ranch dressing mix	1 packet
salt and pepper to taste	

Directions:

1. Slice the venison into 1 inch thick slices.
2. Open the can of cheese cream conjoin it with chicken soup cream, add dressing, salt, and pepper at will, sliced venison at the Crock Pot.
3. Cover and cook on LOW for 5 – 6 hours so the venison must be tender.
4. Stir from time to time during the cooking process.
5. Serve warm.
6. Bon Appetite!

50.Keto awesome pot roast

I like easy and simple recipes but essential ones. They don't need a plenty of ingredients, are tasty and for all the family members. Here is the simple pork roast recipe for morning breakfast for those who work hard during a day! Don't forget about the keto diet rules.

Ingredients (3 servings):

pork roast such as Boston butt roast	4 pounds
Worcestershire sauce	1/4 cup
seasoned salt	1 teaspoon

Directions:

1. Add a half of the Worcestershire sauce to the Crock pot's bottom.
2. Put the pork in the bottom inside.
3. Spread the remaining sauce over the top of the pork roast.
4. Cover and cook on LOW for 8-10 hours.
5. Take off the pork roast, place it on the plate and shred on slices.
6. Bon Appetite!

51.Keto creamy Italian pork chops

Keto creamy Italian pork is one of the easiest recipes to prepare for the breakfast. Simple contents and the tasty dish is on the table. You may put the pork into the Crock Pot late in the evening and serve it warm early in the morning. The Italian mix gives a great taste, the other ingredients keep the pork chops tender and moist.

Ingredients (5 servings):

pork chops	6 whole pcs
Dressing (Italian one)	1 package
yellow onion	1 pcs
cream of chicken soup	10.75 ounces can

ground paprika   2 dashes

salt and pepper at will

Directions:
1. Peel and chop the onion.
2. Spray the bottom and walls of Crock Pot with a little bit of cooking spray.
3. Put down the pork in the Crock Pot, covering it with chopped onions.
4. Take a medium bowl and conjoin there all volume of the envelope of Italian dressing, cream of chicken soup, add salt and pepper, ground paprika.
5. Add the contents over the combination of chopped onions and pork chops in the Crock Pot, supplement a little bit paprika pinches over the top.
6. Cap and cook on LOW for 4-5 hours.
7. Bon Appetite!

52. Keto simple corned beef

I decided to cook for the morning the simple corned beef, I took the package with sugar-free ingredients. Be attentive, the corned beef is rather a salty one, if you want to eat less salt, rinse the beef with water. If you have a smaller package of corned beef (ex. 1 pound) than the mentioned dosage, divide the ingredients in a half and cook.

Ingredients (8 servings):

yellow onion   1 large pcs

corned beef (without sugar)   2-pounds

laurel leaf   1 leaf

garlic   3 - 4 whole cloves

water   3/4 cup

Stevia   2 tablespoons

prepared yellow mustard   2 teaspoons

freshly ground black pepper   1/4 teaspoon

salt and pepper at taste

Directions:
1. Peel and slice the onion. Peel the garlic and mince it.
2. Spray the Crock Pot with cooking spray.
3. Put the sliced onion. Take off the corned beef from the package and wash properly with warm water.
4. Add the beef to the onion pillow. Place the laurel leaf.
5. Take a medium bowl mix there Stevia, water, mustard, salt, pepper and stir together.
6. Pour the mixture over the dish, don't take off the laurel leaf.
7. Cover and cook on HIGH for 5-6 hours.
8. Take off the dish to the place and enjoy!
9. Bon Appetite!

53. Greek eggs breakfast casserole

I'd like to present you here an amazing mixture of vegetables, Feta cheese, and eggs! Try to taste the Greek eggs breakfast casserole and I'm sure it will be among your favorites forever!

Ingredients (9 servings):

eggs (whisked)	12 pcs
milk	½ cup
salt	½ teaspoon
black pepper	1 teaspoon
Red Onion	1 tablespoon
Garlic	1 teaspoon
Sun-dried tomatoes	½ cup
spinach	2 cups
Feta Cheese	½ cup
pepper at will	

Directions:

1. Peel the onion and garlic and cut them (you may also press the garlic). Cut the spinach. Crush Feta cheese in a little plate.
2. Take a bowl, crack the eggs and whisk them thoroughly.
3. Add to the mixture milk, pepper, salt and stir to combine.
4. Add there minced onion and garlic.
5. Add dried tomatoes and spinach.
6. Pour all the mixture into the Crock Pot, add Feta cheese.
7. Cover and cook on LOW 5-6 hours.
8. Bon Appetite!

54. Savory keto bread Crock Pot

If you possess a little bit more time than usual, I advise you to bake this savory keto bread for the morning meal. I have already proposed you to prepare some tasty cheese or seafood dips, or kale, spinach and artichoke dips. The keto bread could be a great base for these dishes! This prescription has the best texture I have ever tried!

Ingredients (9 servings):

almond flour	2.5 cups
coconut flour	1/4 cup
Kerrygold butter	1/2 cup
cream cheese	8 oz

eggs	8 pcs
Rosemary seasoning	1 teaspoon
Sage seasoning	1 teaspoon
Parsley seasoning	2 tablespoon
baking powder	1,5 teaspoon
salt and pepper at will	

Directions:

1. Take a bowl, stir jointly butter, cream cheese. You must get a creamy consistency.
2. Add rosemary, sage, parsley to the mix and proceed to stir.
3. Add cracked eggs and blend up to the smooth consistency.
4. Finally, add baking powder, coconut and almond flour.
5. Spray the Crock Pot with cooking spray. Pour the consistency to the Crock Pot.
6. Cover and cook on LOW 3-4 hours. Keto bread should be golden on top and come out clean.
7. Serve warm and enjoy!

55.Keto Crock Pot Shepherd's pie

The Crock-Pot is great helper both for house women and business ladies. Along with tasty meat dishes, you may prepare cakes and pies that don't need to much time than to bake this in the oven. This recipe of Shepherd's pie is easy and tasty one!

Ingredients (10 servings):

Cauliflower	1 medium head
coconut oil or olive oil	1-2 tablespoon
yellow onion	1 medium
ground turkey	2 lb.
garlic powder	1 tablespoon
dried thyme	2 teaspoons
dried parsley	1 tablespoon
zucchini, chopped	2 medium
tomatoes, chopped	2 medium
grated Parmesan cheese	1/2 to 1 cup
salt and pepper at will	

Directions:

1. Wash and dry the cauliflower.
2. Rice it in a food processor.

3. Peel the onion and slice. Wash and cut zucchini. Chop the tomatoes.
4. Combine everything in a large bowl – riced cauliflower with chopped onions, add turkey, chopped zucchini, and tomatoes, species. Stir to combine. Add pepper and salt.
5. Cover the bottom of the Crock Pot with oil.
6. Transfer the mix to the Crock Pot.
7. Lay one more layer of the cauliflowers (riced) on the top of the mix (in the Crock Pot already).
8. Spread the cheese over the top in a layer.
9. Cover and cook everything on LOW 4-5 hours.
10. Bon Appetite!

56. Keto maple custard

An easy keto maple custard could be cooked using the maple syrup but it could be changed easily to another preferred one. As for me, I prefer Sukrin Gold as a sugar replacement that corresponds to a keto diet. Of course, you may use the other replacement if you want.

Ingredients (8 servings):

Yolks	2 egg
Eggs	2 pcs
heavy cream (Horizon Organic)	1 cup
milk	1/2 cup
Sukrin Gold (or other sugar substitutes)	1/4 cup
maple extract	1 teaspoon
salt	1/4 teaspoon
cinnamon	1/2 teaspoon

Directions:

1. Prepare the eggs' yolks. Conjoin them with heavy cream, Sukrin Gold, salt maple extract, cinnamon. Mix or stir everything carefully.
2. Spread the Crock Pot with cooking spray or grease if you have such one, fill the Crock Pot with the mixture.
3. Cover the mixture and cook on LOW for 2 hours.
4. The maple custard must be jiggly after 2 hours.
5. Enjoy the maple custard with whipped cream!
6. Bon Appetite!

57. Keto bacon cheeseburger pie Crock Pot

One of the delicious and easy keto meal is this bacon cheeseburger pie. There is a mixture of fresh ground beef, roasted bacon, minced garlic, and delicious cheeses/cheddar and Mexican! You must try this!

Ingredients (8 servings):

Bacon	6 slices
ground beef	1 lb
garlic	2 cloves
hot pepper flakes	1/4 tsp
Salt and pepper	
cream cheese	4 ounces
eggs	6 large pcs
Mexican shredded cheese or cheddar cheese	1 1/2 cups

Directions:

1. Spread the cooking spray over the Crock Pot and the sides.
2. Chop the roasted bacon, peel the garlic and mince. Shred the cheese both cheddar and Mexican.
3. Mix in a large bowl ground beef, minced garlic, salt and pepper at will, hot pepper flakes.
4. Take a small bowl, whisk cracked eggs with cream cheese, the mixture must be smooth.
5. Put the mix into the Crock Pot. Put on the top of this chopped bacon, cover with the smooth mixture, add shredded cheese.
6. Cover and cook everything on LOW 5 hours.
7. Remove to a plate and eat warm!
8. Bon Appetite!

58.Keto Mexican Chicken Crock Pot

The chicken breasts could be prepared so delicious using only 5 ingredients. Your breakfast could be easier than you think! I propose you to follow this simple recipe and prepare it for breakfast.

Ingredients (5 servings):

sour cream	1 cup
chicken broth	1/2 cup
tomatoes	1 - 14 oz can
green chilies	1 - 14 oz can
taco seasoning (homemade)	1 batch
chicken breast	2 lbs
pepper and salt at will	

Directions:

1. Spread the cooking spray over the Crock Pot.
2. Combine the sour cream, diced tomatoes, chicken stock, green chilies with taco seasoning. All the ingredients must be combined well.
3. Put the chicken into the Crock Pot.

4. Cap and cook on low for 6 hours.
5. Bon Appetite!

59.Keto ranch chicken Crock Pot

It is amazing boneless chicken with the creamy ranch sauce over the chicken corresponds to your keto diet and could make your breakfast perfect! You may also garnish it with favorite seasonings!

Ingredients (11 servings):

Chicken:

yellow onion	1 whole
chicken breasts	6 whole pcs
table blend seasoning	1 teaspoon
butter	1/4 cup
ranch dressing mix	1 packet
canned cream of chicken soup	10.5 ounces
chicken broth	1/2 cup
onion soup mix	1/2 packet
cream cheese	8 ounces

Salt and pepper at will

Garnish:

green onions sliced	1/4 cup
ground paprika	1/2 teaspoon

Directions:

1. Peel the yellow onion, slice it. Prepare the chicken. It must be skinless and boneless.
2. Cut the cream cheese into very small cubes.
3. Melt the butter in a small bowl.
4. Place the sliced onion on the bottom of the Crock Pot, add a little chicken broth.
5. Put the chicken over the sliced onions and dress it with seasoning. Add salt and pepper at will.
6. Cover and cook on LOW 5-6 hours.
7. While the chicken is cooking, take a medium bowl, mix there cream of chicken soup, onion soup mix, chicken broth, stir all the mixture together.
8. After the time is over, open the Crock Pot and pour the liquid to the chicken and put on WARM.
9. Take the chicken off and serve with green onions, ground paprika and cream cheese cubed.
10. Bon Appetite!

SOUPS AND STEWS

60.Hearty Crock Pot Fish Stew

This fish stew is easy to cook in the Crock Pot. The catfish is better for this recipe but you may also use the other fish if you prefer. Serve it with keto bread, vegetable salad for family dinner or late supper as it is light and delicious.

Ingredients (12 servings):

catfish	1 1/2 pounds
butter	2 Tsp
garlic	1 large clove
onion	1 large
green bell pepper	1 pcs
zucchini squash	1 to 2 small
tomatoes (whole)	1 can/14.5 ounces
dried leaf basil	1/2 Tsp
dried leaf oregano	1/2 Tsp
salt	1 Tsp
pepper	1/8 Tsp
dry white wine	1/4 cup

parsley for garnish

Directions:

1. Wash the fish thoroughly, rinse well. Take off the scales, wipe dry. Take off the skin. Cut into 2-inch pieces.
2. Take a little saucepan and melt the butter.
3. Peel the garlic and mince. Peel the onion, slice it.
   Combine all ingredients in crockpot. Stir gently, but thoroughly.
   Wash the pepper, take off the seeds and cut into 1-inch pieces.
4. Wash and slice zucchini.
5. Open the Crock Pot, spray with cooking spray the bottom and sides of it.
6. Put to the Crock Pot catfish, pour the melted butter. Add garlic, onion, pepper, salt, whole tomatoes, zucchini dried basil and oregano. Stir thoroughly. Add wine.
7. Cover the lid of the Crock Pot and cook on HIGH for 4 hours.
8. Serve with parsley.
9. Bon Appetite!

61. The easy fish stew recipe

Easy fish stew is the best keto version for the Crock Pot that is perfect for any season of the year. If you don't have fresh veggies like tomatoes, you may don't use them at all (remain the tomato paste) or add more Tabasco sauce and clam juice. Eat hot with keto bread.

Ingredients (11 servings):

olive oil	6 Tbsp
onion	1 medium
garlic	3 large cloves
fresh parsley	2/3 cup
fresh chopped tomato	1 1/2 cups
tomato paste (optional)	2 teaspoons
clam juice (or shellfish broth) 8 oz	
dry white wine	1/2 cup
fish fillets	1 1/2 lb
dry oregano at will	
dry thyme if desired	
Tabasco sauce (or more at will)	1/8 teaspoon
ground black pepper to taste	
Salt at will	

Directions:

1. Peel the onion and chop finely.
2. Peel the garlic and mince it.
3. Wash the parsley, chop also.
4. Wash the tomatoes and crush them.
5. Wash the fish fillets. It is better to use a firm fish such as cod, halibut. Cut into 2-inch pieces.
6. Take a medium-sized skillet, add olive oil and saute onion over high heat. It takes about 3 minutes. Add the garlic and cook a little bit more. Add parsley and stir 1 minute.
7. Add tomatoes and tomato paste, stir 8 minutes approximately.
8. Open the Crock Pot, spray with cooking spray the bottom and sides of it.
9. Put fish fillets, add clam juice, wine, the mixture from the skillet.
10. Add seasoning and salt to taste.
11. Add tabasco sauce.
12. Cover the lid of the Crock Pot and put on LOW for 5 hours.
13. Once the cooking time is over, serve with keto bread.
14. Eat hot!
15. Bon Appetite!

62.Crock Pot Portuguese fish stew

This fish Portuguese stew is amazing! Even when I write and remember how I cooked it last time, I feel all the tenderness and flavor of it... The great combination of seafood with veggies is perfectly well here. What could be more delicious for today's dinner?

Ingredients (16 servings):

rapeseed oil	1 Tsp
onion	1 pcs
roasted red peppers, from a jar	2 pcs
garlic	3 cloves
grated fresh ginger	1 Tsp
sweet smoked paprika	1 tsp
cayenne pepper	1/4 tsp
white wine	7 fl oz
chopped tomatoes	2 cans small
sweetener	1/2 Tsp
fresh bay leaves	2 pcs
Pinch saffron	
Clams	1lb 2oz
cod loin	13oz
raw tiger prawns	12oz

Juice of a lime, plus extra wedges, to serve 1 pcs

parsley leaves at will

keto bread if desired for garnish

Directions:

1. Peel and slice the onion, slice the roasted peppers from a jar roughly.
2. Peel the garlic and mince it.
3. Peel and grate the fresh ginger.
4. Cut cod loin into 2-3 cm, cut in cubes.
5. Squeeze the juice of one lime in a cup. Set aside.
6. Take a medium-sized skillet and heat the oil, add the onion and roast for 5 min, until softened.
7. Add garlic, peppers, and spices and continue cooking further 3min. Pour in the wine and let it boil for 7 min.
8. Put in the tomatoes, sweetener, ginger, bay leaves and saffron, cover with the lid and let it simmer.

9. Sprinkle with salt and pepper at will. Remove the skillet from the heat, remove the bay leaves.
10. Use a blender and make the smooth consistency of the stew.
11. Open the Crock Pot, pour the mixture into the Crock Pot. Add the clams, cod, prawns, and juice of a lime put on LOW for 2 hours. Check when the clams are opened otherwise they are overcooked.
12. Season to taste.
13. Serve with remained lime slices, sprinkle with the parsley.
14. Bon Appetite!

63.Crock Pot Greek Fish Stew

This recipe of fish stew is budget friendly as you can use also frozen fish fillets and add the veggies you have in the fridge. Greek fish stew is a super delicious dish that works well both for everyday and parties, nice in the summer and in winter days. It's like enjoying the Greek fish stew version in a little cafe somewhere on the Mediterranean… Drink a glass of wine and enjoy sun… Let the sunny days be at your home today!

Ingredients (11 servings):

Onion	1 large pcs
white fish fillets	5 large pcs
leek	1 pcs
celery	3 sticks
lemon	1 pcs
fish or vegetable stock	8 cups
mint leaves	½ tsp
parsley leaves	½ tsp
garlic	4 cloves
saffron threads	1/2 Tsp
tomatoes	1 can

pepper and salt at will

Directions:

1. Peel the onion and slice. Peel the garlic and mince.
2. Rinse well the fish fillets.
3. Slice the leek and chop the celery.
4. Squeeze the juice of a lemon and gate the rest. Set aside.
5. Wash and chop mint and parsley leaves.
6. Take a large bowl, mix onion, leek, celery, mint leaves, parsley leaves, garlic, saffron, tomatoes, add pepper and salt at will. Add broth.
7. Add lemon juice and a little bit zest. Toss well.
8. Add the fish fillets and cover thoroughly with mixture.

9. . Open the Crock Pot and out the mixture with fish fillets into the Crock Pot, cover the lid and put on LOW for 4 hours.
10. Serve with fresh mint and parsley leaves.
11. Bon Appetite!

64.Crock Pot veal stew

The recipe of keto veal stew is an amazing combination of white wine, veggies, and veal. It is of high importance to cook the veal tender but don't let the veggies be overcooked especially cabbage. Check the tenderness of meat with the fork from time to time. Add your favorite species if you want.

Ingredients (8 servings):

olive oil	1 tbsp
veal blade roast	2 lb
cabbage	1-2 cups
onions	½ pcs
garlic	2 cloves
Herbes de Provence	2 tsp
white wine	¼ cup
water	1/3 cup
ground pepper at will	
salt at will	

Directions:

1. Peel the onion and slice. Peel the garlic and mince.
2. Cut the cabbage. Set aside.
3. Take a large skillet, heat the oil over high heat.
4. Add the veal and sauté until it is little browned (from all sides). It takes usually about 7 min.
5. Open the Crock Pot and put the veal from the skillet to the bottom of the Crock Pot.
6. Add to the Crock Pot cabbage, onions, garlic, white wine, water, salt and pepper at will, season with Herbes de Provence.
7. Cover the Crock Pot with the lid and put on LOW for 7 hours or until meat is fully tender (check with a fork).
8. Season with pepper before serving.
9. Eat hot!
10. Bon Appetite!

65.Old-fashioned Crock Pot veal stew

Some of the recipes don't get old with time. I have remembered this old-fashioned veal stew that was always cooked in my family earlier. At the time when we didn't have the Crock Pot, it took too long to wait for a ready dish, moreover, the meat had to be tender. But now, you don't need to wait all day long in the kitchen. The Crock Pot will do all the work itself.

Ingredients (10 servings):

cooking spray

almond flour	2 Tbsp
table salt	1/2 tsp
black pepper	1/4 tsp
veal shoulder	1 pound(s
onion(s)	1 large
garlic	2 clove(s), medium
ground sage	1/8 Tsp
dried oregano	1/4 tsp
canned beef broth	1/2 cup(s)
diced tomatoes	14 1/2 oz canned

Directions:

1. Peel the onion and slice. Peel the garlic and mince.
2. Take a skillet, spray with cooking spray.
3. Mix in a medium-sized bowl almond flour, salt, and pepper.
4. Rinse the veal and cut into cubes. Coat veal with flour mixture.
5. Put on the skillet and roast about 5 minutes from all the sides.
6. Open the Crock Pot and put veal, onion, garlic, add oregano and sage.
7. Pour the beef broth into the Crock Pot.
8. Add tomatoes with liquid to the Crock Pot.
9. Cover the lid and put on LOW for 7.
10. Bon Appetite!

66.Crock Pot rustic lamb stew

Frankly speaking, I like easy and quick recipes. If I have a good mood I can cook all day long, roast boil, simmer and so on. But if I have too little time but still want to eat delicious dishes I always use this recipe for dinner and cook in my Crock Pot. I'm sure, your family and friends would like this stew also. Good luck!

Ingredients (8 servings):

boneless lean lamb stew meat	1 1/2 lbs
salt divided	1 teaspoon
pepper	1/2 teaspoon
vegetable oil	2 teaspoons

thyme	1/2 teaspoon
rosemary	1 teaspoon
onion	1 large
water	2 cups

Directions:

1. Peel the onion and slice thin. Crush the rosemary.
2. Wash the lamb, remove all the bones, cut into 1-inch cubes.
3. Open the Crock Pot and put lamb pieces, season with salt and pepper at will. Add vegetable oil, thyme, rosemary, water, onion. Cover the lid of the Crock Pot and put on HIGH for 5 hours.
4. Once the cooking time is over, serve the hot stew with fresh parsley and keto bread.
5. Bon Appetite!

67.Crock Pot Moroccan lamb stew

I know that people usually cook stews in the winter months. But sometimes it happens that you just hear the name of the dish and can't stop cooking it! It is all about the keto Moroccan lamb stew. Juicy, delicious, flavor and tender lamb stew melt in your mouth... It is a perfect combination of meat and species!

Ingredients (18 servings):

ground cumin	1 tsp
ground coriander	2 Tsp
red pepper powder	1/4 tsp
turmeric	1/4 Tsp
dried mint	1/2 Tsp
salt	1 and 1/2 Tsp
ground black pepper	1/2 Tsp
lamb shoulder chops	2 and 1/2 lbs.
olive oil divided	2 Tsp
onion	1 medium
garlic	4 cloves
ginger	1 tsp
cinnamon	1/4 Tsp
chicken stock	1 and 1/2 cups
tomato sauce	3 cups

| tomatoes | 1/2 cup |
| spinach | 1 cup |

fresh mint at will

Directions:

1. Wash the meat and cut into 1-inch cubes. Set aside.
2. Peel the garlic and mince it. Peel the onions, chop finely.
3. Wash and cut tomatoes. Peel and grate the ginger. Wash and chop spinach.
4. Take a medium bowl, conjoin together coriander, cumin, red pepper powder, mint, turmeric, salt and pepper at will.
5. Add lamb meat and toss to coat.
6. Take another large skillet, heat olive oil over high heat. Put lamb meat and cook for about 5 minutes (or until browned from all sides).
7. Put the lamb in the Crock Pot.
8. In this skillet, roast quickly onion, minced garlic, ginger, cinnamon. Cook for 4 minutes. Put this mixture in the Crock Pot also.
9. Add tomato sauce and chicken broth.
10. Add tomatoes to the Crock Pot. Cover the lid of the Crock Pot and put on LOW for 7 hours.
11. Serve with fresh mint.
12. Bon Appetite!

68.Crock Pot vegetable and lamb soup

This keto Crock Pot vegetable and lamb soup in perfect winter dish. Hot and easy! You may add other veggies you like – frozen onions, garlic, dill, cabbage etc. Add your favorite species or sour cream by serving!

Ingredients (6 servings):

Onion	1 pcs
Celery	1 stalk
lamb shanks	2 pcs
asparagus	⅛ cup
salt	1 teaspoon
beef stock	4 cups

fresh parsley at will

pepper and salt at will

Directions:

1. Peel the onions, chop finely. Chop the celery.
2. Wash the lamb meat, remove fat, cut into cubes.
3. Open the Crock Pot and put lamb pieces, season with salt, and pepper at will.
4. Add chopped onion, celery, add asparagus, salt, and pepper at will, add beef stock, toss everything well.
5. Cover the lid and put on HIGH for 4 hours.

6. Serve with pepper and fresh parsley at will.
7. Bon Appetite!

69.Crock Pot Authentic Scotch broth

This is the authentic Scotch recipe of the broth cooked of fresh lamb with onions, leek, cabbage. The amount of the species is minimum but you may add dill, chili or other hot species right before eating!

Ingredients (6 servings):

lamb neck	1lb
Water	4 cups
onion	1 large pcs
leek	1 pcs
salt and black pepper at will	
cabbage	1 cup
fresh parsley at will	

Directions:

1. Wash the lamb meat, take off fat, cut into cubes.
2. Peel the onions, chop finely.
3. Chop the leek.
4. Shred the cabbage. Set aside.
5. Open the Crock Pot and put lamb pieces, season with salt, and pepper at will.
6. Add chopped onion, leek, cabbage. Add water.
7. Toss everything well, cover and out on LOW for 5 hours. Until lamb is fully cooked.
8. Season with salt and pepper at will.
9. Add the chopped parsley and serve.
10. Bon Appetite!

70.Keto Crock Pot Reuben soup

The keto Crock Pot Reuben soup full of corned beef, sauerkraut, a bouquet of various seeds for flavor, adding the whipping cream or Swiss cheese the will be melted at the end, makes an excellent fallback to any other common soup. Have just a taste!

Ingredients (10 servings):

beef broth/stock (or your favorite one homemade) 7- 8 cups

onion	1 pcs medium
garlic	3 cloves
butter	2 Tablespoons
corned beef	2 lbs

sauerkraut	1 lb (453 grams)
celery seeds	1/2 teaspoon
coriander seeds	1 teaspoon
dill seeds	1 teaspoon
mustard seeds	1 tablespoon
Swiss or whipping cream cheese	½ cup

Sea salt and pepper at will

Directions:

1. Peel and dice the onion. Peel the garlic and mince it.
2. Wash and dice carefully the corned beef.
3. Take a medium or a little skillet, add there 1 tablespoon of butter and brown there diced onion. It must be translucent. After some minutes add minced garlic, cook not more than 1 - 1.5 minutes. Take the skillet off.
4. Take the Crock Pot, add there beef broth, seeds, sauerkraut, prepared garlic and onion, add there also the remained butter from the skillet. If you don't like to eat the seeds in the prepared dish later, you may put the coriander, dill and celery seeds in a small tea ball, they will soften nicely though.
5. Cover and cook on LOW for 6 hours or on HIGH for 3-4 hours.
6. After the cooking time is over, open the Crock Pot and add cheese, put on WARM.
7. Serve warm, the cheese must be melted!
8. Bon Appetite!

71. Mexican keto chicken soup

For this tasty keto Crock Pot soup, you need just 4 simple ingredients. This extraordinary soup recipe let you leave the kitchen fats and forget about the long cooking process! If you don't want to lose too much time preparing the chicken broth, you may buy it in the store. The «hardest» work here will be taking off the chicken pieces and cut them into cubes. This keto Crock Pot Reuben soup includes only about 400 calories, the fat percent here is about 20 grams per serving. Let the Mexican keto chicken soup prepare when you are away from home!

Ingredients (4 servings):

chicken pieces boneless	1 1/2 pounds
chunky salsa	15.5 ounces
chicken broth	15 ounces
Hard cheese	8 ounces

Pepper and sea salt at will

Directions:

1. Prepare the chicken pieces – wash it thoroughly, take the skin off, cut into pieces.
2. Cut the cheese into small cubes or shred it into the plate.
3. Put the chicken pieces into the Crock Pot.

4. Add there chicken broth (bought at the market or readymade), add the remaining ingredients – chunky salsa, salt, pepper.
5. Cover and cook on HIGH for 4-5 hours, or on LOW for 6-7 hours.
6. After the time is over, take the chicken pieces off, shred them and place in the Crock Pot again. Add cheese and cover.
7. Serve hot. You may dress the soup with your favorite greenery.
8. Bon Appetite!

72.Keto pumpkin and coconut soup Crock Pot

Do you know the recipe how to prepare an easy keto coconut and pumpkin soup? Not yet? I will tell you the easiest and cheapest way to cook it. This soup prepared quickly in the Crock Pot is super winter warmer one! Moreover, you may freeze this tasty soup in small baking dishes (for example for baking of muffins in portions) and re-heat when you wish.

Ingredients (7 servings):

Yellow onion	1 pcs medium
ginger	1 tsp
garlic	1 tsp
butter	55 g
pumpkin chunks	500 g
vegetable stock	500 ml
coconut cream	400 ml

salt and pepper to taste

Directions:

1. Peel and dice the onion, after this garlic and mince it (or press – as you wish).
2. Peel the ginger and crush it.
3. Wash and cut the pumpkin. Take off the seeds.
4. Put all the ingredients into the Crock Pot – diced onions, garlic, butter, vegetable stock, pepper and salt at will, pumpkin chunks, crushed ginger.
5. Cover and cook on LOW for 6-7 hours or on HIGH for 5-6 hours.
6. After the time is over, take the cover off, puree the mixture in the blender until smooth consistency.
7. Put on WARM until ready and serve!
8. Garnish with coconut cream.
9. Bon Appetite!

73.Keto cabbage soup Crock Pot

Never cooked a cabbage soup in the Crock Pot? It is rather easy and tasty dish! You may think: «What is the reason this recipe is included in the cookbook?» This soup is simple to prepare, tasty to eat corresponds to your keto diet, doesn't need great cooking skills, just basic one. Everything you need – to follow the recipe and carry off all the measurements!

Ingredients (8 servings):

Ground beef	2 pounds
Onion	¼ pcs large
Garlic	1 clove
cumin ground	1 teaspoon
cabbage	1 head large
bouillon	4 cubes
Diced tomatoes & green chilies	10 oz can
Water	4 cups

Salt and pepper to taste

Directions:

1. Peel the yellow onion diced it into a bowl. Peel the garlic, press it into the bowl or mince. Chop the cabbage, adding it to the same bowl where the onion is.
2. Brown the ground beef a little over high heat. After some minutes, add the onion, cook in the same skillet until translucent.
3. Put the ground beef in the Crock Pot, add there the browned onion, bouillon.
4. Add to the Crock Pot pressed or minced garlic, chopped cabbage, ground cumin, diced tomatoes, green chilies, water to the Crock Pot.
5. Stir all the ingredients thoroughly, cover the Crock Pot and bring them to boil over the high heat. It takes you about 5 hours.
6. After the time is over (5 hours), reduce it to medium-low, the soup must simmer for 30 minutes on LOW.
7. Add pepper and salt at will.
8. Serve warm.
9. Bon Appetite!

74. Keto Beef Stroganoff soup Crock Pot

For those who have always loved to cook the beef stroganoff at home or to taste it at the restaurants. There is no other better way to taste the delicious and tender beef in a classic variation. Spice the beef with onion and garlic, add paprika or black pepper at will. Warm, flavorful, savory, spoon after spoon... Mmm, it's delicious! I think this soup idea is a great one!

Ingredients (12 servings):

beef rump steaks	2 large pcs
ghee or lard	¼ cup
garlic	2 cloves
white onion	1 pcs medium
bone broth (it may be also chicken or vegetable stock)	5 cups
paprika	2 tsp

Dijon mustard (or homemade)	1 tbsp
juice of lemon	1 pcs
sour cream (it could be also heavy whipping cream)	1 ½ cup
freshly parsley	¼ cup
salt	1 Tsp
ground black pepper	¼ tsp

Optionally, a thickener could be used: take 1 tablespoon ground chia seeds or arrowroot powder at will. Mix everything in a ¼ cup warm water or use cream and egg yolk mixture.

Directions:

1. Prepare two beef rump steaks and put them in the freezer in a single layer (for 40 minutes). This procedure makes the steaks to cut them easily into thin strips. After 40 minutes, take a keen knife and slice the steaks into thin strips. Season them with pepper and salt.
2. Peel the white onion, chop it carefully. Peel the garlic and mince.
3. Squeeze the juice of 1 lemon in a cup (it must be about 4 tablespoons).
4. Wash and chop the fresh parsley into a plate.
5. Take a large skillet with a heavy bottom, grease with a half of lard or ghee. Once the skillet is hot, add the beef slices, but only in a single layer. Fry them over a high heat until brown and take them off to the plate. Do the same with remaining beef slices. Combine them in the plate altogether.
6. Take a bowl with a bone broth, add there paprika, Dijon mustard, salt, and pepper and mix everything. Add the lemon juice, browned beef slices, onion, and garlic. Cover and cook on LOW in the Crock Pot for 3 hours.
7. After the time is over, open the Crock Pot and add sour cream, freshly chopped parsley and ground black pepper. Keep on WARM for 30 minutes.
8. If you use a thickener, add this mixture at the end of the same rule.
9. Eat the dish hot with a slice of keto bread. It could be also cooled in the fridge and stored up to 5 days!
10. Bon Appetite!

75.Keto chicken bacon chowder

The keto chicken bacon chowder is beyond belief! If you are going to strike your relatives and friends, or your lover with your cooking skills, this is the right choice to prepare. This chowder could be well kept in the refrigerator for 4-5 days. A mix of vegetables and chicken make this combination amazing!

Ingredients (15 servings):

Garlic	4 cloves
shallot	1 pcs medium
leek	1 small
celery	2 ribs
sweet onion	1 pcs medium

butter	4 tablespoons	
chicken broth		2 cups
chicken breasts		1 lb
cream cheese	8 oz	
heavy cream		1 cup
bacon, cooked crisp and crumbled	1 lb	
sea salt		1 teaspoon
black pepper		1 teaspoon
powder of garlic		1 teaspoon
thyme dried		1 teaspoon

Directions:

1. Peel the garlic and mince it carefully. Peel the shallot, chop it finely. Clean the leek, trim and slice. Wash and dice the celery. Peel the sweet onion also, wash and slice it.
2. Divide the chicken broth into two cups. Do the same with butter.
3. Prepare your Crock Pot, add there shallot, garlic, celery, leek, onion, 2 tablespoons of butter, chicken broth (1 cup), season with a little bit pepper and salt to taste.
4. Cap and cook on LOW for 1 hour.
5. While the veggies are cooked, prepare the chicken pieces – wash and cut them thoroughly.
6. Open your Crock Pot and add cut chicken breasts, add also cream cheese, cream, black pepper and salt, garlic powder, dried thyme, chicken broth, bacon strips. Mix plenty all the components. Cap and cook on LOW for 6-7 hours.
7. Serve warm.
8. Bon Appetite!

76.Keto Crock Pot cream of broccoli soup

This is the soup season! The easy combination of vegetables with cheddar cheese is amazing! The keto cream of broccoli soup is the best way to add healthy vegetables to your daily life during cold and long winter days. Cauliflower and broccoli are full of vitamins, their superpower is incredible of which you might be not aware!

Ingredients (11 servings):

Ghee (or grass-fed butter, coconut oil)	1 tablespoon
broccoli	4 cups
cauliflower	1 cup
garlic	3 cloves
shallot	1 large pcs
chicken broth or stock	4 cups

sea salt	1.5 teaspoon
black pepper	1/2 teaspoon
turmeric	1/4 teaspoon
coconut milk (you must double this if you don't use the cheese)	1/2 cup
cheddar cheese from pasture-raised cows	4 oz

For garnish (if desired): sliced bacon, parsley, fresh cracked black pepper

Directions:

1. Wash and chop the broccoli and cauliflower into florets. Peel the garlic, slice it. Peel, wash and slice a large shallot.
2. Shred the cheddar cheese onto the plate.
3. Put all the ingredients into the Crock Pot – chopped cauliflower and broccoli, garlic and onion. Add the chicken broth, melted butter or ghee (or coconut oil), mix everything in a Crock Pot. Season with pepper and salt, turmeric.
4. Cover and cook on LOW for about 5-6 hours. The vegetables must be tender and melt in the mouth. You may cook everything on HIGH for 3 hours.
5. When the time is over, add coconut milk, cheddar cheese and blend the soup with a food processor or blender. The soup is hot that's why be very careful!
6. Serve warm, garnish with chopped parsley, bacon slices, cracked black pepper.
7. Bon Appetite!

77.Keto Crock Pot Chicken Soup

This soup is an amazing combination of chicken luscious pieces, mixed with veggies. The Crock Pot saves your precious time as well as the energy in the kitchen. Basically, one should just add the chicken to your Crock Pot, pile the onion, add your favorite vegetables that will make a delicious mixture of the ingredients. Sweet peppers and jalapenos give the more substance to this chicken soup. I usually serve this soup with avocado, black pepper at will. Usually, I begin to cook this dish in the early morning, and then I have it ready for dinner.

Ingredients (13 servings):

boneless skinless chicken breasts	1 1/2 lbs.
yellow onion	1 medium
bell pepper	1 pcs medium
jalapeno	1 pcs
garlic	2 cloves
diced tomatoes	1 15-oz. can
chicken stock	2 cups
chili powder	1 tbsp
cumin	1 tbsp

dried oregano	1 tsp
paprika	1/2 tsp
fresh coriander	2 tbsp
avocado, pitted and sliced	1 pcs medium

Salt and freshly ground pepper, to taste

Directions:

1. Prepare the chicken pieces – take off the bones and skin. Wash the breasts and dry with the paper towel.
2. Peel the onion, wash and dice. Wash the sweet pepper, take off the corns, slice it thinly.
3. Wash the jalapeno, dry it with the paper towel, dice into the bowl. Peel the garlic and mince it. Wash the coriander and mince. Wash the avocado, take off the core, slice.
4. Put the chicken pieces into the Crock Pot, add the onion, sweet pepper sliced, chopped jalapeno, minced garlic on the top of the chicken. After this pour the diced tomatoes as well as chicken broth over the top. Season with chili powder, dried cumin, paprika and oregano, pepper, salt.
5. Cap and cook on LOW for 7-8 hours.
6. Once the preparation time is over, open the Crock Pot and using a fork check if the chicken is ready.
7. Serve with fresh chopped coriander and slices of avocado.
8. Bon Appetite!

78.Pumpkin, chicken and spinach keto soup

I call this keto soup the Shrek soup because of its yellow-green-mustard color. It is an easy and quick meal that is a fantastic one for those mums who are always busy. The mix of sage, pumpkin, sweetener, a little bit nutmeg allows the dish to be delicious and perfect. This consistency is something between stew and soup.

Ingredients (14 servings):

olive oil	2 tablespoons
chicken breast	1 pound
onion	1 large
garlic	3 large cloves
chicken stock	3-4 cups
pumpkin purée	15 ounce can
sweetener	2 teaspoons
fresh sage leaves	1½ teaspoons
salt	1 teaspoon
freshly ground black pepper	¼ teaspoon

freshly ground nutmeg	⅛ teaspoon
bay leaf	1 pcs
fresh baby spinach leaves	4 cups
fresh lemon juice	1 tablespoon

Dressing: crispy bacon strips

Directions:

1. Prepare the chicken breasts: wash them thoroughly, dry with the paper towel, cut into cubes.
2. Peel the onion and garlic, crush them. Wash the fresh sage leaves, mince them (or use the dried sage leaves). You may roast the minced onion and garlic in 2 tablespoons of olive oil or add these ingredients unroasted to the remained ingredients.
3. Put the chicken pieces into the Crock Pot and stir it with 3 cups of chicken broth. Add there the pumpkin puree, sweetener, pepper, and salt, nutmeg, sage, and bay leaf. Stir everything together.
4. Cover, and cook on LOW for 3 hours.
5. Open the Crock Pot after the time is over, add fresh minced spinach leaves, add ground nutmeg, ground black pepper, salt.
6. Cover the Crock Pot again, turn on WARM and let the leaves wilt. (about 1-2 minutes). After this stir in the fresh lemon juice.
7. Serve warm! Dress with crispy bacon strips.
8. Bon Appetite!

79.Jalapeno popper keto soup

When the weather is wet and cool I try to eat warm and delicious dishes to let my soul and stomach get warm. This soup is, in general, a one pot meal, keto-friendly and adapted for my great helper – the Crock Pot. My family always enjoys this one, tasting all spicy and hot ingredients. I'm sure enough you'll like it very much. The great thing about this soup, you may add here your favorite species to make it hotter or vice versa.

Ingredients (17 servings):

boneless skinless chicken breasts	1 1/2 lbs	
butter		3 tablespoons
garlic minced		2 cloves
onion chopped		½ pcs
green pepper	1/2	
jalapenos		2 pcs
bacon crumbled and cooked	1/2 lb	
cream cheese	6 oz	
chicken broth	3 cups	

heavy whipping cream	1/2 cup
paprika	1/4 Tsp
cumin	1 teaspoon
salt	1 teaspoon
pepper	1/2 teaspoon
Swiss Cheese	3/4 cup
Cheddar Cheese	3/4 cup
xanthan gum	1/2 Tsp

Directions:

1. Peel the onion and garlic, mince them and put in a bowl.
2. Prepare the chicken breasts – wash them and cut. Shred the Swiss cheese and cheddar.
3. Wash the green pepper, take off the seeds, dry with a paper towel.
4. Wash and dry with a paper towel jalapenos, take off the seeds. Chop carefully.
5. Put the chicken breasts into the Crock Pot, add chicken broth, butter, onion and garlic, chopped jalapenos, green pepper, salt, cumin, paprika, and pepper.
6. Cover and cook on HIGH for 3-4 hours or on LOW on 5-7 hours.
7. After the cooking time is over, take off the chicken, cut into small pieces, and add to the Crock Pot again.
8. Turn the Crock Pot on WARM, open the cover and add cream cheese, heavy whipping cream, cooked bacon (a half of it). Cheese must be melted.
9. At the end of the preparation, sprinkle xanthan gum on the top of your dish, allow it to simmer a little bit on LOW or on WARM for 10 minutes. Let the soup reach the thick consistency.
10. Serve warm with shredded cheese, bacon strips and parsley at will.

80.Keto cabbage-pork Crock Pot

I like to cook soups because this meal is first, a delicious one, secondly, it is essential one, and third – you don't need to wash too many dishes after it! Moreover, cooking the essential meal like cabbage-pork Crock Pot you don't need to prepare each day the new dish – this delicious one will be enough for 2-3 days. This soup is something fabulous, reach on flavor without carbs. You may also add cauliflower (riced). But it is also great without it.

Ingredients (12 servings):

onion diced	½ pcs medium
garlic minced	2 cloves
pork	1 1/2 lbs
broth (homemade or buy at the store)	3 cups
diced tomatoes	1 14 oz can
tomato sauce	1 8 oz can

Bragg's Aminos	1/4 cup
cabbage chopped	1 small/medium
Worcestershire Sauce	3 Tsp
Parsley	1/2 Tsp
Salt	1/2 Tsp
Pepper	1/2 Tsp

Directions:
1. Peel garlic and onion and slice them thoroughly.
2. Prepare the pork slices – wash and cut them, drain the water.
3. Cut the cabbage. Wash the parsley and chop.
4. Put the pork slices into the Crock Pot, add sliced onion and garlic, tomato sauce, diced tomatoes from the can, broth, Bragg's Aminos, Worcestershire Sauce, pepper and salt, chopped fresh parsley.
5. Cover and cook on HIGH for 6-7 hours, on LOW for 3-4 hours.
6. The cabbage and the pork must reach the desired tenderness it means the soup is ready.
7. Serve with fresh parsley.
8. Bon Appetite!

81.Keto Crock Pot pizza soup

This keto pizza soup is awesome! I have cooked it several times already! It is something amazing on a plate! I use my favorite sausages, pepperoni, Parmesan and mozzarella cheeses, delicious and hot species. You may also add fresh dill or parsley at the end of cooking process.

Ingredients (12 servings):

crushed tomatoes (can use whole or stewed)	1 (16 ounces) can
beef broth	2 (16 ounces) cans
olives	2 (16 ounces) cans
green pepper	1 pcs medium
onion	1 small
Italian sausage	1 lb
Pepperoni	1/2 lb
garlic powder	1 teaspoon
dried oregano	2 teaspoons
Italian seasoning	2 teaspoons
mozzarella cheese	1 cup
Parmesan cheese	1/4 cup

Pepper and salt to taste

Directions:

1. Wash and dry the green pepper, take off the corns. Slice the pepperoni thinly. Peel the onion and crush.
2. Cut the sausages.
3. Grate the mozzarella cheese and Parmesan cheese.
4. Put the sausages into the Crock Pot, add crushed tomatoes, beef broth, crushed olives, crushed green pepper and pepperoni, onion, dried oregano, garlic powder, pepper and salt to taste.
5. Cover and cook on LOW for 6-7 hours.
6. Once the time is over, add crushed or shredded Parmesan and mozzarella cheese.
7. Serve warm and enjoy!

82.Crock Pot Zuppa Toscana soup

If you have ever heard about Zuppa Toscana soup, you must know that the main components are sausages, diced tomatoes, kale, and broth. It is not hard to prepare this soup, the diced tomatoes could be easily substituted with fresh cauliflower florets and vice versa. This soup could be prepared from the frozen cauliflower. I always use the Italian sausage but don't forget to check the sugar consistency in these sausages in the stores.

Ingredients (11 servings):

hot or mild ground Italian sausage	1 pound
olive or avocado oil	1 tablespoon
onion	½ cup
garlic	3 cloves
chicken (maybe also vegetable stock)	36 ounces
cauliflower	1 large head
kale	3 cups
crushed red pepper	¼ teaspoon
salt	1 teaspoon
black pepper	½ teaspoon
heavy cream	½ cup

Pepper and salt at will

Directions:

1. Peel the onion and garlic, dice it finely.
2. Wash the head of cauliflower, dice it into small florets.
3. Cut the kale.
4. Wash and crush the red pepper, take off the seeds.
5. Prepare the sausages – cut them into small pieces.

6. Put the sausage into the Crock Pot, place there olive oil, crushed onion, minced garlic, chicken broth, crushed red pepper, chopped kale, black pepper, and salt at will. Stir everything well.
7. Cover and cook on LOW for 7-8 hours on HIGH for 3-4 hours.
8. Once the time is over, add heavy cream.
9. Serve hot!

83.Keto Crock Pot buffalo chicken soup

This tasty buffalo chicken soup is easy to cook in the Crock Pot. It is keto-friendly, delicious and simple one. You need here just 7 simple ingredients that could be found at the store near your house. I'm sure you will definitely like it for the next dinner!

Ingredients (7 servings):

cooked chicken, shredded	2 cups
cream cheese	4 oz
butter	3 tablespoon
Frank's Red Hot Sauce (or another one)	1/3 cup
chicken broth	4 cups
Celery	¼ cup
blue cheese dressing (optional)	1 tablespoon

Salt and pepper to taste

Directions:
1. Shred the cooked chicken.
2. Chop the fresh celery in cubes. Shred the blue cheese onto a plate.
3. Combine butter, cream cheese, hot sauce, chicken broth, chopped celery, pepper and salt to taste. Puree everything in a blender until smooth consistency.
4. Cover and cook on LOW for 2-3 hours. Don't let the mixture boil.
5. Once the cooking time is over, add shredded cheese, a little bit fresh celery, pepper, salt and the shredded chicken.
6. Taste and season with favorite greenery.
7. Bon Appetite!

84.Crock Pot Chicken Fajita soup

Any soup is a great idea especially when there is a cold time of the year outside. Especially I like the soups that are tasty and flavor, so do the whole my family. The keto chicken Fajita soup is a great combination of vegetables and chicken meat on a plate as well as the mix of flavor species. Don't hesitate to prepare this one for today's dinner.

Ingredients (10 servings):

chicken breast	1 1/2 lbs
chicken stock	32 oz

diced tomatoes	14.5 oz can
yellow bell pepper	1 medium pcs
orange bell pepper	1 medium pcs
onion	1 medium
garlic	4 large cloves
Taco Seasoning	4 tablespoon
fresh cilantro	2 tablespoon
sea salt, more to taste	2 teaspoon

Directions:

1. Wash and dry with a paper towel the peppers, take off the seeds, slice.
2. Peel the onion and dice. Peel the garlic and press it or mince. Chop the fresh and washed cilantro.
3. Put the Crock Pot on LOW, add there all the ingredients – diced tomatoes, chicken pieces and broth, sliced colored peppers, diced onions, minced garlic. Add Taco Seasoning, chopped fresh cilantro, sea salt, and pepper to taste.
4. Cook for 6 hours.
5. Once the time is over, check the readiness with a fork. The chicken pieces should come easily apart.
6. Keep on WARM.
7. Bon Appetite!

85.Keto Italian meatball noodle soup

This recipe includes my favorite vegetable – it is zucchini! Have you known that making noodles from zucchini could be so fun and fantastic!? The great thing about this delicious soup – is that a person could make noodles for almost any veggies you like or you have at your house right now! The meatballs are the integral parts of this soup, cooked from the ground beef or ground pork as you wish. Adding the Parmesan cheese makes it absolutely delicious!

Ingredients (17 servings):

beef stock	32 oz
zucchini	1 medium pcs
celery	2 ribs
onion	1 small pcs
tomato	1 medium pcs
garlic powder	1 1/2 teaspoon
ground beef	1 1/2 lb
Parmesan cheese	1/2 cup

Garlic	6 cloves
egg	1 large pcs
fresh parsley	4 tablespoons
sea salt	1 1/2 teaspoon
onion powder	1 1/2 teaspoon
Italian seasoning	1 teaspoon
dried oregano	1 teaspoon
black pepper	1/2 teaspoon
coconut flour (for meatballs)	1/2 cup

Directions:

1. Wash and dry with a paper towel zucchini. Cut in noodles.
2. Wash and dice the tomatoes.
3. Peel the onion, dice it also. Chop the celery. Peel the garlic and mince it carefully. Chop the fresh and washed parsley.
4. Shred the Parmesan cheese onto a plate.
5. Add to the Crock Pot the beef broth, zucchini, celery, tomato, onion, garlic, salt, pepper to taste.
6. Cover and cook on LOW for 3 hours.
7. While the broth is cooking, combine in a large bowl a half of shredded Parmesan cheese, minced garlic, cracked fresh egg, sea salt, a little bit black pepper, parsley, onion powder, Italian seasoning, oregano. All the components must be well mixed. A form of this mixture the meatballs, it must be approximately 20-25 meatballs. Put them in the coconut flour from all the sides.
8. Add the meatballs into simmering soup carefully (use the long spoon). Don't worry to put them without prior cooking, as they will be cooked in the Crock Pot.
9. Cover and continue to cook for 1-2 hours on LOW or put it after this on WARM.
10. Serve with the rest of shredded Parmesan cheese.
11. Bon Appetite!

86.Crock Pot Andouille sausage cabbage soup

It doesn't matter what kind of climate is appropriate for your area – is it warm, wet or cold, it doesn't matter what season is it now – this dish will be amazing always! You can buy the main ingredients for the preparation of this soup at any time of the year almost at any store – sausages and cabbage are the most widespread ingredients for soup cooking.

Ingredients (13 servings):

andouille sausage sliced (4 links)	12 ounces
extra virgin olive oil	1 tablespoons
shallots	1/2 cup
garlic	4 cloves

cabbage	1 medium head
chicken broth	6 cups
water	4 cups
cider vinegar	1 tablespoon
onion powder	1 teaspoon
celery salt	1 teaspoon
dried thyme	1/2 teaspoon
caraway seeds	1 teaspoon
fennel seeds	1 teaspoon

Pepper, and salt at will

Directions:
1. Peel the shallots, slice it finely. Peel the garlic, mince it. Slice the cabbage thinly.
2. Slice the sausages, heat the olive oil in a medium skillet. Brown the sausages in a skillet from all the sides. Add shallots and cook until softened (translucent).
3. Put the browned sausages together with onions to the Crock Pot, after this add the garlic, sliced cabbage, chicken broth, water (4 cups), cider vinegar, onion powder, celery salt, dried thyme, caraway seeds, fennel seeds, pepper and salt at will.
4. Cover and cook on LOW for 7 hours or on HIGH for 4 hours. The cabbage must be tender.
5. Serve warm.
6. Bon Appetite!

87.Crock Pot celery soup with bacon

This recipe is for those who like celery-bacon combination garnished with bacon. When you don't have too much time to cook complicated dishes following recipes with 15-17 servings, this one is definitely for you. It is so easy that even a kid could prepare it. If you don't like the pale color of this soup on your plate, you may garnish it with fresh bright parsley that will add some spotted colors in it.

Ingredients (9 servings):
celery	1 bunch (about 1 1/2 pounds)
broccoli	1 pound
yellow onion	2 large pcs
Garlic	3 cloves
chicken broth	4 cups
salt	1/2 teaspoon
white pepper	1/2 teaspoon
heavy cream	1/3 cup

bacon   4 to 6 slices

salt and pepper to taste

Directions:

1. Peel the onion, garlic. Chop the celery, onions, and garlic.
2. Cut the bacon into thick slices.
3. Mix the vegetables in the broth (broccoli, celery, onions, garlic), add white pepper, salt. Put everything in the Crock Pot.
4. Cover and cook on LOW 4 hours.
5. Once the time is over, puree the mixture using a food processor or a blender.
6. Stir in cream before serving. Blend once more.
7. Season with bacon slices pepper and salt.
8. Bon Appetite!

88. Wisconsin Cauliflower Soup

Wisconsin cauliflower soup is one of my favorite dishes. It has a creamy consistency with a light version. This version is great for dinner every day or for family parties. I always use the chicken broth to reach the creaminess and lightness, but it may be also turkey broth or another favorite one. In the same way, you could choose cheese.

Ingredients (7 servings):

Butter	1 tablespoon
sweet white onion	1 medium pcs
garlic minced	3 cloves
chicken broth	14.5 oz. can
cauliflower florets	2 lbs.
dry mustard	1/2 teaspoon
pepper cheese	1 cup

Salt and pepper to taste

Directions:

1. Peel carefully onion and garlic, finely dice the onion into a bowl, mince the garlic.
2. Take a medium skillet, melt the butter over medium heat, brown there the diced onion 3-4 minutes, add the minced garlic at the end of the time. Put the mixture into the Crock Pot.
3. Shred the pepper cheese, put it into a cup.
4. Wash the cauliflowers, cut into florets.
5. Add to the Crock Pot dry mustard, salt, paprika or black pepper to taste, cauliflower florets, pour chicken broth.
6. Cover and cook on LOW for 3 hours.
7. Once the time is over, open the Crock Pot and using a food processor or a blender make a smooth mixture of it.
8. Season with black pepper and shredded cheese.
9. Bon appetite!

89.Crock Pot chicken Thai soup

Using the genius invention of the Crock Pot, my dream dinner comes easily true. I don't need to brown some ingredients, using different pans or skillets. This recipe is easily adapted for those who follow keto diet, tries to eat healthy food and vegetables. In your version, change the chicken broth with water if you wish or with vegetable broth.

Ingredients (12 servings):

red curry paste	2 tablespoons
coconut milk	2 12 ounce cans
chicken stock	2 cups
fish sauce	2 tablespoons
sweetener	2 tablespoons
peanut butter	2 tablespoons
chicken breasts	1½ pounds
red bell pepper	1 pcs
onion	1 pcs
fresh ginger	1 pcs
lime juice	1 tablespoon
cilantro for garnish	

Directions:

1. Wash and dry with the paper towel the chicken breasts, cut into 11/2 inch pieces. Set aside.
2. Wash and dry with the paper towel sweet pepper, take off the seeds, slice it into ¼ inch pieces.
3. Peel the onion and slice finely.
4. Peel the fresh ginger, mince it.
5. Wash the lime, squeeze a lime juice into a cup.
6. Take a large bowl, mix there curry paste, chicken broth, coconut milk, fish sauce, sweetener, peanut butter, stir well. Put the mixture into the Crock Pot, add chicken breasts, sweet pepper, ginger, onion. Combine well.
7. Cover and cook on HIGH for 3 hours.
8. Once the time is over, open the Crock Pot, stir in lime juice. Serve with cilantro.
9. Bon Appetite!

90.Crock Pot keto Taco soup

Most of all I like easy and light recipes, that don't need many steps in preparation and too many skills. I think Taco keto soup is one of these recipes. This dish needs 8 simple components, after some hours the dish is ready on your table. I like to use a combination of sausages, it makes the recipe, even more, quicker than usual. When it comes about Taco seasoning, I try to use my homemade one – using garlic salt, chipotle pepper, adobo seasoning, paprika.

Ingredients (8 servings):

ground pork beef (or sausage)	2 lbs
cream cheese	2, 8- ounce package
Rotel	2, 10- ounce cans
Taco seasonings	2 Tablespoons
chicken broth	4 cups
Cilantro - fresh or dried	1-2 tablespoons
cheese (for garnish optional)	1/2 cup
Sea salt and pepper at will	
Dill for garnish	

Directions:

1. Prepare the sausages – slice them finely, or crown the ground pork beef on the skillet using olive oil (ca. 1 – 2 tablespoon). Set aside.
2. Shred cheese into a little plate.
3. Place the cream cheese, Rotel, taco seasonings, all cups of chicken broth, cilantro into the Crock Pot. Mix everything.
4. Add there the ground pork beef or sausages, combine once more.
5. Cover and cook on LOW for 3-4 hours.
6. Season with pepper and salt, add dill to the plate.
7. Garnish with shredded favorite cheese.
8. Bon Appetite!

91. Crock Pot tomato basil Parmesan soup

This keto tomato basil soup is especially for the tomato fans. Creamy tomato-basil soup is the easiest you can cook quickly and that tastes extraordinary! This combination of red tomatoes and flavor basil make me crazy. Shredded Parmesan adds special eating qualities to this keto soup.

Ingredients (13 servings):

diced tomatoes	2 15-ounce cans
tomato sauce	1 10-ounce can
fresh basil	¼ cup
minced garlic	3 teaspoons
salt	1 tablespoon
pepper	1 teaspoon

white onion	1 medium pcs
heavy cream	1 cup
chicken or vegetable broth	4 cups
Parmesan cheese	2 cups
butter	3 tablespoons
almond flour	¼ cup
heavy cream OR half & half	½ cup

Directions:

1. Wash fresh basil, chop it finely.
2. Peel the onion, dice it. Peel the garlic, mince it. Shred the Parmesan cheese into a little bowl.
3. Add to the Crock Pot tomatoes, tomato sauce, garlic, pepper and salt, heavy cream, onion, broth (vegetable or chicken).
4. Cover and cook on HIGH for 2 hours or on LOW for 6 hours.
5. Once the time is over, using a food processor or a blender, make the smooth consistency of the soup. After the mixture is ready, return it to the Crock Pot.
6. Prepare the roux: melt the butter in a saucepan (on a medium heat), add almond flour, stir all the time. Flour clumps up. Add slowly (whisk) the heavy cream (possible also half & half), the mixture must be thickened, smooth. Pour this mixture into the Crock Pot, stir well.
7. Cover and cook on WARM for 1 hour.
8. Serve with shredded Parmesan cheese and remained fresh basil.
9. Bon Appetite!

92.Crock Pot acorn squash soup

Today, I decided finally to cook acorn squash soup. This is delicious, vegan, healthy soup that is rather easy to cook even for beginners. I decided to add a little bit cayenne pepper, just to accent the natural tastes of acorn squashes.

Ingredients (13 servings):

acorn squashes	3 pcs
sea salt	1 Tsp
ground black pepper	1 tsp
olive oil	2 tbsp
shallot	1 pcs
yellow onion	½ pcs
red onion	½ pcs
dried ginger	1/2 tsp

dried sage	1/4 Tsp
cayenne pepper	1/8 tsp
ground allspice	1/8 tsp
vegetable stock	4 cups
water	1 cup

Directions:

1. Peel the shallot, yellow and red onion, wash and chop everything finely.
2. Sprinkle the ready prepared cut acorn squashes with salt and pepper, put them into the Crock Pot, add a cup of water, cover and cook on LOW for 5 hours.
3. Remove the squash once the time is over, let it cool.
4. Remove flesh from acorns' skin using a spoon into the medium bowl.
5. Mix everything in a large bowl:
   Chopped onions, shallot, ginger, olive oil, cayenne pepper and stir everything. Add squash flesh and vegetable broth.
6. Cover and cook on LOW for 2 hours. Add dried sage.
7. Using a food processor or a blender make a puree mixture.
8. Once the puree is ready, add pepper and salt to taste. Eat warm.
9. Bon Appetite!

93.Keto Crock Pot Chicken Cordon Bleu soup

If you would like to surprise your family with silky and creamy soup texture, the chicken Cordon Blue soup is the right choice for today! Vegetables, ham, tarragon definitely help you to make a bouquet of flavors adding something amazing in your daily routine. The main part of preparation that is done in the Crock Pot let you leave home and don't wait until your dish is ready.

Ingredients (12 servings):

chicken broth	6 cups
ham	1 cup
chicken	2 pcs
white onion	1/2
garlic	2 cloves
Kosher salt	1 teaspoon
black pepper	1/2 teaspoon
tarragon	1 teaspoon
Swiss cheese	1 cup
Almond milk	1 cup
Butter	2 tablespoon

| almond flour | 2 tablespoons |

Directions:

1. Peel and dice the onion, peel the garlic and mince.
2. Prepare the chicken – take off the skin and bones, dice it.
3. Grate the Swiss cheese into the plate. Dice the ham.
4. Add the chicken broth, diced ham, chicken pieces, chopped onion, minced garlic, pepper and salt at will, tarragon in the Crock Pot.
5. Cover and cook on LOW for 5 hours.
6. At this time, heat the milk in a little bowl and whisk it in the cheese until everything is melted. Using a fork, stir together flour and softened butter. Whisk into the soup in the Crock Pot, stir until creamy and well mixed.
7. Put on WARM and cook for 1 hour.
8. Serve warm and season with pepper.
9. Bon Appetite!

94.Keto Crock Pot BBQ chicken soup

The flavor BBQ chicken soup appeared in my memory at once as I saw the barbecue sauce in the store. This recipe of BBQ soup is easy to prepare, isn't too watery, but tasty one. It would be a fantastic way to use chicken, combining it with sauce and cheddar cheese. You just need to have 8 servings to prepare this dish.

Ingredients (8 servings):

boneless skinless chicken breast	2 lb
onion	1/3 cup
garlic	3 cloves
chicken broth	5 cups
barbecue sauce (sugar-free)	1 cup
salt	1 teaspoon
pepper	½ teaspoon
Cheddar cheese	½ cup

Directions:

1. Wash the chicken breasts, cut them into pieces.
2. Peel the onion and garlic, chop and mince it finely.
3. Put in the Crock Pot the chicken breasts, minced garlic and chopped onion. Mix well everything together.
4. Take a medium bowl, combine there chicken broth, pepper, barbecue sauce, and salt. Pour this mixture into the Crock Pot.
5. Cover and cook on LOW for 6 hours.
6. Serve with shredded cheese.
7. Bon Appetite!

95.Spring Soup with a poached egg

This soup recipe I prepare all the time. It is the quickest one, easy to prepare when you need just three ingredients. Tender romaine lettuce and poached eggs make a great composition of light taste! Don't hesitate to cook it right now!

Ingredients (3 servings):

Poached eggs	2 pcs
chicken broth	32 oz (1 quart)
romaine lettuce	1 head
salt, pepper to taste	

Directions:

Bring the chicken broth (bought one or homemade) to the Crock Pot, let it boil for 1 hour.

1. Peel the poached eggs, cut into 2 parts.
2. Wash the romaine lettuce, chop it carefully. Add to the broth and let it cook for some minutes in the Crock Pot. The romaine lettuce must be slightly tender.
3. Add pepper and salt to the broth.
4. Serve warm with poached eggs.
5. Bon Appetite!

96.Spicy shrimp and chorizo soup

This spicy shrimp and chorizo soup is a perfect one for a cozy and warm family dinner. There is one big reason to love this soup – it is delicious and easy one! If you are a keto Crock Pot soup-lover, this dish must be in your soup collection! Try to cook it with your favorite species.

Ingredients (14 servings):

avocado oil divided	2 tablespoons
onion	1 medium pcs
celery ribs	3 pcs
yellow bell pepper	1 pcs
garlic sliced	4 cloves
Spanish-style dry-cured chorizo	12 ounces
tomato paste	1 tablespoon
smoked paprika	1½ teaspoons
ground coriander	1 teaspoon
sea salt	1 teaspoon
shrimp or chicken broth	1 quart
shrimp	1 pound

minced fresh cilantro   2 tablespoons

avocado   1 pcs

fresh cilantro for garnish

salt and pepper to taste

Directions:

1. Peel the onion and cut into slices. Wash the celery ribs and slice also. Peel the garlic, mince it.
2. Wash the pepper, dry with the paper towel, take off the corns and slice. Wash the cilantro and mince it. Wash the avocado, slice or dice for serving.
3. Peel the shrimps, wash and chop.
4. Take a medium pot, add avocado oil, heat it. While the oil is simmering, add the celery, onion, sweet pepper and stir everything. It takes you 6-7 minutes. The mixture must be translucent.
5. Add to the same pot minced garlic, chorizo (three-quarters), tomato paste, coriander, smoked paprika, and stir a little bit.
6. Put everything in the Crock Pot, add tomatoes, pour broth and cover. Cook on LOW for 1-2 hours.
7. Once the time is over, open the Crock Pot, add there more smoked paprika, salt, shrimps, coriander, cover and let it WARM for half an hour.
8. Season with fresh minced cilantro and black pepper, slices of avocado.
9. Bon Appetite!

97.Southern keto soup recipe

The traditional southern keto soup is enjoyed on New Year's Day, but, you may also cook it all year long! You may add here your favorite veggies, mustard greens, species and so on! I think, among the huge number of recipes, this soup must be definitely be cooked in your kitchen. I used here Sriracha – my favorite one, you may choose the other one preferred.

Ingredients (10 servings):

ghee or organic butter   3 tablespoons

onion   1 large pcs

fully-cooked ham steak   1 pound

garlic   2-3 cloves

celery stalks   2 pcs

chicken or veggie broth   6 cups

chopped kale   4 cups

chopped collards   6 cups

cider vinegar   1 tablespoon

Sriracha (or another hot sauce)   1 tablespoon

sea salt and ground pepper at will

Directions:
1. Peel and dice the onion, peel the garlic and mince it.
2. Cut the cooked ham steak into cubes.
3. Wash and chop the celery stalks.
4. Chop the kale into a cup. Chop the collards.
5. Add to the Crock Pot butter, diced onion, minced garlic, cut ham, celery, six cups of broth (veggie or chicken), chopped kale, collards, pepper and salt, cider vinegar. Mix everything. Add hot sauce and stir once more.
6. Cover and cook on LOW for 3 hours.
7. Add more pepper and salt if necessary.
8. Enjoy it warm!

98.Thai Tom Saap Pork Ribs Soup

One of the appetizing soups from Thailand is the Tom Saap pork ribs keto soup. This one is cooked usually with a plenty of chilies, but if you don't like it, you may exclude. It is amazing unusual soup, where the pork spare ribs could be changed for your favorite meat without losing the taste!

Ingredients (8 servings):

pork spare ribs		1 lb
red shallots		2 small
lemongrass stalks		3-4 small
slices of galangal (or use ginger)		10 thick
water		8 cups
kaffir lime leaves (or cilantro)	10 pcs	
Juice of 1 lime	1 pcs	
fish sauce		2 Tablespoons

Salt to taste

Optional: chili, green onions for garnish

Directions:
1. Wash the pork spare ribs, dry with the paper towel. Cut them into 2-inch chunks. Set aside.
2. Pell the red shallots, chop them into large pieces.
3. Chop the lemongrass stalks.
4. Tear the galangal up (or cut the ginger).
5. Press the juice of 1 lime into a cup.
6. Put the pork spare ribs into the Crock Pot, add water, add shallots, galangal, lemongrass, pepper, and salt if desired.
7. Cover and cook on LOW for 3 hours.

8. Once the time is over, open and put the lime juice, kaffir lime leaves, fish sauce, salt added to taste.
9. Cover and put on WARM.
10. Eat warm, season with green onions or chilies.
11. Bon Appetite!

99.Turmeric chicken soup

Nothing could be easier and quicker than this chicken turmeric soup! Let's think about the number of soups and the total time that you spend in the kitchen. It is not easy to prepare dinner, breakfast and supper, seven days a week. This soup recipe is your life-line. If you don't want to spend too much time in the kitchen or maybe you even hate this work, turmeric chicken soup is an inviting and warm bowl of goodness at your table, full of veggies and species.

Ingredients (13 servings):

turmeric powder	2 and 1/2 Tsp
cumin powder	1 and 1/2 Tsp
cayenne powder	1/8 teaspoon
boneless chicken thighs	3 small
coconut oil or butter	2 tablespoon
onion	1 small pcs
vegetables	4 cups
broth	4 cups
water	1 cup
bay leaf	1 pcs
grated fresh ginger	1 Tsp
chard	2 cups
full fat coconut milk	1/2 cup
fresh cilantro for garnish	
pepper and salt to taste	

Directions:

1. Peel and dice the onion.
2. Chop the vegetables (it is preferred to use broccoli and cauliflower). Grate fresh ginger.
3. Take a small bowl, combine cumin, salt, pepper, turmeric, cayenne.
4. Prepare the chard – slice it into thin ribbons,
5. Prepare the chicken things, cut them into small pieces, place into a bowl.
6. Melt one tablespoon of ghee or butter in a little skillet. Add there chopped onions. The mixture must be translucent. Put a half of the turmeric mixture, add a little bit broth (1 cup). Continue to stir.

7. Add to the Crock Pot water, broth (remaining), bay leaf, vegetables, ginger. Put the chicken things. Add also turmeric mixture there.
8. Cover and cook on LOW for about 2 hours.
9. Once the time is over, add milk.
10. Cover and put on WARM for an hour.
11. Serve warm, garnish with fresh cilantro, black pepper.
12. Bon Appetite!

100. Italian meatball soup

The Italian Meatball Soup is full of beef meatballs in a tasty broth! I usually prepare this soup as a one pot. The frozen cooked meatballs are rather tasty and tender. They rich the wished tenderness during the cooking time in the Crock Pot, savory broth makes them even more appetizing. Of course, you can make homemade meatballs from your favorite meat, frozen them and use when necessary. Diced tomatoes in a combination with oregano, garlic, and basil add the meatballs and the whole soup special relish. Season this soup with fresh basil leaves, remained shredded Parmesan cheese and keto bread!

Ingredients (5 servings):

frozen cooked Italian meatballs	1 bag (16 oz)
beef broth	1 ¾ cups
1 cup water	1 cup
diced tomatoes with basil, garlic and oregano	1 can (14.5 oz)
Parmesan cheese	1/3 cup
salt and pepper to taste	

Directions:

1. Unpack the frozen Italian meatballs, let them thaw.
2. Open the can with diced tomatoes.
3. Shred the Parmesan cheese into a small plate.
4. Put in the Crock Pot meatballs, beef broth, one cup of water, tomatoes undrained, pepper and salt to taste.
5. Cover and cook on LOW 8 hours.
6. Once the time is over, put the dish in a bowl and garnish quickly with shredded Parmesan cheese.
7. Bon Appetite!

101. Roasted red pepper smoked Gouda soup

If you are looking to cook something new and tasty for the dinner, this roasted red pepper smoked Gouda soup is a real discovery for today's dinner! Have you ever combined roasted red peppers with Gouda? Not yet? Except the removing of the skins from the pepper, this soup is rather easy to cook. Season with your favorite species and smoked Gouda!

Ingredients (11 servings):

large red peppers	6 pcs

olive oil	3 tablespoons
celery	2 stalks
onion	1 medium pcs
garlic	2 cloves
bay leaf	1 pcs
ground cumin	1 and 1/2 teaspoons
smoked paprika	1 and 1/2 teaspoons
chicken stock	3 cups
heavy cream	1/2 cup
grated smoked gouda	2 cups
salt and pepper to taste	

Directions:

Wash the large red peppers, dry them with a paper towel.

1. Take a large skillet, add the olive oil, place the peppers, roast them quickly, turn from all the sides, cover with a lid. All the peppers should be soft and charred. Let them cool. Set aside.
2. Once the peppers are cool enough, remove the seeds, chare the skin. Cut the peppers into strips.
3. Grate the Gouda.
4. Dice the celery stalks. Peel the onion and garlic, chop finely.
5. Add to the Crock Pot celery, chopped onion, and minced garlic, smoked paprika, bay leaves, cumin, pour the chicken broth, salt, and pepper.
6. Cover and cook on LOW for 2 hours.
7. Using a food processor or a blender, blend the soup to smooth consistency.
8. Add to the soup heavy cream and grated Gouda slowly.
9. Season with pepper and salt.
10. Bon Appetite!

102. Keto salmon head soup

Once the fishing season is opened, it is high time to cook this amazing, unique, tender soup. It means you can buy salmon or another fish you prefer. But salmon is the most proper one for today's dinner. This soup could be also cooked only with tails and heads if you just use heads or ties you have to double the portion. The soup prepared in the Crock Pot is so tender!

Ingredients (9 servings):

salmon head	1 pcs
salmon tail or other remaining pieces	1 pcs
onion	1 small pcs
green garlic	1 clove

wakame	1 cup
ginger	1 3 inch pieces
coconut vinegar	1/4 cup
coconut aminos	1/4 cup
zucchinis, spiraled into noodles	3 pcs
water	2 cups
chilies for garnish	
pepper and salt to taste	

Directions:
1. Peel the onion, slice it finely.
2. Peel the garlic, mince it.
3. Peel the ginger and grate.
4. Wash the zucchinis, spiralizer into noodles.
5. Add to the Crock Pot salmon heads on the bottom of it, tails (or other parts), add ginger, salt.
6. Add water, cover and cook for 2 hours on LOW.
7. Once the time is over, pick the meat apart, add them into the Crock Pot again.
8. Add there garlic, onion, ginger, wakame, coconut aminos, vinegar, stir.
9. Cover and cook on LOW 1 hour.
10. Once the time is over, add spiralized zucchinis.
11. Cover and put on WARM. Zucchinis must be tender.
12. Garnish with chilies.
13. Serve warm and enjoy!
14. Bon Appetite!

103.Keto butternut squash soup

Have you ever heard about butternut keto squash soup? The butternut squash is actually a fruit. But to prepare tasty soup is possible! Mix chicken broth, butternut squash, roasted golden onions, coconut oil and finally you have an amazing soup. Use a food processor or a blender to make the consistency smooth.

Ingredients (4 servings):
onion	1 medium sized
chicken broth (other broth)	32oz (4 cups)
butternut squash	1 pcs
coconut oil	1 tablespoon
salt to taste	
nutmeg and pepper at will	

Directions:

1. Peel and chop the onion.
2. Take a medium pot, add there one tablespoon of coconut oil, heat on medium high. Add the onions. Stir well.
3. Chop the butternut squash. Cut into 1-inch thick slices.
4. Take off the skillet, remove the onions to the Crock Pot, add the broth, add chopped butternut squash. Salt and pepper to taste.
5. Cover and cook on LOW 2 hours.
6. Once the time is over, open, pour the mixture into the food processor and blend. Puree the mixture.
7. Season soup with pepper and salt, nutmeg.
8. Eat warm.
9. Bon Appetite!

104.Keto Thai broccoli beef soup

One of my last creations is this keto Thai broccoli beef soup. It is a flavorful, savory, easy soup, a great mix of coconut aminos, fish sauce, Thai curry paste, species. I prefer to use in this recipe a rather large amount of broccoli, but you may use less. I would like to say, broccoli is rather «comfortable» vegetable, you may easily change boring potatoes with broccoli following your keto diet. The mixture of the soup is silky and colorful.

Ingredients (14 servings):

avocado oil or other oil	2 tablespoons
onion	1 pcs
Thai green curry paste	2 tablespoons
Ginger	2-inch
garlic	2 cloves
serrano pepper	1 pcs
ground beef	1 pound
coconut aminos	3 tablespoons
fish sauce	2 teaspoons
salt	½ teaspoon
black pepper	½ teaspoon
beef bone or chicken broth	4 cups
broccoli	2 large stalks
canned coconut milk	1 cup
Cilantro (for garnish)	

Directions:

1. Peel the onion and chop it. Peel the garlic and mince.
2. Mince the peeled ginger. Mince serrano pepper.
3. Add to the Crock Pot avocado oil on the bottom of it, put there chopped onions, minced garlic, Thai paste, serrano pepper, salt. Combine everything well.
4. Add ground beef, fish sauce, coconut aminos, pepper.
5. Pour the broth, cover and cook on LOW for 4 hours.
6. Once the time is over, open the Crock Pot, add broccoli and milk, put on WARM and cook another 1 hour.
7. Season with cilantro.
8. Bon Appetite!

105.Keto Southwestern pork stew

This recipe of Southwestern pork stew will fill you with best feelings and let you warm on cold and windy days. Here is the right amount of species, chili coaxes the taste buds without suppressing them fully. Ground cumin works rather well with dried oregano, garlic, and onion. The dish gets a special note! This pork stew is pretty colorful!

Ingredients (10 servings):

medium onion	1 pcs
cloves garlic	3 pcs large
boneless pork	2 lb
almond flour	¼ cup
ground cumin	2 teaspoons
dried oregano leaves	a ½ teaspoon
salt	½ teaspoon
chili in sauce	1 can (15 to 16 oz)
diced tomatoes with mild green chilies	1 can (14.5 oz)
chicken broth	1 cup
pepper and sea salt at will	

Directions:

1. Peel onion, after this peel garlic, mince carefully.
2. Prepare the pork: take the boneless part, wash it and dry with the paper towel. Cut it into 1 1/2-inch pieces.
3. Take the Crock Pot, add there chopped onion, minced garlic that you already prepared.
4. Place the pork pieces on the top of the mixture (from the onion and garlic).
5. Take a small bowl, mix here flour, cumin, salt, pepper, oregano, pour over the pork.
6. Take another bowl, mix chicken broth, chili in sauce (you may add undrained), tomatoes (the same) and stir to combine. Pour this also over the pork.
7. Cover and cook on LOW for 7-8 hours.
8. Take the pork stew off the Crock Pot, season with pepper and salt.

9. Bon Appetite!

106.Crock Pot spicy chicken stew

Chili powder and salsa make this recipe of chicken stew extra tasty! Probably, it will be too much chili powder for you, in this way you may reduce the amount of this, taking into account that your kids would also like to taste this delicious dish! You may add ground pepper or chili right to your plate during the dinner. Don't hesitate to cook it and enjoy!

Ingredients (10 servings):

Celery	2stalks
onion	1medium
garlic	2cloves
Thick 'n Chunky salsa	1 cup
ground cumin	1 1/2teaspoons
chili powder	1teaspoon
freshly ground pepper	1/2teaspoon
skinless chicken breasts	1lb
boneless skinless chicken thighs	1/2lb
chicken broth	2 1/2cups

Chopped fresh cilantro, if desired

Pepper and salt if desired

Directions:

1. Peel the garlic, mince it. Peel the onion and cut into 1/2-inch-thick slices. Chop the celery. Chop the cilantro and set aside.
2. Take a medium bowl, stir there salsa, chili powder, cumin, minced garlic and chopped onion, ground pepper.
3. Wash the chicken breasts, cut them into pieces.
4. Put all these ingredients in the Crock Pot, put the chicken on the top of the mix and pour the chicken broth over the ingredients.
5. Cover and cook on HIGH for 4 hours.
6. Remove chicken stew to the plate once the time is over, garnish with chopped fresh cilantro and parsley (if desired).
7. Eat warm.
8. Bon Appetite!

107.Keto Crock Pot beef stew

The keto Crock Pot beef stew recipe is one of the favorite meals of whole my family! All family members could eat this one all day long, instead of breakfast, dinner, and supper. This recipe is a so-called culmination of tastes, the beef stew mix is an absolutely great addition to the meat! This meal is essential one, easy and quick. Can you imagine – you need here just 4 servings! Amazing! Cook this recipe, and you won't regret it definitely!

Ingredients (4 servings):

Beef stew	2 pounds
Onion	1 medium
beef stew mix	1 package
(green vegetables – it could be a package of broccoli, Brussels sprouts, celery, leeks – this is the best mix of them)	4-6 cups
Water	1 cup

Pepper and salt at will

Directions:
1. Prepare the beef stews, cut them into bite-sized pieces.
2. Peel the onion and cut it into large chunks.
3. Mix the beef stew with chopped onion, add the cups of beef stew mix, stir everything in the Crock Pot, add water. Combine everything once more.
4. Cover and turn on LOW for 8 hours.
5. Season with salt and pepper.
6. Serve with mashed cauliflower or cauliflower rice.
7. Bon Appetite!

108.Crock Pot caramelized onion beef stew

An amazing combination of caramelized golden onions and meat. What could be more delicious than this meal? I would like to use in this recipe beef meat, but if you prefer the other one, just do it. Pay attention that it may take you more or less time at the Crock Pot (for meat cooking). Serve this amazing one with black pepper, parsley or dill if you eat them with pleasure.

Ingredients:

butter	2 tablespoons
sweet onions	4 cups
sweetener	2 teaspoons
fresh thyme leaves	2 teaspoons
beef stew meat	1 ½ lb
beef flavored broth	1 cup
onion gravy mix	1 package (87 oz)
parsnips	1cup

salt and pepper at will

Directions:

1. Peel the onion, slice it thinly. Chop the fresh thyme leaves. Cut the parsnips into 1-inch pieces diagonally
2. Take a medium skillet, melt the butter over high heat. Place the onions there, add sweetener (Splenda) and roast 5 minutes. Stir it frequently, onions must get a golden color and be caramelized.
3. Put this mixture in the Crock Pot.
4. Prepare the beef stew meat – wash it, dry with the paper towel, cut into pieces.
5. Put the beef stew meat into the Crock Pot also, add thyme.
6. Take a little bowl, mix here onion gravy mix, flavored broth, combine well. Pour this mixture over the meat, top with parsnips.
7. Cover and cook on LOW for 7 hours. Meat and vegetables must be tender.
8. Serve with black pepper, eat warm!
9. Bon Appetite!

109. Bacon-cabbage chuck beef stew

Have you known earlier that cabbage is one of the healthiest foods a person consumes? Cabbage is the best spring of sinigrin, Vitamin C, and K, B6, copper as well as manganese, fiber. It also contains such healthy ingredients like niacin, iron, calcium, protein. Add to this perfect vegetable a little bit bacon strips, chunk beef, some species and you'll get a perfectly well beef stew!

Ingredients (8 servings):

Bacon	½ pound
chuck roast	2 to 3 pound
red or yellow onions	2 large pcs
garlic	1 clove
cabbage green or Savoy	1 small
fresh thyme	1 teaspoon
broth (beef or chicken or made at home)	1 cup
sea salt	
ground black pepper, chopped parsley at will	

Directions:

1. Prepare the organic bacon – slice or cut in strips. Set aside.
2. Cut the chuck roast into pieces (approximately 2-inch pieces).
3. Peel the onion, garlic, mince the garlic and slice the onion.
4. Slice the green cabbage (or Savoy cabbage).
5. Put into the Crock Pot bacon strips, chuck roast, sliced onion, pressed or minced garlic, fresh thyme, sliced cabbage, broth, season with pepper and some pinches of sea salt.
6. Cover and cook on LOW for 7 hours.
7. Serve warm!
8. Bon Appetite!

110Keto Crock Pot Korean Beef Stew

A flavorful and delicious beef stew that crocks slowly up to get the tenderness and begin to melt in your mouth! This is one of the best dishes you could cook following the keto diet in the Crock Pot. Cooking the beef is so easy in the Crock Pot. It is one of the favorite ways to prepare the beef meat of hundreds of women, I'm sure you'll love it also! The Korean sauce covers all the beef pieces, the sesame seeds in a combination with green onion don't leave you half-hearted.

Ingredients (10 servings):

beef stew meat	2 lb
green onions	6 pcs
garlic	2 cloves
tomato juice	½ cup
spicy sauce	¼ cup
xanthan gum	3 tablespoons
sesame or vegetable oil	2 tablespoons
pepper	¼ teaspoon
cold water	4 teaspoons
cooked cauliflower rice (optional)	3 cups

pepper and salt to taste

sesame seeds and green onion for garnish

Directions:

1. Prepare the beef stew meat –cut into 1-inch pieces. Set aside.
2. Peel the onion, cut into 1-inch pieces. Peel the garlic and press it or chop finely.
3. Add the vegetable or sesame oil in the Crock Pot.
4. Combine there beef stew meat with chopped onions and garlic, add tomato juice, xanthan gum, spicy sauce, pepper (dried), the rest of oil, water.
5. Cover and cook on LOW 9-10 hours, or on HIGH 4-5 hours.
6. Season with fresh chopped parsley, black pepper, salt. Add chopped green onion and sesame seeds.
7. Enjoy this dish with cooked cauliflowers rice (optional).
8. Bon Appetite!

111.Keto sausage and kale stew

This keto sausage and kale stew put a little bit Italy taste on your plate. Sweet Italian sausages are a perfect combination of garlic and species. Kale, diced tomatoes, and tomato paste add bright colors to the dish. This stew is tasty for lunch or dinner, it lets you breeze the light Italian wind in the air!

Ingredients (11 servings):

bulk Italian sausage	1lb

white or yellow onion	1 pcs
diced tomatoes, organic	1can (28 oz)
tomato paste	2 tablespoons
minced garlic	2 teaspoons
salt	½ teaspoon
pepper	½ teaspoon
water (vegetable broth)	1cup
kale	1bunch
milk (use more if needed)	¼ cup 1/3 cup
butter	2 tablespoons
almond flour	1 tablespoon

Additional salt and pepper at will

Directions:

1. Prepare ready the Italian sausages – cut them into small or medium pieces.
2. Peel and chop the onion, peel the garlic and mince it. Set aside.
3. Remove the stems from kale, chop it coarsely.
4. Put into the Crock Pot cut sausages, chopped onion, minced garlic, diced tomatoes, tomato paste. Mix everything well. Add vegetable broth or water, pepper, and salt at will. Add chopped kale on the top of the mixture.
5. Cover and cook on LOW 4 hours.
6. While the main dish is cooking, melt butter in a little pan, add the milk, flour and stir well. Add pepper, salt to taste. The texture must get smooth.
7. Pour this mixture into the main dish almost when the general cooking time is over. Put on WARM for 15 minutes.
8. Serve warm and enjoy!

112. African groundnut keto stew

The peanuts are always eaten as snacks, we add them to salads or prepare the peanut butter paste. But for some people, this has been an essential food for centuries. They use peanut butter in different ways for the dishes you couldn't even imagine one may add it there! The most widespread way to use it – to add to flavor sauces, stews, and soups. Today I would like to present you a delicious groundnut African stew. A delicious mix of the grated ginger root, onion, peanut butter is a rich source of flavor combination.

Ingredients (10 servings):

boneless skinless chicken thighs	6 pcs (about 1 lb)
boneless skinless chicken breasts	3 pcs (about 3/4 lb)
onion	1 medium pcs

peanut butter	¾ cup
organic diced tomatoes, undrained	1 can (28 oz)
grated gingerroot	2 tablespoons
tomato paste	2 tablespoons
curry powder	2 teaspoons
red pepper flakes	1 teaspoon
cauliflower	1 ½ lb
pepper, and salt to taste	

Directions:

1. Peel the onion and chop it finely.
2. Prepare for the large bowl chicken things (boneless and skinless) as well as chicken breasts (also boneless and skinless).
3. Grate the gingerroot.
4. Crush the red pepper carefully.
5. Cut the freshly washed cauliflower in florets.
6. Put the chicken breasts and things into the bottom of the Crock Pot, add chopped onion, diced tomatoes with drain, grated gingerroot, tomato paste, red pepper flakes, curry powder, pepper and salt to taste.
7. Stir everything well.
8. Add on the top of the mixture peanut butter.
9. Cover and cook on LOW 8 hours.
10. Serve warm and enjoy!

113.Crock Pot keto Hungarian beef stew

What could be easier than cooking keto recipes with this cookbook having a great technical achievement like a Crock Pot!? Traditional Hungarian beef stew! No problems! This recipe is an amazing flavor combination of paprika, beef stew, caraway seeds. Following the keto diet, I used here broccoli instead of usual potatoes. Try to cook it right now!

Ingredients (9 servings):

beef stew meat	2 pounds
broccoli	6-8 pcs (about 3 cups)
frozen small whole onions	1 cup
almond flour	¼ cup
paprika	1 tablespoon
peppered seasoned salt	½ teaspoon
caraway seed	¼ teaspoon
beef flavored broth	1 ¾ cups

| sour cream | ½ cup |

pepper and dill at will

Directions:
1. Wash the broccoli, dry with the paper towel, set aside.
2. Open the bag with frozen onions and put them on a plate.
3. Spray the Crock Pot with cooking spray a little bit, add beef, broccoli, frozen onions from the plate, almond flour, paprika, seasoned salt, black pepper (optional), caraway seeds. Mix well everything.
4. Add on the top of the mixture sour cream and broth.
5. Cover and cook on LOW for 7-8 hours.
6. Serve with the rest of sour cream, eat warm.
7. Bon Appetite!

114.Crock Pot Cuban seafood stew

This easy traditional Cuban dish includes a variety of fresh seafood products, species, vegetables. It doesn't take too much time to cook everything but is like a big and hot hug from sunny Cuba. This low carb recipe combines bay leaves, onion, green pepper in a junction of cod and shrimps. It is the healthy choice for today's dinner. You may also use your favorite tender seafood products if you don't prefer cod or shrimps. The more seafood the better!

Ingredients (13 servings):

olive oil	1 tablespoon
onion	1 large pcs
green pepper	1 large pcs
garlic	3 cloves
ground cumin	½ teaspoon
dried oregano	½ teaspoon
sea salt	½ teaspoon
bay leaves	2 pcs
Roma or plum tomatoes	3 medium pcs
tomato paste	2 tablespoons
chicken broth or stock	2½ cups
cod cut in half	1 pound
shrimp	½ pound

Toppings (optional) - lime wedges, cilantro

Directions:
1. Peel one large onion and slice it finely.

2. Peel the garlic, mince it.
3. Wash the green pepper, take off the seeds and dice it. Wash the fresh tomatoes. Dice them or quarter.
4. Prepare the shrimps – wash them and peel.
5. Take a large skillet, add the olive oil, add sliced onion and cook on medium heat for 3-5 minutes. After this add green pepper, continue cooking 5 minutes. The vegetables must be softened (light golden color).
6. Put to the Crock Pot minced garlic, dried oregano, ground cumin, pepper and salt, the mixture from the skillet. Mix well.
7. Add there bay leaves, tomato paste, quartered tomatoes. Gently mix all the components. Pour the stock or chicken broth.
8. Cover and cook on LOW 3 hours.
9. Once the cooking time is over, add shrimps and cod cut in half to the mixture, cover (they must be cover fully with liquid), put on WARM. Cook another 30 minutes.
10. Season with chopped cilantro and lime wedges at will.
11. Bon Appetite!

115.Crock Pot vegetable beef stew recipe

This is a great vegetable beef stew. It is a tasty dish both for adults and kids, no matter is it a daily meal or a dish prepared for the special occasion. I think it could taste better even for the next day, you may keep it in the refrigerator for some days.

Ingredients (14 servings):

cauliflower	2 cups of florets
celery ribs	2 pcs
roasted bacon strips	3 pcs
almond flour	1/4 cup
pepper	3/4 teaspoon
1/2 teaspoon salt	1/2 teaspoon
beef stew meat	2 pounds
onion	1 large pcs
garlic	2 cloves
vegetable oil	1 tablespoon
beef broth	1 can (14-1/2 ounces)
bay leaf	1 pcs
dried thyme	1/8 teaspoon
condensed tomato soup	1 can (10-3/4 ounces)
pepper and salt at will	

Directions:

1. Thinly slice the celery ribs.
2. Dice the roasted bacon strips.
3. Cut the beef stew meat into 3/4-inch cubes.
4. Peel the onion and chop. Peel the garlic and mince it.
5. Add to the Crock Pot cauliflower, celery, pepper, and salt.
6. Take a large bowl, mix the flour, pepper (1/4 teaspoon), salt (1/4 teaspoon). Add the meat and shake it to coat. Take a medium skillet, spread a little bit vegetable oil, brown the beef, minced garlic and sliced onion. Put everything in the Crock Pot.
7. Add to the Crock Pot broth, thyme, tomato soup, bay leaf, bacon, pepper and salt to taste.
8. Cover and cook on LOW 7 hours.
9. Discharge bay leaf before eating.
10. Serve warm.

LUNCH

116.Avocado Toad in the Hole

Such a cute name for a simple lunch. First time when I heard this recipe I thought it must be something with bread. But I think eating avocado is healthier than eating bread. Moreover, you get a great quantity of fat at the first part of the day, set of vitamin and good mood.

Ingredients (6 servings):

avocados	3 medium pcs
eggs	6 medium
garlic powder	1 tsp
sea salt	1/2 tsp
black pepper	1/4 tsp
Parmesan cheese	1/4 cup

Directions:

1. Wash and cut in half avocados, remove the pits. Scoop out about 1/4 of the meat from each part. You must create enough space to fit the egg inside.
2. Open the Crock Pot and spray the cooking spray over the bottom.
3. Place the halves of avocado into a bottom of the Crock Pot.
4. Sprinkle each part with salt, garlic powder, and black pepper.
5. Grate the Parmesan cheese.
6. Crack the fresh egg into each part of the avocado and sprinkle with cheese over the tops of the eggs.
7. Cover the Crock Pot and put on HIGH for 1 hour.
8. The egg whites must be no longer jiggles.
9. Eat warm.
10. Bon Appetite!

117.Japanese pumpkin dip

Today I say «Hello» to this delicious and tasty Japanese pumpkin dip. You don't need to rise to Japan or Thailand to taste this amazing and colorful dip. Everything you need – to follow my instructions strictly, be patient and get a super tasty, light dip for lunch!

Ingredients (11 servings):

Japanese pumpkin	3 lbs
olive oil	1/4 cup
sea salt	1 tsp
white onion	1 medium
unsalted butter (or ghee)	2 tbsp

heavy cream (or coconut cream)	2 cups
garlic powder	1 tbsp
sea salt	1 tsp
fresh rosemary	4 sprigs
water or broth	1/2 - 1 cup
pumpkin seeds	1/3 cup

Directions:

1. Wash the Japanese pumpkin and remove the seeds.
2. Chop into 2-inch cubes.
3. Open the Crock Pot and spray the cooking spray over the bottom.
4. Put the cubes on a bottom of the Crock Pot, drizzle with olive oil and season with salt. Cover and put on HIGH for 2 hours.
5. Peel chop finely the white onion cook it until golden in a little saucepan with unsalted butter.
6. Once the onion is translucent, put it into a bowl. Set aside.
7. Blend heavy cream in a food processor for about 5 minutes.
8. Add the cooked onion, garlic powder, salt and fresh rosemary. Blend everything well.
9. Once the pumpkin is ready, let cool a little and peel the skin off. Blend the peeled pumpkin into the food processor until creamy.
10. Transfer the pumpkin soup to the Crock Pot and put on LOW for 1 more hour.
11. Serve with pumpkin seeds!
12. Enjoy warm!

118.Blackberry Egg Keto Bake

This recipe is absolutely for those why are lazy but still, like to enjoy something tasty and unusual. It requires very little time to make and is pretty delicious. This recipe includes an unusual flavor combination and the texture. The rosemary, lime zest and ginger combined together with a little bit vanilla give the eggs a refreshing backdrop to the fresh blackberries.

Ingredients (9 servings):

Eggs	5 large
butter (melted)	1 tbsp
coconut flour	3 tbsps
grated fresh ginger	1 tsp
vanilla	1/4 tsp
fine sea salt	1/3 tsp
zest of lime	1/2 tbsp
fresh rosemary	1 tsp
cup fresh blackberries	1/2

Directions:

1. Open the Crock Pot and spray the cooking spray over the bottom.
2. Melt the butter in a little saucepan.
3. Chop finely fresh rosemary.
4. Place freshly cracked eggs, melted butter, coconut flour, freshly grated ginger, vanilla, salt, zest into a blender and process about two minutes on high. The mixture must be fully combined and smooth.
5. Add the rosemary and pulse a few times until rosemary is just combined.
6. Put the egg mixture into the Crock Pot add blackberries there.
7. Cover the Crock Pot and set on HIGH for 1 hour, until the egg mixture puffs and is fully cooked through.
8. Let it cool for some minutes once the cooking time is over. Add chopped rosemary.
9. Bon Appetite!

119.Quick Sausage lunch for two

Quick sausage lunch is great because you put all the ingredients in the Crock Pot and let it cook. Today I decided to combine the robust flavors of Italian sausages with full of carbs with species, ketchup, and veggies. A plenty of melted cheese will never damage your dish!

Ingredients (9 servings):

sausage	5 pcs
white onion	1 tbsp
ketchup	1/2 cup
Parmesan cheese	1/4 cup
shredded mozzarella	1/4 cup
oregano	1/2 tsp
basil	1/2 tsp
salt	1/4 tsp
red pepper	1/4 tsp

Directions:

1. Open the Crock Pot and spray the cooking spray over the bottom.
2. Cut the sausages into rounds (about 1/2 inch) and put them to the Crock Pot.
3. Shred mozzarella and Parmesan cheese.
4. Peel and finely dice the onion. Add to the Crock Pot also.
5. Pour the ketchup and Parmesan cheese. Stir to combine everything well.
6. Add onion, oregano, pepper, and salt. Cover the Crock Pot and set on LOW for 2 – 3 hours.
7. Once the cooking time is over, open the Crock Pot and sprinkle with mozzarella cheese.
8. Sprinkle with basil.
9. Bon Appetite!

120.Shakshuka keto Crock Pot

This dish can be enjoyed together with all your family and friends or you may eat it alone. It's essentially a sauce made of tomatoes and finely chopped chili peppers. If you are bored of the usual scrambled eggs prepared for lunches, this can be a great alternative. Enjoy preparing your sauce if you have a plenty of time and a really awesome recipe. This time I decided to use one of my favorite marinara sauces.

Ingredients (7 servings):

marinara sauce	1 cup
pepper	1 chili
eggs	4 pcs
feta cheese	1 oz
cumin	1/8 tsp
salt	
pepper	
fresh basil (at will)	
or fresh oregano (if desired)	

Directions:

1. Finely chop the chili. But be careful!
2. Take a medium-sized bowl and add a cup of marinara sauce, chopped chili. Whisk everything together
3. Crack fresh eggs to the marinara and chili mixture, continue whisking.
4. Crumble the feta cheese and sprinkle it over the marinara-eggs mix, season this with pepper and salt at will. Add cumin.
5. Open the Crock Pot and spray the cooking spray over the bottom.
6. Pour the mix into the Crock Pot, cover and set on LOW for 2 hours. Check the dish from time to time, it must seem not cooked enough rather to heat itself.
7. Once the time is over, the eggs must be still runny a little. Transfer the shakshuka from the Crock Pot on a plate carefully, helping with spoon or blade.
8. Wash and chop fresh basil, sprinkle it over the ready dish.
9. Enjoy!

121.Keto Feta & Pesto Omelet

This keto omelet is absolutely great for a season of fresh and flavor basil. This time pesto must be on the menu, of course, if you like it. That's why I decided to cook this quick Italian lunch and namely pesto and feta omelet. The end result I became after mixing all these simple and delicious ingredients was really great. I don't want even describe this sunny, delicate and herby pesto omelet but wish you cook it quickly.

Ingredients (5 servings):

Butter	1 tbsp

Eggs	5 pcs
heavy cream	1 tbsp
feta cheese	1 oz.
pesto	1 tbsp
salt	
pepper	

Directions:

1. Take a medium-sized saucepan and heat it up. Melt a tablespoon of butter.
2. Take another little bowl, crack the fresh eggs, add melted butter and put a tablespoon of heavy cream. (If you want to get your omelet fluffy).
3. Open the Crock Pot and spray the cooking spray over the bottom.
4. Pour the eggs mix into the Crock Pot and put on LOW for 1-1,5 hours until fully cooked.
5. Once the time is almost over, open the Crock Pot and sprinkle pesto on the top of the dish.
6. Shred the feta cheese and spread it over the top of the omelet also.
7. Cover the Crock Pot and wait until the feta cheese is fully melted over the omelet.
8. Once the feta is melted, transfer the ready dish on a plate carefully and season with salt and pepper.
9. Garnish with more feta at will and fresh basil leaves if desired or cherry tomatoes.
10. Bon Appetite!

122.Egg Clouds & Bacon Weave

Have you ever tried the egg clouds? It is awesome! You just whisk them into a foamy peak and bake. When I firstly whisked the egg whites into foam I was rather skeptical as I could do this creation only using eggs and blender. I couldn't believe it happened so quick and so easy. The egg whites made a cloud-like creation that is a rather beautiful creation of mine. Finally, I added egg yolks that stayed rather fluffy inside. If you like to get bacon crispy, prebake the strips for about 7 minutes before you add the egg whites.

Ingredients (6 servings):

Bacon	6 – 9 strips
Eggs	2 pcs
Salt	1/2 tsp
garlic powder	1/2 tsp
pepper	1/4 tsp
cayenne	1/4 tsp

Directions:

1. Firstly let's prepare the bacon waves: take three strips of bacon per cloud and fold them in half lengthwise. Ensure that both halves have the same length. They must create a perfect square bed.

2. Lay three long strips of bacon parallel to each other and fold the middle strip over. Put a strip perpendicular to the three, fold back over. Take the two outer strips and fold over.
3. Put another bacon strip in the center perpendicularly. Turn over the middle strip on the weave.
4. Put the final strip and tuck up. If you like to get bacon crispy, prebake the strips for about 6-7 minutes before you add the egg whites.
5. Take a medium-sized bowl, separate eggs and leave the yolks in a bowl. Do not break the yolks it is of high importance.
6. Put the egg whites in another deep bowl, whisk the egg whites with blender for about 7 minutes. The egg white must be thick, white foam.
7. Add salt and garlic powder and whisk all together. Be attentive, if you add these ingredients earlier, the eggs could take longer to form the cloudiness.
8. Open the Crock Pot and spread the cooking spray on a bottom and sides of the Crock Pot.
9. Place the bacon waves on the bottom of the Crock Pot, using a spoon place your seasoned egg whites onto the weave and create a little cloud.
10. Carefully make a little dip in a cloud (in each one) and place the egg yolk there.
11. Season the tops of the egg clouds with paprika and cayenne pepper.
12. Cover the Crock Pot and set on HIGH for 1 hour, until the egg clouds have become golden.
13. Once the time is over, transfer your creation carefully on a plate and sprinkle with some coarse salt!
14. Bon Appetite!

123.Avocado fries Crock Pot

Have searched for amazing quick lunch recipes? You have found the recipe you must cook for sure! Simple to make, keto-friendly, quick and flavor! Crispy outside and tender inside. Every beat of this tasty lunch is full of fat, so you will not feel hunger the rest of the day! If you don't like sriracha hot sauce, feel free to prepare the other one like garlic dip or cilantro lime dip.

Ingredients (8 servings):
Fries

Avocados	3 pcs
Egg	1 pcs
almond meal	1 1/2 cups
sunflower oil	1 1/2 cups
cayenne pepper	1/4 tsp
salt	1/2 tsp

Spicy Mayo

homemade mayo	2 tbsp
sriracha	2 tbsp

Directions:
1. Take a medium-sized bowl, crack a fresh egg into this bowl, whisk it thoroughly.

2. Tae another medium bowl, join the almond meal with a little bit salt and cayenne pepper.
3. Wash and slice avocados in half, carefully take out the seeds.
4. Peel off the skin off every half.
5. Slice each slice of avocado 4 or 5 pieces (if it is rather big).
6. Open the Crock Pot and sunflower oil to the bottom of the Crock Pot.
7. Coat each of avocado slices the egg mixture.
8. Put each avocado slice in the almond meal carefully, do this until you will not fully see the avocado green.
9. Place each covered slice of avocado into the Crock Pot.
10. Cover and put on HIGH for 2 hours. Turn the slices from time to time.
11. Once the cooking time is over, transfer slices quickly to a plate.
12. In a little bowl, mix sriracha sauce and mayo and deep the avocado slices before eating!
13. Enjoy hot!

124.Spicy Shrimp Omelet Crock Pot

This healthy and quick lunch idea is easy to cook and amazing to eat. If you have never tried shrimp in the omelet or with eggs, I think this recipe will be great for opening new tastes. I was very pleased with the result I got finally.

Ingredients (8 servings):

Shrimp	10 large
Eggs	6 pcs
grape tomatoes	4 pcs
spinach	1 handful
onion	1/4
sriracha salt	1 tbsp
parsley	1 sprig
cayenne	1/4 Tsp

Directions:

1. Peel and chop the onion.
2. Take a medium-sized saucepan, put it over medium heat and place onions. Season this with salt. Cook for some minutes.
3. Wash and slice the tomatoes in half lengthwise.
4. Add the grape tomatoes to onions and, cut side down and cook a little.
5. Wash and chop the spinach.
6. Once the onions are translucent, add spinach and let it cook for some minutes.
7. Open the Crock Pot and pour the mix of tomatoes, onions, and spinach into the Crock Pot. Add cayenne. Cover and put on HIGH for 2 hours.
8. Add shrimp and brake fresh eggs. If you wish to whisk them for a little.
9. Once the omelet is ready, transfer your dish on a plate!
10. Garnish with some parsley and enjoy!
11. Bon Appetite!

125.Keto Crock Pot lunch balls

I know a lot of people who prefer to have essential lunch during their busy working day. I think this recipe of the quick and essential meatballs it that recipe they could look for. Lunch balls are great in a combination of caramelized onions. It is something like a burger if you eat this with keto bread.

Ingredients (15 servings):

ground beef	1/2 lb
bacon	1 strip
jalapenos	1 tbsp
mayo	1 tbsp
tomato	1/2 plum
onion	¼ pcs
sriracha	1 tbsp
egg	1 pcs
butter	2 tbsp
lettuce	2 leaves
Spices	
Salt	1/2 Tsp
crushed red pepper	1/2 tsp
cayenne	1/4 Tsp
basil	1/2 Tsp

Directions:

1. Knead the meat for about 4-5 minutes. This makes it sticky and keeps it together when you add all the ingredients to it.
2. Chop the bacon.
3. Chop finely jalapenos. Crush the red peppers.
4. Wash and slice tomatoes. Pell the onion and cut.
5. Take a large bowl, combine the onion, mayo, sriracha, freshly cracked egg, salt, red pepper, basil, and cayenne. Stir everything well. Add this to the ground beef. Knead it again once more.
6. Make balls from the meat.
7. Open the Crock Pot, sprinkle the bottom with oil or ghee.
8. Put the meatballs on the bottom.
9. Cover and put on HIGH for 3 hours. Turn balls from time to time.
10. Once the dish is ready, combine it with caramelized onions.
11. Bon Appetite!

126.Healthy breakfast spaghetti squash

This recipe of the dish doesn't have to be rather exact. I would say, you may add also other ingredients to the spaghetti squash. Add another kind of cheese or another mix of veggies. Make your own breakfast!

Ingredients (8 servings):

spaghetti squash	1 pcs
salt and pepper at will	
tomato sauce	2 - 3 Tbsp
spinach	1 - 2 handfuls
ham	2 slices
red onion	1 - 2 thin slices
Cheddar cheese	1 handful
green onions	1 handful
eggs	2 pcs

Directions:
1. Wash and chop the spinach. Set aside.
2. Chop the ham into slices.
3. Peel the onion and slice the onion.
4. Shred the Cheddar cheese. Set aside.
5. Chop the green onions.
6. Wash and slice the squash in half, take off the seeds.
7. Sprinkle the squash with pepper and salt to taste.
8. Spread a little bit tomato sauce into the squash.
9. Put the spinach, cheese, ham, red onion.
10. Open the Crock Pot and spray with cooking spray the bottoms and the sides.
11. Put the filled spaghetti squash in the Crock Pot.
12. Crack two eggs into the spaghetti squash. Cover the lid and set on HIGH for 4 hours.
13. Once the time is over, dress with pepper and salt.
14. Serve warm.
15. Bon Appetite!

127.Canadian bacon, asparagus, and cheese mix

Try this new asparagus, cheese, Canadian bacon mix for lunch. Add a little bit lemon zest for flavor and tenderness. Be sure, you will surprise your guests with this lunch recipe!

Ingredients (8 servings):

Eggs	5 large
Parmesan cheese	4 Tbsp
Milk	2 Tbsp

lemon zest	¼ tsp
kosher salt	1 Tsp
black pepper at will	
olive oil	1 Tbsp
asparagus	4 oz stalks
Canadian bacon	4 medium slices

Directions:

1. Shred the cheese. Grate the lemon zest.
2. Cut the asparagus into halves.
3. Take a medium-sized bowl, whisk freshly cracked eggs, add shredded cheese, add milk, zest, salt, and pepper at will.
4. Open the Crock Pot and cover the bottom and walls with cooking spray.
5. Add the asparagus, Canadian bacon, pour the mixture of the eggs and cheese into the Crock Pot.
6. Cover the lid of the Crock Pot and put on HIGH for 2 hours.
7. Serve the dish warm or room temperature. Season with dill or parsley at will.
8. Bon Appetite!

128.Italian sausage and egg bake

This is the mix of eggs and Italian sausage made in the Crock Pot, low-carb. If you don't know how to prepare the keto bred, I recommend you to follow the instructions of the cooking the keto bread. Eat this dish for a lunch today!

Ingredients (11 servings):

keto bread	½ small loaf (about 1 1/2 cups)
olive oil	2 Tbsp
onion	1 medium
Italian turkey sausage	1 lb(s)
spinach	1 (10 to 12-oz) package
sun-dried tomatoes	1 (6.5-oz) jar
fresh basil	2 Tbsp
kosher salt	½ tsp
black pepper	¼ tsp
goat cheese	1 (5-oz)
large eggs	6 pcs

Directions:

1. Peel the onion and dice it finely. Peel garlic and mince it.
2. Drain the liquid from tomatoes and chop finely.
3. Wash leaves of basil, chop.
4. Crumble the goat cheese.
5. Open the Crock Pot and spread the spray for cooking.
6. Toss the keto cubes with oil and put in a medium-sized skillet. Roast until golden, it takes 5minutes.
7. Take a medium-sized skillet, had the rest of oil, add onion, garlic, sausage, prepare until sausage is almost cooked through.
8. Add spinach, stir frequently, about 2 minutes.
9. Add tomatoes and basil.
10. Season with salt, add pepper if desired.
11. Put the ingredients in the Crock Pot, add the keto cubes. Add the goat cheese.
12. Cover the lid and set on HIGH for 2 hours.
13. Bon Appetite!

129.Crock Pot Yorkshire Pudding

Cooking a keto Yorkshire pudding in the Crock Pot? Not a problem! Flavor, tender and fully amazing! Perfect meal for lunch is today on your table! Enjoy immediately once the pudding is ready.

Ingredients (15 servings):

refined avocado oil	¼ cup
eggs	4 large
whole milk or 2% milk	2 cups
almond flour	2 cups
salt	½ tsp
grated nutmeg	⅛ tsp
Filling	
Roma tomatoes	2 pcs
mozzarella	12 mini
eggs, any size	5 pcs
Topping	
Avocado	1 pcs
green onion, diced	1 pcs
olive oil	1 Tbsp
lemon juice	2 Tsp

| chili flakes | ¼ tsp |
| salt | ¼ tsp |

Directions:

1. Take a large bowl, whisk freshly cracked eggs with milk. Season with salt, flour, and nutmeg. Mix thoroughly. Set aside.
2. Place the oiled base in the Crock Pot (it must be covered with cooking spray previously) and bake for 2 hours until softened.
3. While the base is cooking prepare the filling: wash the tomatoes, take off the seeds and cut into pieces.
4. Cube the mozzarella cheese.
5. In the hole of the prepared base, put diced tomatoes and mozzarella. Crack fresh eggs.
6. Put the pudding again into the Crock Pot and set on LOW for 1 hour or until yolks are still a little bit runny.
7. Prepare the topping: take a small bowl, peel and dice avocado, green onion, salt, chili flakes, olive oil, lemon juice.
8. Once the pudding is ready, remove it from the Crock Pot and top with the avocado mix.
9. Serve immediately.
10. Bon Appetite!

130.Keto egg bread bowl

This keto bowl is full of sausages and chopped roasted veggies, herbs, sweet pepper, and tasty cheese. This recipe is great for several days, you might keep it in the fridge. Add preferred types of cheese if you want.

Ingredients (11 servings):

keto bread	1 loaf (round)
avocado oil	2 Tbsp
salt and black pepper	
Italian sausage	8 oz
Yellow onion	1 small
Green sweet pepper	1 pcs
red sweet pepper	1 pcs
Calabrian chilies	2 jar
parsley	¼ cup
basil leaves	2 Tbsp
eggs	10 large pcs
Parmesan cheese	¼ cup

Directions:
1. Peel the onion and cut finely.
2. Wash sweet pepper and thinly slice.
3. Thinly slice chilies. Set aside.
4. Wash the parsley, fresh basil, and chop.
5. Grate the Parmesan cheese.
6. Slice the top (approximately 1 inch) of the keto bread. Remove the insides carefully of the loaf, leave about 2/4-inch of keto bread to make a shell.
7. Place the keto bread on the bottom of the Crock Pot, sprinkle with avocado oil, season with salt.
8. In a little skillet heat avocado oil.
9. Add sausage, continue cooking until light brown. Take off the sausage.
10. Add onion to the same skillet, both peppers, and cook, stirring carefully, about 3 minutes. Add chilies, parsley, sausage, basil. Toss to combine.
11. Stir the eggs. Pour the ingredients into the inside of the keto bread.
12. Top with grated cheese.
13. Cover the lid of the Crock Pot and put on LOW for 2 hours.
14. Transfer the loaf to the cutting board and then slice.
15. Bon Appetite!

131.Crock Pot Scrambled Eggs with Green Herbs

I cook these eggs in the Crock Pot to get them a velvety and delicious, tender texture. This recipe is great – I put all the ingredients into the Crock Pot, set on LOW and do my private business. Once the cooking time is over I have a perfect light lunch!

Ingredients (8 servings):

Eggs	10 extra-large
whole milk	6 Tbsp
kosher salt	1 tsp
black pepper	½ tsp
parsley leaves	2 Tbsp
scallions	2 Tbsp
fresh dill	2 Tbsp
unsalted butter	2 Tbsp

Directions:
1. Wash fresh parsley leaves. Chop them finely and set aside.
2. Peel the scallions, cut finely.
3. Wash the fresh dill and mince it also.
4. Take a medium-sized bowl, whisk together milk, eggs, salt, pepper, scallions, parsley, and dill.
5. Melt the butter in an omelet pan.
6. Mix the egg mix with butter and pour into the Crock Pot.
7. Cover the lid of the Crock Pot and put on LOW for 1-2 hours.

8. Serve hot.
9. Bon Appetite!

132.Crock Pot Tart with Butternut Squash and Kale

I don't know the lighter tart prepared in the Crock Pot following all the keto rules than this one! The base is tender and delicious, despite the butter in the base, it is far less than the traditional type. It is in crumbly, flavor and amazing!

Ingredients (11 servings):

Base cooking:

almond flour	1 cup
sea salt	1 Tsp
sprigs fresh thyme	
butter, cold	½ cup
ice-cold water	4 - 6 Tbsp
beaten egg	1pcs

Filling

olive oil	2 tbsp
red onion	1pcs
butternut squash	1 pcs
kale	1 cup
sea salt and black pepper	
organic eggs	3 pcs
whole milk	1 cup
nutmeg, for grating	
Gruyere cheese	½ cup

Directions:

Base:

1. Prepare the base using hands: mix the flour, salt, thyme altogether.
2. Add butter and continue mixing thoroughly.
3. Add water, whisk all the time, until all the ingredients come together.
4. Make a circle with the same diameter as your Crock Pot, and put into the refrigerator for 1 hour.
5. Once the time is over, roll the base, sprinkle the bottom and the walls of the Crock Pot with cooking spray and put it inside.
6. Prepare the filling: peel and cut finely the onion.

7. Peel and grate the squash, take off the stalks from kale and chop the leaves. Grate the cheese on a plate.
8. Take a medium-sized skillet, heat the oil and add onion, cook until soft and sweet.
9. Add squash, kale, season with salt and pepper. Stir well. Set aside.
10. Take a little bowl, break the eggs and whisk them. Pour the milk over the eggs and whisk all together, then add salt and pepper, nutmeg. Mix together.
11. Once the veggies are cool, add the egg mixture and whisk well.
12. Pour the mix into the base and set on HIGH for 2 hours.
13. Serve hot!
14. Bon Appetite!

133.Ginger and turmeric keto dip

The tender and healthy dip with broccoli, ginger, and turmeric is full of healthy components and rather warm for a windy day. It is amazing for lunch, busy day when you don't have time to cook the amazing dishes consisting of a huge amount of the components.

Ingredients (8 servings)

Butter	2 tsp
leeks	4 cups
ginger	2 tsp
broccoli florets	8 cups
ground turmeric	1 tsp
salt	1 tsp
pinch of black pepper	
sesame oil	1 tsp
stock	6 cups

Directions:
1. Wash and chop the leeks.
2. Peel and grate the ginger.
3. Chop the broccoli florets.
4. Take a large saucepan over high heat, melt the butter.
5. Add the leeks, cook, toss well, leeks must be cooked through.
6. Put the leeks in the Crock Pot, add grated ginger, broccoli florets, turmeric, pepper, salt, sesame oil.
7. Add broth and toss well.
8. Cover the lid of the Crock Pot, cook on HIGH for 2 hours. Broccoli must be tender.
9. Use a blender, mix until smooth.
10. Serve with yogurt.

134.Crock Pot Sausage and Fennel

When I wrote this recipe I decided that you don't need to pre-cook the sausages as you have enough time in the Crock Pot to be cooked fully. I like to eat this keto Crock Pot with watercress salad. It is a light, simple and colorful dish.

Ingredients (11 servings):

Cooking Sausage and Fennel:

fresh chorizo links	1-1/2 pounds
garlic	4 cloves
fennel	2 bulbs
yellow onion	1/2 large pcs
chicken stock	2/3 cup
vinegar	3 tsp
salt	1/2 Tsp
pepper	1/4 Tsp

Salad:

vinegar	2 tsp
grain mustard	1 tsp
salt	1/4 Tsp
Pinch of ground pepper	
olive oil	1/4 cup
watercress	2 cups

Directions:

1. Peel the garlic, chop roughly.
2. Peel the onions and cut.
3. Core and chop the fennel.
4. Mix garlic, add fennel, onion, stock, sausages, season with salt, add vinegar, pepper to the Crock Pot and put on LOW for 4 hours.
5. While the sausages are cooking, prepare salad: take a medium-sized bowl, conjoin mustard, vinegar, dress with salt at will.
6. While whisking, add carefully oil. Add watercress to the mix, toss well.
7. Arrange sausage, fennel on a large plate. Serve at once.
8. Enjoy!

135.Crock Pot Turkey Noodle Bowls

Today I would like to surprise you with my new lunch recipe of turkey prepared in my lovely Crock Pot and a mix of colorful veggies. I have chosen the soy sauce sugar-free, you may also add your favorite hot species or sauce.

Ingredients (8 servings):

coconut milk	1/2 cup
creamy peanut butter	1/4 cup
soy sauce	2 tablespoons
organic Turkey Breast Tenderloin	1 package (24 ounces)
zucchini noodles	2-3 cups
English cucumber	½ pcs
red cabbage	1/2 small

Chopped cilantro and mint for serving

Directions:
1. Wash and shred the cucumber. Shred the cabbage.
2. Mix together peanut butter, coconut milk, soy sauce in a large bowl.
3. Add turkey, toss until combined.
4. Put the mix into the Crock Pot, cover and set on HIGH 4 hours.
5. Once the time is over, remove the turkey from the Crock Pot, cut coarsely.
6. Place shredded turkey in a large bowl and keep warm.
7. Mix zucchini noodles, cucumber, cabbage, liquid from the Crock Pot, toss until combined. Add to the ready-cooked turkey.
8. Serve with cilantro and mint.
9. Bon Appetite!

136.Crock Pot keto kale Gratin

When it comes to lunch dishes I usually prefer to cook this keto kale gratin and taste it hot. I place all the ingredients early in the morning and let my Crock Pot work a little. I have a super tender gratin for the lunch!

Ingredients (11 servings):

whole milk	1 cup
mascarpone	1/4 cup
unsalted butter	1 tablespoon
kale	1 to 2 medium
coconut flour	1/2 cup
salt	1/2 teaspoon

pepper	1 teaspoon
dried thyme	1 teaspoon
garlic powder	1 teaspoon
vegetable broth	1 cup
shredded gruyere	1 cup

Fresh parsley at will

Fresh chives if desired

Directions:
1. Shred the cheese and set aside.
2. Take a small bowl, whisk together mascarpone with milk.
3. Melt the butter in a saucepan.
4. Add chopped kale, flour, salt, pepper at will, thyme and garlic powder. Mix everything in a bowl. Add butter melted.
5. Pour in milk with mascarpone mixture, add the vegetable broth.
6. Add shredded gruyere. Mix well everything.
7. Pour the mix into the Crock Pot and set on HIGH for 3 hours.
8. Serve with fresh chopped parsley at will and chives if desired.
9. Bon Appetite!

137.Crock Pot Teriyaki Chicken

When I need to feed my housemates I always choose chicken Teriyaki. This meal might seem not as habitual lunch, but the soft texture of chicken makes it unforgettable. I prepare keto variation of Teriyaki – I don't need sugar, soy sauce or cornstarch. This is a simple compound of ginger, tamari, onions and garlic, vinegar, pepper. Try this extraordinary meal during your lunchtime!

Ingredients (8 servings):
chicken thighs	2 pounds (about 5-6 thighs)
yellow onion	1/2 medium (about 1 cup)
garlic	2 cloves
tamari	1/2 cup
Splenda	1/2 cup
vinegar	1/4 cup
ground black pepper	1/4 teaspoon
ginger	1 tablespoon

salt and pepper to taste

For serving: cauliflower rice, sesame seeds, red pepper flakes.

Directions:

1. Peel yellow onion and dice, peel the garlic and mince.
2. Peel the ginger and grate it.
3. Wash the chicken pieces (skinless and boneless), dry them with a paper towel, cut into smaller pieces if necessary.
4. Put the chicken pieces on the bottom of the Crock Pot.
5. Take a small bowl and mix there minced garlic and onions on the top of the chicken. Pour tamari, Splenda, vinegar, pepper, salt, grated ginger. Pour over the chicken.
6. Cover and cook on LOW for 3 hours or on HIGH for 2 hours. Chicken pieces must get tenderness.
7. Serve with red pepper flakes, sesame seeds, cauliflower rice.
8. Bon Appetite!

138.Crock Pot Chicken Tikka Masala

As soon as I remembered about Chicken Tikka Masala I decided to cook it at once at the Crock Pot. What could be easier than cooking in the Crock Pot? I call this innovation «smart cooking». If you have some possess extra time today I advise you to rickle the chicken breasts in the mixture from this recipe, adding a little bit yogurt to the bowl. Another way is to follow the directions of my recipe and add heavy cream (or milk if you wish) at the end of cooking time. I'm sure you'll be pretty happy having this tasty chicken for lunch.

Ingredients (11 servings):

onion	1 large
chicken pieces	7-8 pcs
garlic	3 cloves
whole ginger	1-inch piece
tomato paste	2 tablespoons
garam masala	1 to 2 tablespoons
paprika	2 teaspoons
kosher salt	2 teaspoons
diced tomatoes	1 (28-ounce) can
heavy cream or coconut milk	3/4 cup
cooked cauliflower rice, to serve	2 cups
cilantro for garnish	
Salt and pepper at will	

Directions:

1. Peel the onion and slice it finely.
2. Peel the garlic, mince into a bowl.
3. Peel and grate whole ginger. Chop the fresh cilantro

4. Wash the chicken pieces (breasts), cut them into slices, put into the Crock Pot.
5. Mix in a medium bowl garlic, onion, salt and pepper, tomato paste, grated ginger, garam masala (one tablespoon). Put this mixture into the Crock Pot too and combine with chicken until it will be covered fully with species.
6. Add diced tomatoes together with juice.
7. Cover the Crock Pot and cook on LOW 4 hours.
8. Twenty minutes before cooking time is over, open the Crock Pot and stir coconut milk or heavy cream. You may also add a little bit garam masala or salt and pepper to taste.
9. Serve with cauliflower rice, season with fresh cilantro on the top of the chicken.
10. Enjoy!

139.Keto Crock Pot Brisket Chili

Some people think that keeping a keto diet means you are hungry all the time. Is it really so? I don't think. The flavored keto brisket chili is great to try. Species, beef broth, tomatoes appear almost all the time in old traditional chili recipes. Beef brisket must be cooked rather slowly, at a low temperature to get the wished tenderness. You might also serve it without if this lunch would be eaten by kids. This dish corresponds to the broccoli or rice (keto cauliflower). If somebody prefers hot sauce, chili, you may add fresh chili to the plate. Enjoy it warm!

Ingredients:

beef brisket	1.5 lbs
olive oil	4 Tablespoons
onion	1 pcs
garlic	2 cloves
green sweet pepper	1 pcs
Jalapeño pepper	1 pcs
ground cumin	2 Tablespoons
chili powder	1 Tablespoon
beef stock	2 cups
diced tomatoes	1 can

Salt and freshly ground black pepper

Directions:
1. Peel the onion, garlic and mince carefully.
2. Wash the bell and jalapeno pepper, remove the seeds, chop finely.
3. Take a medium pan, add the olive oil, roast the beef briskets from all sides. Put on a plate. Set this aside.
4. At the same pan golden the onions, garlic, pepper (both jalapeno and sweet pepper). Add here chili powder and cumin.
5. Put the briskets of the beef, add the browned mixture to Crock Pot. Pour diced tomatoes with liquid, broth, pepper, salt.
6. Cover and cook on LOW for 6 hours.

7. Turn the beef briskets from time to time.
8. Season the dish with black pepper, salt.
9. Bon Appetite!

140. Artichokes with lemon tarragon dipping sauce

My magic Crock Pot always controls my keto diet as well as allows me more time for my family. All its functions allow preparing incredible dishes combining uncommon products getting amazing eating qualities! You don't need to spend too much time in the kitchen to prepare lunch or dinner. If you eat artichokes with pleasure, everything you need is two small lemons, broth, and some species, like salt, tarragon, and pepper if you wish. Following my instructions, you could make two things at the same time – prepare the quick lunch that is beyond compare and spend the remaining time with family members.

Ingredients (7 servings):

Artichokes	4 pcs
Lemons	2 pcs
poultry broth	2 cups
tarragon	1 Tbsp
celery	1 stalk
olive oil	1/2 cup
sea salt	1/4 tsp

black pepper at will

Directions:

1. Cut the stalk of artichokes, they must be the one-inch length. Trim off one inch of the «petals». Chop the stalks, petal tips.
2. Peel the lemon zest. Slice it into four pieces, remove the seeds.
3. Chop finely the tarragon leaves.
4. Put lemon slices to the bottom of the Crock Pot, top each piece with artichokes, pour the bone broth around the artichokes.
5. Cover and cook on LOW for 1-2 hours.
6. At the time while artichokes are cooking, prepare the dipping sauce. Chop the tarragon leaves, chop celery into small pieces. Throw the seeds from the remained lemon, chop it finely.
7. Put the lemon slices, zest, tarragon leaves, olive oil, celery, salt to the blender or a food processor. Blend until smooth texture.
8. Once the cooking time of artichokes is over, serve them topped with prepared sauce.
9. Enjoy your lunch time!

141. Keto garlic butter chicken

One of the fastest ways to prepare appetizing and dainty lunch is to make it in the Crock Pot. This easy recipe doesn't need too many ingredients; it is perfectly well with hot sauce that could be added right to the plate or without it! Don't be surprised if using too many cloves of garlic, they make this recipe special. Enjoy this keto recipe today!

Ingredients (4 servings):

chicken breasts   4 pcs

turmeric ghee   ¼ cup

salt   1 teaspoon

garlic   10 cloves

pepper and salt to taste

Directions:

1. Prepare the chicken breasts, cut them into pieces. Put them into the Crock Pot.
2. Peel the garlic and dice.
3. Put the ghee in the chicken, season with pepper and salt, add garlic.
4. Cover and cook on LOW for 2 hours.
5. Once the cooking time is over, take off the chicken and shred the breasts into small pieces.
6. Serve warm with additional pepper, salt and ghee if needed.
7. Bon Appetite!

142.Curried lemon coconut chicken

When I don't have time at all I realize that I have one «emergency»-recipe. I need just some ingredients, quickly put them into the Crock Pot, push the button, add delicious species, my favorite coconut milk, dress it with salt and pepper and my problem is solved! I think, such situation happens almost with every busy woman today and even not one time during a busy weekend.

Ingredients (6 servings):

full fat coconut milk   1 can

zest and juice from 1 lemon   1 pcs middle size

curry spice   1 tbsp

turmeric   1 tsp

sea salt   1/2 tsp

chicken breasts or thighs   5-6 things

Directions:

1. Wash the chicken breasts or thighs, dry with a paper towel. Cut into pieces.
2. Zest the lemon.
3. Put to the Crock Pot chicken breasts, add coconut milk full of fat, season with pepper and salt, turmeric, curry spice.
4. Cover and cook on LOW for 4 hours.
5. Dress with black pepper if desired.
6. Eat warm.
7. Bon Appetite!

MEAT CHICKEN AND BEEF

143.Crock Pot White Chicken Chili

This is a simply delicious chicken with spicy chilies. I have heard too many varieties of this recipe, but this is the best recipe I have tried. You just have to put everything in the Crock Pot, prepare easy dressing and pour the chicken breasts. That's all. I have garnished this dish with grated cheese, fresh cilantro, and sour cream. This mix tastes the best.

Ingredients (17 servings):

chicken breast fillets	6 pcs	
cumin		1 Tbsp
coriander		1 Tbsp
oregano		2 tsp
paprika		½ tsp
pepper flakes	½ tsp	
celery		4 stalks
garlic		4 cloves
green chiles		2 cans
onions		2 pcs
green bell peppers		2 pcs
jalapeno		1 pcs
chicken broth	4 cups	
whole milk		1 cup
flour (almond)	¼ cup	
Juice of 1 lime	1 pcs	
shredded cheese		½ cup
Sour cream, cilantro		
Black pepper, salt at will		

Directions:

1. Prepare the breasts, take off skin and bones.
2. Peel onion, garlic. Chop celery, onion, cut garlic.
3. Chop green chilies from cans and green peppers. Slice jalapeno. Grate the cheese.
4. Place breasts into the Crock Pot.

5. Take a bowl of a medium-sized, combine there coriander, cumin, oregano, pepper flakes, paprika, pepper, salt. Combine everything together. Put the mixture over the breasts.
6. Add the top garlic, onions, and celery, chilies, sweet peppers, jalapeno. After this spread the broth over the chicken.
7. Cover and put on LOW for 6hours, the vegetables must be tender.
8. Take a small bowl, stir milk with flour, whisk together carefully. Pour this liquid into the Crock Pot, go on cooking one hour additional.
9. Check the chicken with fork or knife if is it ready. Take off the chicken from the Crock Pot on the plate. Add the lime juice, shredded cheese on the top of the chicken pieces.
10. Serve with chopped cilantro, sour cream. Add pepper and salt additional at will.
11. Eat warm. Bon Appetite!

144.Crock Pot creamy salsa chicken

I have adapted this creamy salsa chicken recipe to my keto diet. It's perfectly well. The creamy texture of this dish is provided by both sour cream and creamy soup. I prefer to use mild salsa here, but hot salsa will be also rather tasty. Everything depends on the preferences of your family or guests. You can use the Taco seasoning or prepare it at home if you have enough time. The cauliflower rice helps to create a full essential plate for dinner.

Ingredients (6 servings):

chicken breasts   3 pounds

salsa   1 cup

taco seasoning (homemade) 1.25 ounces

cream of celery soup   10.5 ounces

sour cream   1/2 cup

For Serving

Cauliflower rice   2 - 3 cups

Salt and pepper to taste

Directions:
1. Take off the skin and bones from the chicken breasts. Wash them and slice.
2. Spray the bottom of the Crock Pot with the cooking spray. Add there the chicken breasts cut into slices.
3. Season with the taco seasoning. Add salsa and cream soup over it, mix everything with a long spoon.
4. Cover and cook on LOW for 6 hours.
5. Once the time is over, take off the chicken slices together with a mixture, add sour cream and serve with cauliflower rice.
6. Bon Appetite!

145.Crock Pot sweet garlic chicken

What could be easier than sweet garlic chicken? I always look for cooking chicken in different ways. This recipe combines the flavors of minced and browned garlic together with a sweetener that makes chicken special savory. This mixture makes chicken tender and juicy. You need just four simple ingredients and the whole family will love it. As soon as I found this recipe I decided to cook it without hesitation. You will cook this chicken again and again!

Ingredients (4 servings):

chicken breasts   2 pounds

garlic minced   4 cloves

olive oil   2 tablespoons

Splenda   1/2 cup

Salt and pepper at will

Directions:
1. Peel the garlic and mince it. Take a medium skillet, add there olive oil and brown there minced garlic. It takes you not more than 2 minutes. It must be little browned and translucent.
2. Add Splenda to the same skillet, stir all the time.
3. Take off the skin and bones from the chicken, cut it into pieces of wished size.
4. Put the chicken into the medium bowl, cover with the mixture of Splenda and garlic. Mix everything well with hands.
5. Put the covered chicken into the Crock Pot, cover and cook on LOW 3 hours.
6. Season with pepper and salt.
7. Bon Appetite!

146.Crock Pot herb chicken and veggies

Sometimes, it happens that I don't have any time at all. I don't have time to peel pounds of veggies, buy 13-15 ingredients and cook delicious and complicated dishes. An easy set of chicken breasts (or whole chicken) that is in my refrigerator almost all the time, seasoning mix, some onions, and garlic – everything I need to cook quickly and tasty dinner. Herb chicken and veggies prepared in the Crock Pot, what could be easier? Everything you need, to know how much seasoning mix you should use. Add fresh herbs to your plate just before serving, it could work even better than after cooking process. My relatives have found this dish very delicious.

Ingredients (7 servings):

olive oil   5 tablespoons

herb chicken seasoning mix   1 packet

chicken breasts   4 pounds

salt   1/2 teaspoon

yellow onions   2 whole pcs

garlic   4 cloves

Roma tomatoes   4 whole

pepper to taste

Directions:

1. Peel yellow onions, chop them, divide into two parts. Peel the garlic, chop and do the same as with onions.
2. Wash and dry with a paper towel Roma tomato, dice them.
3. Take a medium bowl, mix the seasoning mix with olive oil. Set aside.
4. Spread the bottom of the Crock Pot with cooking spray, add the chicken breasts, add pepper, salt. Top the mixture from the bowl over chicken breasts (using a spoon).
5. Add also half of onion and garlic.
6. Lay the rest of the chicken breasts and do the same like the first layer – top with seasoning mix, onions and garlic. Finally, put the diced tomatoes on the top. Dress with the remaining seasoning mix, olive oil, garlic, pepper, onions.
7. Cover and cook on LOW for 7 hours. Chicken breasts must be fully cooked. Check it with a fork.
8. Serve warm. Bon Appetite!

147.Keto chicken curry Crock Pot

When it comes to cooking delicious and appetizing dishes using chicken, I always prepare this chicken curry in my Crock Pot. I have learned that it is my best friend in the kitchen! Cooking meat slowly allows you to reach the desired tenderness, save a juicy chicken. You may prepare curry chicken together with butternut squash, it is a rather great addition. Just peel and add it into the Crock Pot together with chicken pieces. So, your fork is waiting for you!

Ingredients (11 servings):

vinegar	2 Tbsp
almond flour	1 Tbsp
tomato paste	1 Tbsp
garam masala	2 tsp
curry powder	2 Tsp
garlic	2 cloves
tomatoes	1 (14.5-oz) can
ginger	1 (1-inch) piece
chicken thighs	2 lb(s)
spinach	1 (5-oz) pkg
fresh cilantro	½ cup

salt, black pepper at will

chutney, Greek yogurt (optional)

Directions:

1. Peel ginger, grate finely. Do the same with garlic. Chop the fresh cilantro. Wash spinach and set aside.
2. Take a medium bowl, mix there tomato paste, flour, vinegar, garam masala, curry powder, garlic, grated ginger, tomatoes with liquid, pepper, salt, and mix in a blender. It must get the compact structure.
3. Remove the skins from the thighs, wash and dry with a paper towel.
4. Put the thighs into the Crock Pot, add on the top of it the smooth mixture.
5. Cover and put on HIGH for 4 hours.
6. Once the time is over, open the Crock Pot after this put spinach. It must be tender. Add also pepper, salt.
7. Serve this dish with chopped cilantro, chutney, Greek yogurt at will.
8. Eat warm.
9. Bon Appetite!

148.Crock Pot Italian chicken zucchini

This dish matches to that season of the year when our gardens are rich in vegetables and you can buy all veggies you want at the markets. When there some zucchinis in your garden or refrigerator, I think, I know what to cook today. One of the integral components of this recipe is spaghetti sauce (if you prefer, you may cook it yourself). I used two zucchinis (squash is also possible). At the end of cooking time, I used my favorite Parmesan cheese, but mozzarella or Swiss cheese is also possible. I think, I'll cook this dish again soon, as we have a great harvest this season.

Ingredients (11 servings)

chicken breasts	3 pounds
garlic	2 tablespoons
yellow onions	2 small pcs
onion powder	1 teaspoon
zucchini's sliced	2 whole pcs
spaghetti sauce	24 ounces
Italian seasoning	2 tablespoons
Salt	1/2 teaspoon
Pepper	1/4 teaspoon
green onions	1 bunch
Parmesan cheese	2 cups

Directions:

1. Peel the onions and chop them finely. Chop the green onions. Peel the garlic and mince it. Shred the cheese into a bowl. Wash and dry with a paper towel zucchinis and slice.
2. Take off the skin and bones from the chicken breasts. Wash and cut.
3. Spread the cooking spray on the bottom and sides of the Crock Pot.

4. Take a medium bowl, mix here spaghetti sauce, chopped onions, zucchinis, garlic, onion powder, Italian seasoning, pepper. Add salt.
5. Put the chicken into the Crock Pot, spread the vegetable mixture and sauce.
6. Cover and cook on LOW 6 hours.
7. Once the time is over, remove chicken to the plate, garnish with shredded cheese and green chopped onions.
8. Enjoy!

149.Crock Pot Asian-style drumsticks

The Crock Pot recipes are becoming more common nowadays, it is just too simple to use. Of course, chicken breasts are rather tasty, but sometimes they are too expensive and even boring! The Asian-style drumsticks are cheaper and taste as well as other parts. The chicken meat on the bone is more flavor and is cooked quicker.

Ingredients (9 servings):

hoisin sauce	¼ cup
sweetener	¼ cup
ketchup	3 Tbsp
hot sauce	2 Tbsp
garlic	2-3 cloves
chili flakes	¼ tsp
chicken drumsticks	8 pcs
Chinese five-spice powder	2 Tsp
scallions	3 pcs

Salt and black pepper at will

Directions:
1. Peel the garlic and mince. Slice the scallions thinly.
2. Take a medium bowl, add hoisin sauce, sweetener, hot sauce, ketchup, minced garlic, spice powder, chili flakes. Combine everything with a spoon.
3. Put the washed and dried with a paper towel the drumsticks and put them into the mixture. Toss everything with a spoon to cover.
4. Put the drumsticks in the Crock Pot, cover and cook on LOW 5-6 hours. Check with a fork if the drumsticks are ready after 5 hours. The sauce must be thickened slightly.
5. Remove chicken to the plate, season with scallions and pepper, salt at will.
6. Bon Appetite!

150.Crock Pot keto Pesto chicken

I have never cooked meat with pesto before, but one of my friends showed me this great idea. Just think a little bit, how tasty could be a real Italian classic! First time I used pesto that was bought at the store. Of course, you may prepare it yourself if you have enough basil in your garden. I absolutely loved this flavor recipe and advise you to cook it always with more pesto.

Ingredients (4 servings):

cream of chicken soup	21.5 ounces
pesto	1/2 cup
sour cream	1/2 cup
chicken	2 pounds

pepper and salt to taste

Directions:

1. Prepare the chicken – take off the bones and skin, cut into cubes or strips.
2. Spread the cooking spray over the bottom and sides of the Crock Pot. Put the chicken pieces.
3. Combine in a small bowl cream of chicken soup, sour cream, and pesto. Dress with salt and pepper.
4. Add the mixture to the chicken, stir well.
5. Cover and cook on LOW for 5 hours. Chicken must be tender.
6. Serve with cauliflower rice.
7. Bon Appetite!

151.Chicken sliders with an Indian twist

This recipe is the favorite one of the children mostly, of those who like to eat the chicken sliders with keto bread. If this is a classic Indian combination of species, is a question for real experts. These chicken sliders are easy to prepare. I advise you to follow all the measurements that I highly recommend in my recipe. I'm sure you'll like it definitely.

Ingredients:

butter or oil	2½ tbsp
onion	1 large pcs
garlic	4 cloves
ginger root	2 thumb-size pieces
garam masala	2 tsp
cumin	2 tsp
turmeric	1 tsp
cayenne pepper	½-1 Tsp
coconut milk	14 oz
tomato paste	5½ oz
chicken thighs	3 lb

whipping cream   ¼ cup

salt and pepper, to taste

Directions:
1. Peel the onion and slice it. Peel garlic and crush. Peel gingerroot and grate it.
2. Take a medium skillet, heat the oil or butter and add garlic and onion there. Cook until softened. Onions must be brown (golden). Stir all the time.
3. Add there cumin, gingerroot, masala, cayenne pepper, turmeric, stir all the time.
4. Pour the coconut milk, tomato paste. Let it boil some minutes. Remove.
5. Wash and dry with a paper towel the chicken thighs. Remove bones and skin.
6. Pour this mixture into the Crock Pot, add the chicken thighs there. Add pepper, salt at will.
7. Cover and cook on LOW for 6-7 hours.
8. Remove the chicken once the cooking time is over. Shred the chicken.
9. Serve the chicken with whipping cream and cucumbers.
10. Bon Appetite!

152.Crock Pot chicken and broccoli

I think this recipe is a successful combination of chicken and broccoli where both ingredients supply each other. The creamy texture of chicken perfectly blends with the broccoli that couldn't be over-cooked here. I also advise you to use all the species and sauce that are mentioned in this recipe, it is the best combination that could be.

Ingredients (10 servings):

chicken thighs   12 pcs

five-spice powder   1 Tsp

broth (chicken)   2 cups

soy sauce   ½ cup

ginger (fresh)   2 Tbsp

sriracha (sugar-free)   1 Tbsp

garlic   4 cloves

sesame oil   1 Tsp

broccoli florets   2 cups

sweet pepper   1 pcs

Sesame seeds (optional)

sliced scallions for garnish

Directions:
1. Peel the garlic and chop finely. Chop the fresh ginger into a medium bowl. Wash sweet pepper, and slice it.
2. Prepare the chicken thighs – remove skin and bones, cut them into chunks.
3. Put the chicken thighs into the Crock Pot and add there spice powder, pepper, and salt.

4. Mix together broth, chopped ginger, sauce, sriracha, garlic. Pour this mixture over the chicken thighs.
5. Cover and put on LOW for 4 hours.
6. After the mentioned 3 hours are over, open the Crock Pot add sesame oil, slices of sweet pepper, broccoli. Go on cooking for another 1 or put on WARM.
7. Serve with sliced sesame seeds.
8. Add sliced scallions.
9. Bon Appetite!

153.Crock Pot keto BBQ chicken legs

What can you add to the recipe for BBQ chicken legs? – Everything! Everything you wish! BBQ chicken legs recipe is one of the eldest classic versions of the cooking the chicken legs! So tasty as nowhere else. I like hot sauces and eat them well. If you don't like the hot sauces or chili like me, you may reduce the proposed amounts.

Ingredients (8 servings):

chicken legs	2 lb(s)
BBQ sauce	1 ½ cup
cider vinegar	¼ cup
onion	1 medium
garlic	3 clove
Chili powder	1 Tbsp
Paprika	2 tsp
mustard powder	1 Tsp
Worcestershire sauce	
pepper and salt to taste	

Directions:
1. Peel the onion, garlic, chop them finely.
2. Put the chicken legs to the Crock Pot, add chopped garlic and onion, pour the sauce and vinegar, stir together.
3. Add also paprika, mustard as well as chili powder, Worcestershire sauce, salt.
4. Combine everything thoroughly.
5. Cover and cook on LOW 6 hours.
6. Serve with cauliflower rice.
7. Bon Appetite!

154.Crock Pot keto whole chicken in a hot sauce

This recipe of whole chicken in a hot sauce prepared in the Crock Pot is tender and moist. Once the whole chicken is ready, I remove it to the big plate, shred it in pieces take off the remained liquid and add the prepared hot sauce. Remove the skin of the chicken and let the rest of the chicken juice run out... You don't need to cook the other additional dishes (like cauliflower rice or etc.) and other seasonings. It is perfectly well. Enjoy it!

Ingredients (16 servings):

sweet paprika	2 ½ tsp
garlic powder	1 ½ tsp
freshly ground pepper	1 ½ tsp
coriander	½ tsp
caraway	½ Tsp
whole chicken	1 4- to 5-lb

Hot Sauce

Ketchup	1 cup
vinegar	¼ cup
sweetener	½ cup
mustard	2 Tbsp
sea salt	1 Tsp
chili powder	1 Tsp
onion powder	1 Tsp
garlic powder	¾ Tsp
cayenne	¼ Tsp
ground pepper	¼ Tsp

Directions:

1. Spread the cooking spray over the bottom and sides of the Crock Pot.
2. Wash the chicken, take off the insides. Take a middle pan and join there garlic powder, salt, caraway, coriander, and paprika.
3. Put the chicken into the Crock Pot and add this mixture on the top of it. Thoroughly spread this along with the chicken. Be sure that both sides are perfectly covered with mixture.
4. Over cover and put on LOW for 8 hours. Check readiness of the whole chicken with a fork.

Preparing for a hot sauce

1. While the chicken is prepared in the Crock Pot, make ready the hot sauce: join the ketchup, vinegar, mustard, salt, chili powder, onion powder, garlic powder, cayenne and pepper in a bowl. Stir everything well. Let the mixture boil, add the sweetener, stir once more.
2. When the chicken is almost cooked (once the time is over), take off the liquid from the Crock Pot, pour the sauce with a hot sauce, over cover and put on WARM. Leave it in the Crock Pot for 1 hour.

3. Serve additionally with hot sauce. Eat warm.
4. Bon Appetite!

155.Crock Pot keto butter chicken

Today I would like to introduce you a healthy and light version of classic Indian chicken. This tender chicken is rich in fragrant species and creamy sauce consistency, garam masala and curry powder make the base of the classic Indian version. To keep the sauce flavor and creamy I usually add to the sauce heavy cream and tomato paste. This fragrant dish challenges the best flavors of India, keeping your chicken thighs with full of juice.

Ingredients (14 servings):

almond flour   3 Tbsp

garam masala   1 Tbsp

ground cumin   1 tsp

curry powder   1 Tsp

chicken thighs   3 lb(s)

cashews   ½ cup

onion   1 pcs

garlic   4 cloves

jalapeno pepper   1 pcs

fresh ginger   1 Tbsp

tomatoes   2 pcs

heavy cream   ¾ cup

tomato paste   2 Tbsp

Greek yogurt   ¾ cup

Cilantro leaves at will

Salt and pepper

Directions:

1. Prepare the thighs – remove skin and bones from the chicken thighs. Cut each of them into 4 -5 pieces.
2. Peel the onion and garlic, chop them plenty.
3. Wash and dry with a paper towel the peppers. Remove the seeds, slice. Chop fresh ginger.
4. Wash the tomatoes, take off the seeds, slice or quarter them.
5. Take a little pan, join flour, species. Stir finely. Toss chicken thighs with flour mixture.
6. Grind the cashews in a blender.

7. Put the chicken thighs in the Crock Pot, add there masala, cumin, curry, nuts, peppers, onions and garlic, grated ginger, sliced tomatoes and tomato paste, heavy cream. Toss everything.
8. Dress additional with salt and pepper.
9. Cover and put on LOW for 5 hours.
10. Dress with cilantro. Add Greek yogurt at will.
11. Bon Appetite!

156.Crock Pot Thai curry chicken

This delicious recipe was introduced me some years ago by my old friend. I'm sure this recipe should be definitely included in your cookbook. The base of this amazing dish is the Thai sauce cooked from coconut milk, curry paste, sauce, ginger, peanut butter, garlic, lime, a sweetener that makes this sauce at the same time both sour and sweet. The contradiction of the tastes is amazing. Don't be confused when you read lime and sweetener in this recipe, the chicken is perfectly tasty. Be sure, you'll surprise your guests with a rainbow of tastes!

Ingredients (13 servings):

peanut butter	⅓ cup
light coconut milk	14 oz
sauce (your favorite one)	3 Tbsp
ginger (from a jar)	1 Tbsp
garlic (from a jar)	2 Tsp
red curry paste	1 Tbsp
onion	1 pcs
sweetener	2 tbsp
lime juice	1 pcs
red pepper (optional)	1 pcs
fresh cilantro	½ cup
chicken breasts	4 pcs
mussels	10 pcs medium sized (7 oz)

Directions:

1. Take a medium pan, combine there peanut butter, spicy sauce (your favorite one), ginger, coconut milk, ginger from a jar, lime juice, curry paste, sweetener. Stir everything and put this paste into the center of the Crock Pot. Wash red pepper, dry it with a paper towel, remove the seeds and slice. Set it aside.
2. Peel the onion and chop it, add to the Crock Pot also.
3. Wash and dry with a paper towel the chicken breasts. Cut them into pieces and add to the Crock Pot also.
4. Cover and cook 4 hours on LOW.

5. Once the chicken is ready remove it to the plate, add mussels with liquid, fresh chopped cilantro, and sliced pepper.
6. Dress with black pepper at will.
7. Bon Appetite!

157.Crock Pot Creamy Chicken and Veggies

For this recipe, you need only chicken thighs and broccoli, cauliflower as for the veggies. Once the dish is ready, you need just to mix the juice of the chicken, lemon juice, and cream cheese! You can't even imagine how easy, tasty and delicious is the texture! It is a luscious sauce. You'd better eat this creamy chicken and veggies with eggs noodles. Don't hesitate to go to the kitchen and follow the directions you may find below.

Ingredients (11 servings):

olive oil	1 teaspoon
chicken thighs	6 pcs(about 1½-2 pounds)
salt	¼ teaspoon
black pepper	¼ teaspoon
cauliflower florets	1 pound
broccoli florets	1 pound
oregano	1 teaspoon
garlic powder	½ teaspoon
lemon	1 pcs
cream cheese	4 ounces
lemon juice	1 teaspoon

Directions:

1. Wash and chop the fresh parsley. Set aside. Slice the lemon into ¼ inch slices.
2. Scale the skin and bones from the chicken thighs.
3. Spread the olive oil on the bottom and side of the Crock Pot. Put the chicken thighs on the bottom.
4. Season with pepper and salt. Top the florets of the broccoli and cauliflower on the chicken pieces.
5. Add garlic powder and oregano. Top the lemon slice over the florets.
6. Cover and put on LOW for 5 hours. Check the tenderness with a fork.
7. Remove lemon slices at the end of cooking time. Remove firstly the florets of broccoli and cauliflower, then chicken pieces and the rest of liquid.
8. Add the cream cheese and the lemon juice into a small pan, add also the remained juice of chicken from the Crock Pot and stir everything well.
9. Pour this cream cheese over the chicken pieces that are already on your plate.
10. Serve warm and enjoy!

158. Whole Tuscan chicken Crock Pot

I must say, I love my Crock Pot very much. It is my right arm in the kitchen. I can't imagine how I could cook my favorite recipes without it!? Tuscan chicken prepared in the Crock Pot is something amazing and appetizing for me and whole my family. Everything I need here it is just to prepare the seasoning mix, wash the chicken, remove the insides, make a «massage» to the chicken using the readymade seasoning mix and that's all! The remained work is for my right arm. It cooks Tuscan chicken super tasty! I like to enjoy this chicken with fresh tomatoes and cucumbers. Let's try to cook a whole chicken in a Tuscan-style!

Ingredients (13 servings):

Salt	3 teaspoons
Paprika	2 teaspoons
thyme	1½ teaspoons
garlic salt	½ teaspoon
rosemary	½ teaspoon
oregano	¼ teaspoon
ground black pepper	¼ teaspoon
lemon (zest and juice from it)	1 pcs
garlic	8 cloves
onion	1 pcs
olive oil	2 tablespoons
whole chicken	3½ to 4½ pounds
lemon	1 pcs

Directions:

1. Take a middle pan and mix together salt, paprika, thyme, garlic salt, oregano, rosemary, black pepper. Set aside.
2. Peel the onion and chop. Peel garlic and mince it (or press). Wash the lemon and slice.
3. Grate the lemon zest and add to the mixture. Add also minced garlic and combine everything once more.
4. Put the chopped onions in the Crock Pot, squeeze the lemon juice into the Crock Pot at once, add also one spoon of olive oil to the onions and garlic in the Crock Pot.
5. Wash the chicken, dry with a paper towel. Take off the insides, fold-down the wings. Place the readymade seasonings on the chicken and worm. Add the remained olive oil, add also the seasoning inside the chicken. Place the chicken in the Crock Pot.
6. Cover and cook on LOW for 9 hours.
7. Serve the cooked chicken on a large plate together with veggies from the Crock Pot.
8. Bon Appetite!

159.Crock Pot chicken with 40 garlic cloves

If you are a fan of garlic and chicken but haven't ever tasted chicken with garlic cloves, you have been really missing out. But! You are on the right side of the post if you are reading this recipe. Everything you need here – to buy garlic, some species, chicken legs. The hardest work here is… to peel the 40 garlic cloves! Yes, it is really complicated a little bit. But don't be scared of this work, the result worth it! It is a rather comforting dish at any time of the year!

Ingredients (7 servings):

chicken legs	10-12 pcs
garlic	40 cloves
onion	1 small
fresh lemon juice	2 tablespoons
thyme	4 sprigs
bay leaves	2 pcs
paprika	2 teaspoons
Salt and pepper	

Directions:
1. Peel all the garlic cloves. Peel the onion and slice thinly.
2. Squeeze the lemon juice into a cup.
3. Spread the cooking spray of the Crock Pot, add on the bottom of it the half of the onion and a half of the garlic cloves.
4. Wash the chicken legs, season them with paprika, salt, pepper, place them over the onion-garlic bed.
5. Top with bay leaves and thyme. Add the remained onion and another half of the garlic cloves.
6. Add the chicken legs again, the remained thyme.
7. Spread the lemon juice over the dish. Cover and cook 7 hours.
8. Bon Appetite!

160.Crock Pot Creamy Buffalo Chicken

The creamy Buffalo chicken cooked at the Crock Pot tastes tender and amazing. It is so easy to prepare! This recipe must be a crowd pleaser, delicious and remarkably simple. I don't know somebody, who dislikes this recipe of the creamy chicken. Let the chicken pieces be cooked until the chicken parts fall apart. Add the cream cheese at the end of cooking time as well as the bounding mixture of flour and water. Enjoy each piece of this creamy chicken.

Ingredients (13 servings):

chicken breast	2 pounds
salt	½ teaspoon
Buffalo wing sauce	½ cup
chicken broth	½ cup

sweet onion	½ cup
celery	½ cup (about 2 ribs)
almond flour	¼ cup
water	3-4 tablespoons
cream cheese (softened)	1 (8 ounces) package
dried parsley flakes	¼ teaspoon
dried dill	¼ teaspoon
garlic powder	¼ teaspoon
onion powder	⅛ teaspoon
black pepper at will	

Directions:

1. Wash the chicken, dry it with a paper towel. Remove the bones and the skin. Cut into large pieces.
2. Peel the sweet onion and chop. Chop the celery.
3. Spread the pepper and salt over the chicken and put it into the Crock Pot.
4. Mix the Buffalo wing sauce with broth. Top the chicken with this mixture, chopped onions, and celery.
5. Cover and put on LOW for 6 hours. Check the chicken with a fork if it is tender.
6. While chicken is prepared, take a little pan, add flour with water, stir this to the Crock Pot at the end of the cooking time.
7. Take another little pan, combine here dill, parsley flakes, onion powder, garlic powder, cream cheese. Pour this into the Crock Pot also at the final of cooking time. Put on WARM.
8. Serve warm.
9. Bon Appetite

161.Keto chicken and sausage mix

This recipe of keto chicken and sausage mix is indispensable in your daily life. What could be easier than to put chicken thighs into the Crock Pot, add there Italian or andouille sausages, stir with species that you prefer most of all and wait some hours until the Crock Pot cook this delicious addition to the veggies or cauliflower rice?

Ingredients (16 servings):

chicken thighs	8 pcs
sausages andouille or Italian	6 pcs
almond flour	½ cup
chicken broth	3 cups
tomatoes	26 ounces canned or boxed
yellow onion	1pcs

celery ribs	5 pcs
bell pepper	1 pcs
red bell pepper	1 pcs
garlic	4 cloves
dried oregano	1½ teaspoons
dried thyme	1½ teaspoons
smoked paprika	1½ teaspoons
salt	1 teaspoon
cayenne pepper	¾ teaspoons
black pepper	¼ teaspoon

Directions:

1. Peel the onion and chop. Chop the celery ribs. Peel the garlic and mince.
2. Wash and dry with a paper towel bell pepper. Slice it.
3. Wash the chicken thighs, remove the skin. Put them into the Crock Pot.
4. Cut the sausages (optional – you may fry them at the pan). Add them to the Crock Pot too.
5. Add chicken broth, almond flour, chopped tomatoes from a can, chopped celery, sliced pepper, onions, red pepper, oregano, garlic, thyme, salt, paprika, black and cayenne pepper.
6. Toss everything finely.
7. Cover and put on LOW for 6 hours.
8. Serve with cauliflower rice or your favorite veggies. Bon Appetite!

162. Crock Pot Chicken Cacciatore

What do you know about Italian chicken cacciatore? Cacciatore means a «hunter-style» dish cooked from chicken, tomatoes, onions, vegetables, vinegar. This is one of the recipes I have found many years ago. I have tried too many versions of Italian cacciatore, but this one is the best one. Following this name «hunter-style», I hunted at the nearest supermarket, bought all necessary ingredients and returned home with a spoil. Now, I invite you to prepare the real chicken cacciatore together with me. Let's try to do it!

Ingredients (15 servings):

sweet onion	1 large
chicken thighs	6 pcs (roughly 1¾-2 pounds)
bell peppers	3 pcs
garlic	8 cloves
tomato paste	2 ounces
roasted diced tomatoes with juice	2 (14½ ounce each) cans

small artichoke hearts	2 (14-ounce cans each)
chicken broth	1 cup
bay leaf	1 pcs
fresh parsley	2 teaspoons
red pepper	½ teaspoon
dried rosemary leaves	a ½ teaspoon
salt	½ teaspoon
ground black pepper	¼ teaspoon
fresh basil leaves	10 pcs

Directions:

1. Peel and slice the sweet onions. Wash and dry with a paper towel bell pepper. Slice them.
2. Peel and half the garlic.
3. Put the onions on the bottom of the Crock Pot. Put the chicken thighs, add on the top of the garlic, pepper slices, tomato paste, diced tomatoes, salt, artichokes without liquid.
4. Add ground black pepper, rosemary leaves, parsley, chicken broth, bay leaf.
5. Cover and put on LOW for 5 hours.
6. Serve with black pepper and fresh basil leaves. Remove the bay leaf before serving.
7. Bon Appetite!

163.Keto Raspberry-Chipotle Chicken Tacos

From my point of view, this recipe of the raspberry-chipotle chicken tacos prepared in the Crock Pot is great for a crowded party. A delicious meal without a huge of ingredients and an impressive amount of hard work. What do you need more? When I have a crowd of guests I always try to use this recipe, it works great! My Crock Pot makes all possible work so, preparing this dish makes fun. The sweetness of raspberry gets a new taste to a habitual chicken. I like to add to the ready-made dish shredded cheese (I can't imagine the most part of the dishes without cheese!), slices of avocado, sour cream. It tastes great!

Ingredients (8 servings):

chicken breasts	2 pounds
raspberry	⅓ cup
peppers in adobo sauce (sugar-free)	2 chipotle
garlic	1 clove
adobo sauce (from chipotle peppers)	1 tablespoon
kosher salt	1 tablespoon
cumin	½ teaspoon
roasted tomatoes	1 (15 ounces) can

Salt and pepper

Optional: shredded cheese, cilantro, slices of avocado, sour cream.

Directions:
1. Prepare the chicken breasts, remove the skin and the bones. Wash them and cut into halves. Put the chicken breasts on the bottom of the Crock Pot.
2. Peel the garlic, mince it.
3. Take a little pan, mix there.
4. Raspberries, minced garlic, chipotle peppers, salt, adobo sauce, cumin, pepper, blend until smooth consistency.
5. Pour the mixture over the chicken breasts in the Crock Pot, add roasted tomatoes on the top together with juice.
6. Cover and put on LOW for hours.
7. Remove the chicken breasts once they are ready together with the sauce, shred the breasts with the knife. Before serving add shredded cheese, some slices of avocado, two tablespoons of sour cream and enjoy!
8. Bon Appetite!

164.Crock Pot Strawberry-Habanero Pulled Chicken

The main ingredient of this dish is sauce… Yes, the strawberry-habanero sauce. Maybe, you think, it sounds strange, but you must taste it. Habanero peppers combined with the strawberry puree create a flavored sauce for the tender chicken. I usually add avocado slices to this chicken, it adds the sour-sweet-hot combination of sauce and chicken. Don't be scared of habanero peppers, the Crock Pot does it best – during the preparation time the pepper brings its natural sweetness.

Ingredients (12 servings):

fresh or frozen strawberry purée	1 cup
onion	¼ small
garlic	2 cloves
pepper	1 habanero
Sweetener	1 tablespoon
vinegar	1 tablespoon
molasses	1 tablespoon
tomato paste	1 teaspoon
liquid smoke	½ teaspoon
salt	1 pinch
chicken breasts	1 pound
avocado, sliced (optional)	1 pcs

Directions:

1. Peel the onion and chop it finely. Peel the garlic and smash. Wash and dry with a paper towel habanero pepper, mince it carefully. Wash and slice the avocado.
2. Take a medium pan, mix there strawberry puree, chopped onions, smashed garlic, minced pepper, salt, sweetener, vinegar, tomato paste, molasses, liquid smoke. Stir well everything.
3. Remove the skin and the bones from the chicken breasts, wash them thoroughly. Toss the chicken breasts in the mixture and place them into the Crock Pot.
4. Cover and cook on HIGH for 3-4 hours.
5. Remove the chicken, shred it, pour the sauce and add the avocado slices.
6. Bon Appetite!

165.Crock Pot Chicken Korma

Spicy and creamy chicken Korma is an old Indian dish that you can cook at home. Chicken Korma is usually served in the Indian restaurant's menu. But this is my Crock Pot version where I combine chicken and the species together and cook everything for 6 hours, after this I also add Greek yogurt to get the creamy light texture of the dish. Following the rules of a keto diet, you may serve it with cauliflower rice for your guests or with keto bread.

Ingredients:

Tomatoes	5 medium (about 1½ pounds)
onions	2 medium
garlic	3 cloves
fresh ginger	1 tablespoon
curry powder	2 teaspoons
garam masala	2 teaspoons
salt	½ teaspoon
red pepper flakes	¼ teaspoon
chicken drumsticks	8 pcs
Greek yogurt	½ cup
cilantro	¼ cup

Directions:

1. Wash the tomatoes, dry them with a paper towel. Take off the seeds, cut into quarters. Chop the fresh cilantro into a little bowl. Set aside.
2. Peel the onion and chop; peel the garlic and mince. Grate the fresh ginger into a plate.
3. Put in the Crock Pot tomatoes, chopped onions, minced garlic, grated ginger, salt, curry powder, masala, pepper flakes. Mix everything well.
4. Add chicken drumsticks in the mixture at the Crock Pot and toss everything.
5. Cover and put on LOW for 6 hours until chicken is tender. Check it with a fork.
6. Remove the chicken drumsticks to the plate, separate the meat from the bones and skin and return it to the Crock Pot.

7. Pour Greek yogurt, dress with pepper and salt at will.
8. Serve with chopped cilantro.
9. Eat warm.
10. Bon Appetite!

166.Crock Pot chicken and asparagus

The simple Crock Pot chicken recipe with tender asparagus makes a fragrant meal for whole your family. If you don't like the cream of onion soup, you might change it with cream of celery soup. The frozen asparagus is also OK for this recipe. My friend has replaced some ingredients with cream of broccoli, it was also great. So, you can vary a little bit here. You will not stain the dish, be sure! I would better say, be free to adapt this recipe to the preferred ingredients of your family. If you need an extra color, add some tomatoes or basil leaves.

Ingredients (12 servings):

chicken breasts	1 1/2 pounds (about 4 to 6 halves)
chicken stock	1/2 cup
cream of onion soup	1 (10 1/2-ounce) can
tarragon	1/4 to 1/2 teaspoon
lemon pepper seasoning	1 teaspoon
salt	1/4 teaspoon
asparagus	1 bunch
almond flour	1 tablespoon
milk	1 tablespoon
black pepper	
toasted almonds (optional)	
grated or shredded Parmesan cheese (optional)	

Directions:
1. Wash the breasts, take off the skin. Cut them into pieces. Put into the bottom of the Crock Pot.
2. Take a medium pan, mix there condensed soup, broth, seasoning, tarragon. Blend everything well.
3. Add this mix on the top of the chicken, cover and put on LOW for 5 hours. Put there also pepper and salt if needed.
4. While the chicken is in the Crock Pot, cut the asparagus into a 1-inch length. Add them almost at the end of the cooking time to the breasts.
5. Take a small pan, whisk there milk and flour, add this mixture to the Crock Pot also.
6. Continue cooking (put on WARM) for 1 hour. The asparagus must get tenderness.
7. Garnish the ready-made chicken with grated Parmesan cheese and toasted almonds optional.
8. Bon Appetite!

167.Crock Pot cashew chicken

This cookie of the cashew chicken prepared in the Crock Pot needs just 10 minutes of preparation and I think you could find these 10 minutes easily. It is a flavorful and super easy dish that doesn't need special ingredients that couldn't be found on the shelves of the supermarkets. Everything you need could be found at the nearest shop. Let's try to do it!

Ingredients (11 servings):

chicken thighs	2 lbs
almond flour	1/2 Tsp
canola oil	1 Tbsp
hot sauce	1/4 cup
vinegar	2 Tbsp
ketchup	2 Tbsp
xanthan gum	1 Tbsp
garlic	1 clove
grated fresh ginger	1/2 Tsp
red pepper flakes	1/4 tsp
cashews	1/2 cup

Green onions (optional, for garnish)

black pepper

Directions:

1. Peel the onion and mince. Grate the fresh ginger.
2. Chop green onions.
3. Prepare the chicken, take off the skin and the bones, cut into 6-7 pieces.
4. Take a storage bag, mix the flour with pepper flakes, add the chicken thighs. Shake the mixture and the chicken together. Chicken must be covered with the mixture.
5. Spread the cooking spray over the Crock Pot, put there coated chicken thighs.
6. Take another medium bowl, mix the vinegar, sauce, xanthan gum, minced garlic, pepper flakes (the rest of them), grated ginger, top over chicken.
7. Cover and put on LOW for 4 hours. Stir in the nuts and continue cooking 15 minutes more.
8. Serve hot! Add chopped green onions.

168.Crock Pot chicken gizzard recipe

Have you ever cooked or eaten the chicken gizzards prepared in the Crock Pot? Chicken gizzards prepared on this recipe will thaw in your mouth. They are tender, flavor, delicious. The special sauce mix gets an amazing addition to the chicken gizzards. Moreover, this recipe needs the ingredients that are rather cheap. That's why this appetizing dish could be found almost every day on your table.

Ingredients (7 servings):

organic cilantro	1 bunch
garlic	3 large cloves
onion	1 small pcs
chicken gizzards	1 pound
sauce (Passata di Pomodoro)	¼ cup
Wine (white)	½ cup
water	¼ cup
sea salt at will	

Directions:

1. Wash cilantro, take off the seeds.
2. Peel garlic after this slice it. Peel onion, slice also.
3. Put in the Crock Pot chicken gizzards, sliced garlic, onion, add cilantro, sauce, water, wine, salt. Toss everything together.
4. Cover and put on LOW for 5 hours.
5. Eat chicken gizzards with cauliflower rice!
6. Bon Appetite!

169.Crock Pot balsamic chicken

This recipe of the keto balsamic chicken is nothing that a special combination of flavor species that make your chicken breasts unforgettable! It's amazing! I always say that the easier is the recipe, the better it tastes. This is the balsamic chicken recipe. Everything is simple and brilliant. Just buy chicken breasts, wash and cut and join them with species.

Ingredients (9 servings):

garlic powder	1 teaspoon
basil	1 teaspoon
salt	1/2 teaspoon
pepper	1/2 teaspoon
onion	2 teaspoons
garlic	4 cloves
olive oil	1 tablespoon
balsamic vinegar	1/2 cup
chicken breasts	7- 8 pcs
pepper and salt at will	
fresh parsley at will	

Directions:

1. Take the skinless and boneless chicken breasts and chop them into slices.
2. Join garlic powder, salt, basil, onion, and pepper in a medium bowl.
3. Add the olive oil on the bottom of the Crock Pot. Put the chicken breasts into the Crock Pot, add species mix, toss everything. Add balsamic vinegar.
4. Cover and put on LOW for 5 hours.
5. Season with fresh parsley.
6. Bon Appetite!

170.Keto Crock Pot Chicken Parmesan

I like hard cheese and most of all I like Parmesan or Swiss cheese and mozzarella. I don't have a plenty of time to cook the dishes that need many steps. I used my right arm - the Crock Pot to cook this keto recipe, it turned out amazing! Parmesan and mozzarella are great in their combination. It is so delicious! This is step by step instruction that will help you in cooking this chicken Parmesan.

Ingredients (8 servings):

chicken breasts	4- 5 pcs
spaghetti sauce	1 jar
tomatoes	1 can
tomato paste	1 can
garlic	4 cloves
Italian seasoning	1 Tsp
Parmesan cheese	½ cup
mozzarella cheese	2 cups

pepper and salt to taste

Directions:

1. Wash the chicken breasts and take off the skin and bones. Put them into the Crock Pot.
2. Peel the garlic, dice. Shred the Parmesan cheese, cut mozzarella.
3. Add to the Crock Pot sauce, diced tomatoes, tomato paste, diced garlic. Stir everything.
4. Cover and put on LOW 5 hours.
5. Open the Crock Pot, add Italian seasoning. Add shredded Parmesan and mozzarella. Cover for up for half an hour. The cheese must be melted.
6. Serve hot.
7. Bon Appetite!

171.Crock Pot crack chicken

This recipe of crack keto chicken is going to be your favorite one. It is healthy, full of protein, you can add to this crack chicken any fixings. Do you know why I call this recipe «crack chicken» - I can't stop eating it. This dish has only 4 servings! Ranch seasoning, cream cheese, breasts, and bacon! It looks like really delicious and I plan to cook it right now. What about you?

Ingredients (4 servings):

boneless chicken breasts	2 lbs
cream cheese	2 (8 oz) blocks
dry Ranch seasoning	2 (1 oz) packets
bacon (crisply and crumbled)	8 oz

Salt and pepper at will

Directions:

1. Take off the skin and the bones of the chicken breasts, wash them.
2. Take a medium pan, join chicken breasts, cream cheese with dry seasoning, add pepper, salt. Toss everything well.
3. Cover and cook on HIGH 3 hours. Check the chicken with a fork.
4. Once the chicken is ready, serve it hot, add shred bacon.
5. Serve hot.
6. Bon Appetite!

172. Crock-Pot Beef Tips Recipe

I have already told you, I think the Crock Pot is one of the best cooking achievements. I prefer to cook meat and the Crock Pot allows me to make it tender and keep the natural juicy. The keto beef tips are great for salads, veggies, and eggs. It could be eaten for dinner or supper, you can save it in the fridge for some days, it is both well for daily meal and for parties.

Ingredients (9 servings):

almond flour	1/4 cup
black pepper	1/4 teaspoon
garlic powder	1/4 teaspoon
olive oil	3 tablespoon
beef stew meat	1 - 2 pounds
onion	1 medium pcs
beef broth	2 cups
balsamic	1 cup
brown gravy mix	0.87 ounce

salt at will

Directions:

1. Peel the onion and chop it.
2. Take a medium pan, combine pepper, flour, garlic powder. Stir everything finely.
3. Take the beef meat and put in the mixture from all the sides.

4. Take a large skillet, add olive oil and put on medium heat. Add there beef meat and roast from all the sides (all the beef pieces). Let it brown about 5 minutes.
5. Remove the beef from the skillet into the Crock Pot, add to the same skillet chopped onions. Let it brown until translucent. It takes you approximately 10 minutes. Add prepared onions to the Crock Pot also.
6. Add the beef broth, balsamic, gravy mix, salt and stir everything well.
7. Cover and put on LOW for 6 hours.
8. Serve with broccoli or cauliflower rice.
9. Enjoy it!

173.Crock-Pot Homemade Italian Beef Recipe

The recipe of the Italian beef is actually a beef roast prepared for some long hours in the Crock Pot adding Italian dressing mix (you may use also the other one if preferred), beef broth and pepperoncini peppers. I'm not actually a fan of hot and spicy food, but the pepperoncini give this beef a special «bite», the beef is in reality not too hot. I really like such recipes, when you need just to «gather» all the ingredients in the Crock Pot and push a button. You may let this meat cook all day long and be ready only to a finished meal. I always prefer the beef broth homemade, but the bought can of it is also possible. Serve this Italian beef with keto bread and you'll get an appetizing «sandwich».

Ingredients (5 servings):

beef roast	3 pounds
onions	1 pcs medium
Italian dressing dry mix	1-ounce
pepperoncini peppers	16 ounces (1 jar, sliced)
beef broth	28 ounces

pepper and salt to taste

Directions:
1. Peel the onions and ring. Set aside.
2. Spread the cooking spray over the bottom of the Crock Pot and the sides.
3. Place the beef into the Crock Pot.
4. Add there onions, dry mix dressing, peppers, salt, beef broth.
5. Cover and put on HIGH for 5 hours. Check if the beef is ready once the cooking time is over.
6. Remove the beef from the Crock Pot, place it on a plate and shred with a fork.
7. Season with black pepper and juice (sauce) from the Crock Pot.
8. Serve with keto bread.
9. Bon Appetite!

174.Keto Mississippi roast beef

The first time I used the au jus gravy in ajar was a real surprise for me. My previous dish has got a new taste and flavor. The other novel ingredient in this recipe is pepperoncini peppers that could be also bot in a jar whole or sliced. If the chuck roasts that you are going to use are definitely fat, you may use the half of the butter mentioned below. I think, in this way, there will be enough liquid and fat to rich the tenderness of the chuck roasts. You have to avoid pre-cooking through browning it in the skillet (optional), you must just give a nice darkness to the chuck roast. But I actually skip the browning and put my chuck roast beef in the Crock Pot at once. I don't care about the color here, I care about the taste. Add mashed cauliflower and this dish will be fabulous!

Ingredients (7 servings):

beef chuck roast	2 pounds
yellow onion sectioned	1 large pcs
ranch dressing mix	1 packet
bistro au jus gravy	1 cup
salted butter	1/2 cup
pepperoncini peppers whole 4 - 8 jar	
olive oil	2 - 3 tablespoons
salt and pepper to taste	

Directions:

1. Sprinkle the chuck roast beef with pepper and salt from all the sides finely. (If you prefer to have the browned slices you may roast the beef in the skillet for some minutes additionally).
2. Cover the bottom of the Crock Pot with olive oil.
3. Peel the onion and cut it.
4. Pour the bistro au jus gravy. You may use jarred or canned gravy, both variants are possible.
5. Add the ranch mix over the chuck roast, sliced onions, add butter slices on the top of the chuck roast. Put the pepperoncini peppers.
6. Cover and put on LOW for 7 hours. Check the readiness of the chuck roast with a fork.
7. Season the ready-made dish with black pepper (optional) and salt. Put the beef over veggies or zucchini noodles.

175.Crock Pot simple corned beef

At this recipe, I decided to use the corned beef in a seasoning packet that I bought at the grocery store. This time I really wanted to carry out experiments and to taste something new (new variation of meat). It has appeared that corned beef is rather salty meat. So, if you would like to have less salt, you should rinse the beef thoroughly. You could have the larger package of the corned beef than I have in my recipe. In this case, I advise you not to cook all the corned beef from the package at once, but divide it and follow the instructions and mentioned measurements. It is cooked in the Crock Pot perfectly well.

Ingredients (8 servings):

yellow onion	1 large
corned beef	2 pounds (package)
bay leaf	1 whole

garlic	3 - 4 whole cloves
water	3/4 cup
sweetener	2 tablespoons
yellow mustard	2 teaspoons
black pepper	1/4 teaspoon

salt at will

Directions:

1. Peel the onion, slice it and set aside. Peel the onions, slice also.
2. Cover the Crock Pot (the bottom and the sides) with cooking spray, put there sliced onions.
3. Take out the meat from the package, rinse with cold water and put on the top of the onions in the Crock Pot.
4. Add the bay leaf on the top of the meat, spread the sliced onions on the meat pieces also.
5. Take a little pan, mix sweetener, warm water, black pepper, and mustard, stir everything.
6. Pour this mixture over the meat. Cover and cook on HIGH for 5 hours.
7. Once the time is over, remove the beef and slice.
8. Return it to the Crock Pot and put on WARM for some minutes more.
9. Bon Appetite!

176.Keto spicy beef curry

As soon as I recognized such species like curry I began to get full satisfaction of meat. First time I was scared of the texture of the curry but then I realized that it was actually appetizing! I have experimented with many dishes, cooked chicken, pork, beef, turkey. And all the time I got perfectly amazing dishes! Curry dishes are great in a cold weather, but I eat them also the whole year around. This time I advise you to cook the beef chuck curry. Maybe it will take you a little bit longer time, but be sure, it is worth it.

Ingredients (8 servings):

beef chuck	2.5 lbs
white onion	1 medium pcs
curry powder	2 Tbsp
garlic	3 cloves
ginger	1/2" piece
whole fat coconut milk	2 cups
salt	1 tsp
chili sauce	2 Tbsp

black pepper at will

Directions:

1. Peel the onion, garlic, slice them finely.

2. Pee the ginger, slice also (or grate).
3. Cut the beef chuck into 1-inch slices.
4. Cover the Crock Pot with cooking spray. Place the beef slices there.
5. Place the sliced onions and garlic on the meat, add grated or sliced ginger. Toss together.
6. Pour there the coconut milk, combine.
7. Add curry powder, salt, chili sauce. Toss once more, the beef must be coated thoroughly.
8. Cover and put on HIGH for 4 hours.
9. Once the beef is done, serve with cauliflower rice.
10. Bon Appetite!

177.Keto meaty paleo chili

Some years ago I tried to cook a vegetarian variation of chili (it was full of beans). But as I began the keto diet I understood, it wasn't real chili. Meat chili is much better than you can imagine! This recipe includes an interesting combination of ground beef plus chunks of beef, onions, garlic, peppers, and species. Here you may use dried chili flakes or chilies that are finely chopped. Sometimes I stir onions and other ingredients in coconut milk, but today I decided to do this using the traditional olive oil.

Ingredients (11 servings):

ground beef	1 pound
chunks of beef	1 pound
onions	2 pcs
green pepperoncini	2 pcs
bell pepper	2 pcs (red and green)
garlic	6 cloves
tomatoes	1 can (8oz)
chili powder	2-3 Tablespoons
Thai chilies finely chopped	3 pcs
bone broth	1 cup
olive oil	2 tbsp
salt to taste	

Directions:

1. Peel the onions, chop finely. Peel the garlic, do the same.
2. Wash and dry with a paper towel bell peppers. Take off the seeds. Chop the green pepperoncini
3. Take a large skillet, add there olive oil and brown onions, add chopped pepperoncini, sliced bell peppers, and garlic before ending. Pour these ingredients into the Crock Pot after some minutes.
4. At the same skillet brown, a little the ground beef put into the Crock Pot also.
5. Put the beef chunks in the same place.

6. Pour the can of tomatoes, chili powder, broth, salt.
7. Cover and put on HIGH for 3 hours.
8. Serve hot with avocado slices, sour cream or onion slices.
9. Enjoy!

178.Crock Pot beef Barbacoa

This Mexican style is prepared in the Crock Pot with species, vegetables like onions and garlic. You don't need special ingredients to cook the beef in this style, just combine the mentioned ingredients, add species and you'll get the desired result. The more your meat is cooked, the better it will be.

Ingredients (8 servings):

beef chuck roast	3 pounds
onion	1 pcs
bay leaves	3 pcs
ground black pepper	1/2 teaspoon
garlic powder	2 tablespoons
white vinegar	1/4 cup
tomato sauce	1 (14 ounces) can
chili powder	1/4 cup
salt to taste	

Directions:

1. Peel the onion and chop it finely.
2. Take the boneless beef chuck, chopped onions, garlic powder, black pepper, vinegar and toss everything in the Crock Pot.
3. Cover and cook on HIGH for 3-4 hours. The meat must be tender and fall apart.
4. Once the time is over, remove the meat on the plate, shred it. Add to the liquid tomato sauce, salt, chili powder, stir everything. Put the shredded meat again in the Crock Pot.
5. Cover and cook on LOW additional 1 hour.
6. Serve warm.
7. Bon Appetite!

179.Crock Pot easy meatballs

I think, everyone has parties both at home and at work and has to prepare some delicious but easy and quick one dish. I will give you a recipe how to cook the meatballs in the Crock Pot quick and simple. These meatballs might be spicy, sweet-sour, depending on what taste would you like to get and what species you will add. To serve the meatballs on the toothpicks and garnishing them with chives is the best way to present them for a party. They could be eaten as an appetizer or dinner. Either way, they are delicious!

Ingredients (10 servings):

ground beef	1 lb
almond flour	1/2 c
Worcestershire sauce	1 tbsp
Egg	1 pcs
chives	2 tbsp
garlic	2 cloves
ketchup	½ cup
chili sauce	1/2 cup
sweetener	1/2 cup
vinegar	2 tbsp

pepper and salt to taste

Directions:

1. Peel the garlic and press it. Chop the chives and set aside.
2. Take a medium bowl, mix thoroughly ground beef, chopped chives, cracked egg, pressed garlic, Worcestershire sauce. Stir everything well. Add pepper and salt to taste.
3. Roll into meatballs from the mixture. Cover them with almond flour.
4. Add to the Crock Pot ketchup, chili sauce, sweetener, vinegar and stir everything.
5. Place the prepared meatballs to the mixture. Cover the Crock Pot and put on LOW for hours. The meatballs must be cooked through.
6. Toss the meatballs before serving in the sauce (that is right at the Crock Pot). Serve on the toothpicks and garnish with remained chives.
7. Bon Appetite!

180.Crock Pot Korean beef

It is not necessary to go to the restaurant or to travel to Korea just to taste the appetizing, juicy, flavor Korean meat. You may cook it at home! Yes! It is incredible, delicious meat of bright brown color. You may serve this meat with additional green chopped onions and sesame seeds. This will add some contrast colors to your plate. Don't hesitate to immerse in Korean cooking habits.

Ingredients:

rump roast	1 small (3 to 4 lbs.)
beef broth	3 cup
soy sauce	1 cup
sweetener	1/2 cup
garlic	4 cloves

sesame oil	3 tbsp.
Juice of limes	3 pcs
sriracha	2 tbsp
Green onions, for serving	
Pepper salt at will	

Directions:
1. Peel the garlic and press it. Set aside.
2. Squeeze juice of 3 limes into a cup.
3. Combine in the Crock Pot the rump roast, broth, sweetener, soy sauce, pressed garlic, sesame oil, lime juice, salt, sriracha. Toss everything.
4. Cover the Crock Pot and put on LOW for 8 hours or on HIGH for 4 hours.
5. Once the meat is ready, remove it to the plate and shred with fork and knife.
6. Serve with black pepper, green onions (chopped, optional).
7. Bon Appetite!

181.Crock Pot Burgundy beef

This recipe is absolutely amazing. It is a traditional classic French recipe that is waiting for you to be cooked at once. I usually don't roast the meat pieces before putting to the Crock Pot I don't think it is necessary. The Crock Pot does its best and at the result, you get tender, juicy, flavor meat at the plate. I also don't add any potatoes or carrots as at the classic French Burgundy beef, because I follow the ketogenic diet and I'm sure the meat doesn't need some garnishing.

Ingredients (10 servings):

beef chuck	2 pounds
salt	1/2 teaspoon
black pepper	1/4 teaspoon
cooking oil	2 tablespoons
tapioca	2 tablespoons
frozen small onions	1/2 16 - ounce package (2 cups)
garlic	2 cloves
beef broth	1 14 - ounce can
Burgundy wine	1 cup
Bacon strips	4 slices
pepper to taste	

Directions:
1. Wash the boneless meat pieces, trim fat of it and cut into 1-inch pieces. Season the meat with pepper and salt.

2. Peel the garlic and mince.
3. Sprinkle the Crock Pot with cooking oil, place the meat pieces there.
4. Sprinkle them with tapioca. Add small onions, garlic (minced). Pour the broth over the meat in the Crock Pot.
5. Cover and put on LOW for 7 hours.
6. Remove the meat, season with black pepper and crumbled, drained bacon strips.
7. Bon Appetite!

182.Crock Pot classic French Dips

The easy-to-cook delicious classic French dips are usually eaten with keto-bread in my family. This variant of sandwiches is absolutely perfect for busy moms. Prepared sandwiches at home are always healthier than bought ones. A mix of the flavor species, good pieces of meat and broth make healthy dinner for the whole your family and especially for kids!

Ingredients (9 servings):

sweet onion	2 large pcs
boneless beef	1 2 - 2 1/2 - pound
garlic	2 cloves
thyme	1 teaspoon
black pepper	1/2 teaspoon
beef broth	1 1/4 cups
water	1/2 cup
Worcestershire sauce	1 tablespoon
green sweet pepper	1 medium

marjoram or oregano (crushed, optional)

Directions:
1. Peel the onions and cut them into ½-inch slices. Peel the garlic and mince also. Wash and dry with a paper towel sweet pepper. Slice it thinly.
2. Place the onions in the Crock Pot.
3. Take the boneless beef pieces or fresh beef briskets free from fat and place them in the Crock Pot.
4. Season them with pepper, thyme, minced garlic. Pour also the broth, add Worcestershire sauce and ½ cup of water.
5. Cover and cook on LOW for 9 hours or on HIGH for 5 hours.
6. Once the cooking time is almost over, open the Crock Pot and add slices of bell pepper. Cover for some minutes more.
7. Remove the ready beef to a plate, slice the pieces. Add to your meat onions and peppers from the Crock Pot using a long spoon.
8. Serve with crushed oregano or marjoram at will.
9. Bon Appetite!

183.Lemon Herb veal Crock Pot

This is the great recipe where I have made some simple modifications. I would like to add wine (or chicken broth if you don't like wine) and a little bit leeks just to make this dish more flavor. When you put your Crock Pot on LOW (if you have enough time) turn on 6-7 hours. The meat must be very tender.

Ingredients (12 servings):

leek	1 pcs
garlic	3 cloves
dried tarragon	1 tablespoon
lemon zest	1⁄2 teaspoon
dried thyme	1⁄2 teaspoon
white pepper	1⁄2 teaspoon
dried sage	1⁄4 teaspoon
veal	2 1⁄2-3 lbs
almond flour	1⁄3 cup
dry white wine	3⁄4 cup
lemon juice	1⁄4 cup
whipping cream	1⁄4 cup

Salt

Pepper at will

Directions:

1. Wash the leek, slice thinly (only white and pale green parts).
2. Peel the garlic and press.
3. Peel the lemon zest in a small bowl.
4. Wash the veal, dry with a paper towel, trim fat, cut into cubes.
5. Squeeze the juice of one lemon in a cup.
6. Take a large bowl, conjoin leek, garlic, tarragon, lemon zest, white pepper and sage, thyme.
7. Coat the veal cubes with almond flour. Add them to the large bowl with a mix.
8. Pour in wine, add lemon juice from a cup. Pour the mix with veal into the Crock Pot.
9. Cover the Crock Pot and put on HIGH for 3 hours, until veal is tender.
10. Take another small bowl, mix whisk cream. Pour to the veal once the time is over. Put it on WARM for a half an hour.
11. Season with salt and pepper at will.
12. Dress with lemon slices.
13. Bon Appetite!

184. Veal Pot Roast recipe Crock Pot

The recipe of the veal roast with vegetables is perfect for the Crock Pot – both ingredients (vegetables and veal) get extra tender and, of course, juice. You can't even imagine how tasty is this! Serve with black pepper or gravy!

Ingredients:

veal pot roast	3 to 4 pounds
oil (vegetable)	2 Tsp
onions	2 medium
celery	4 stalks
water	1/4 cup
butter	3 Tsp
coconut flour	3 Tsp
white wine	1/3 cup
salt and pepper	

Directions:

1. Wash the veal, dry with a paper towel, trim fat, cut into cubes.
2. Peel the onion and finely cut into quarters.
3. Peel carefully celery and cut into chunks
4. Take a large skillet, add oil, put the veal on it and brown from all.
5. Put meat into the bottom of the Crock Pot, add vegetables to it also.
6. Cover the lid and put on LOW for 8 hours.
7. Take off the veal with vegetables from the Crock Pot and keep warm.

For Gravy

1. Take a medium-sized pan, melt the butter, add flour.
2. Prepare over a medium heat until smooth texture.
3. Add a little bit water if needed, stirring constantly. Add a little bit wine and continue cooking for 3 minutes.
4. Season pepper at will, pour over vegetables and veal.
5. Bon Appetite!

185. Crock Pot Veal Marengo Keto

Despite the fact, this Veal Marengo recipe includes 17 servings it is rather easy and tasty! You may prepare it and keep in the refrigerator for some days. It is perfect for both dinner, supper and lunch! Tender pieces of veal, golden onions and mixture of tomatoes and species will make a great combination that is simple to prepare in the Crock Pot.

Ingredients (17 servings):

boneless veal	1.5 lbs cut into 1 1/2 inch cubes
almond flour	1/2 cup

salt	1 teaspoon
ground pepper	1/2 Tsp
garlic powder	1/2 tsp
paprika	1/2 Tsp
canola oil	5 tablespoons
onion	2 cups (1 large)
garlic	3 cloves
tomato paste	1 tablespoon
tomato	1 1/2 cup (1 large)
dried thyme leaves	1 teaspoon
salt	1/2 teaspoon
beef or chicken broth	3 cups
lemon zest	1/2 teaspoon
salt	1 teaspoon
parsley	1/4 teaspoon

Directions:

1. Cut the veal into cubes, wash it and dry with a paper towel.
2. Place the almond flour into a small bowl, add salt, pepper, paprika, add garlic powder. Mix everything thoroughly.
3. Mix this with the veal cubes finely. Set aside.
4. Take a large skillet, pour oil and put it over medium heat. Add coated veal pieces to the skillet and roast a little for about 4 minutes from all sides. (Toss the pieces all the times!). Veal must be of golden color. Put the pieces into the Crock Pot.
5. Peel the onions and chop finely. Peel the garlic and mince. Wash tomato and cut in cubes.
6. Take the previous skillet, add a little bit oil, add garlic and onions. Cook for some minutes until soften.
7. Add tomato, salt, thyme, tomato paste and continue cooking other 3 minutes.
8. Add broth. Let the mixture stir for some minutes.
9. Pour the mixture into the Crock Pot, on the top of the veal. Add lemon zest. Cover the lid and set on LOW for 6 hours.
10. Serve with pepper if desired.
11. Garnish with parsley.
12. Enjoy warm.
13. Bon Appetite!

186.Veal Paprikash Crock Pot

This is a flavorful dish with fresh parsley, chives and a lot of vitamins. I remember I cooked this Hungarian dish for the first time last year. My friends were really surprised! This one could delight the taste buds. Don't hesitate to cook it today!

Ingredients (15 servings):

lean boneless veal	1 (2 1/4-pound)
onion	1 cup
fresh parsley	2 tsp
garlic	4 cloves
bay leaves	2 pcs
almond flour	2.25 ounces (about 1/2 cup)
Hungarian sweet paprika	1 tsp
Salt	3/4 Tsp
dried thyme	1/2 tsp
black pepper	1/2 tsp
dry white wine	1/4 cup
sour cream	1/2 cup
egg noodles	5 1/4 cups
fresh parsley	3 1/2 teaspoons
fresh chives	7 teaspoons

Directions:

1. Cut the veal into cubes, wash it and dry with a paper towel.
2. Peel the onions and chop finely. Wash fresh parsley and chop finely, chop fresh chives. Peel garlic and mince.
3. Take a large bowl, mix cubes of veal with chopped onion, minced garlic, paprika, parsley.
4. Put this mixture in the Crock Pot. Toss well.
5. Mix in another little bowl bay leaves, salt, dried thyme, black pepper. Carefully add wine, blended well.
6. Add flour mixture to the Crock Pot; toss well.
7. Cover the lid and cook on LOW for 7 hours, until veal is tender.
8. Take off the bay leaves.
9. Add sour cream.
10. Serve the ready-made veal over the egg noodles.
11. Season with parsley and chives.
12. Bon Appetite!

187.Keto Veal With Cabbage Crock Pot

The recipe of the veal roast with cabbage could be eaten as a main dish or a stew. Both adults and kids like it at winter time and in autumn. Full of vitamin C, minerals, and good mood, of course! Only 5 main servings! Could you imagine this? Enjoy it today!

Ingredients (5 servings):

veal pot roast	4 pounds
olive oil	3 tsp
onions	2 medium
cabbage	4 cups
water or broth	1/4 cup
salt and pepper	
parsley for garnish	

Directions:

1. Wash the veal, dry with a paper towel, trim fat, cut into slices.
2. Peel carefully the onion and finely chop it.
3. Chop the cabbage. Set aside.
4. Take a medium skillet, add olive oil, put the veal on it and brown from all.
5. Put it into the bottom of the Crock Pot, add a little bit water or broth at will, add cabbage and onions to it also.
6. Cover the lid and put on LOW for 8 hours.
7. Take off the veal with vegetables from the Crock Pot and keep warm.
8. Wash and chop fresh parsley for garnish.
9. Season pepper at will, pour over vegetables and veal.
10. Bon Appetite!

188.Crock Pot veal with winter veggies

You may be surprised that I have chosen the veal shank to cook for this recipe. This part is frequently a tough cut of any meat. But be sure, after preparing this dish in the Crock Pot following my instructions you'll be also surprised at how tender the veal shank could be!

Ingredients (12 servings):

veal shanks	4 (10- to 12-ounce)
bone broth	1/2 cup
butter	3 tablespoons
salt	2 teaspoons divided
onions froze	24 pearl
garlic	4 cloves
parsnips	2 pcs

leeks	2 pcs
celery ribs	2 pcs
fresh thyme	1 sprig
fresh rosemary	1 sprig
freshly ground pepper	1/2 teaspoon
salt and pepper at will	

Directions:
1. Wash the veal, dry with a paper towel, trim fat, cut into slices of medium size.
2. Cut the parsnips into eighths.
3. Halve the leeks and chop.
4. Chop celery ribs. Peel garlic and mince it.
5. Mix in a pan veal shanks, broth, a little bit water and place it over high heat. Let it boil until the liquid is mostly reduced. Let in a pan a little.
6. Add butter and continue cooking all this over a low heat. Toss all the time.
7. Remove veal from a pan, and place in the Crock Pot.
8. Season with salt.
9. Put in the Crock Pot also garlic, frozen onion, parsnips, leeks, celery, thyme, fresh rosemary and black pepper.
10. Cover the lid and put on HIGH for 5 hours.
11. Bone Appetite!

189.Crock Pot veal shoulder

There are many variations how to cook the veal tender and what parts are better to use. Now, I would like to present you my recipe for cooking the veal shoulder. I will show you how to make it tender, delicious and flavor. Don't forget to follow the instructions as I think this is the best mix of veal with veggies. Good luck!

Ingredients (12 servings):

Veal shoulder	1 pcs
Olive oil	3 Tsp
Red wine merlot	3 Tsp
Onion	½ cup
Celery	½ stick
Garlic	4 cloves
Tomato	4 big pcs
Bay leaves	4 pcs
Thyme	1 bunch

Vegetable stock	3-4 cups
Flaked sea salt	
Ground black pepper	
Parsley	1 bunch
Sage	1 bunch

Directions:
1. Wash the veal shoulder, dry with a paper towel, trim fat, cut in slices.
2. Peel an onion and cut finely.
3. Cut celery, wash the tomatoes, take off the seeds and chop.
4. Peel garlic and mince it.
5. Wash and chop fresh thyme, parsley, and sage.
6. Put a large pan over medium heat. Add oil and roast veal shoulder finely.
7. Take off the shoulder and set aside.
8. Sautee tomatoes, parsley, onion, garlic. Add herbs, deglaze with red wine.
9. Add vegetable stock. Let it simmer for 10 minutes.
10. Put the veal shoulder and the ingredients from a pan to the Crock Pot.
11. Cover the lid and put on HIGH for 5 hours.
12. Once the veal shoulder is ready, serve it warm with favorite species!
13. Bon Appetite!

190.Crock Pot veal meatballs with tomato sauce

Veal meatballs recipe need just one word: AMAZING! Cook it for dinner, supper or breakfast! This recipe is great for the party and also is so delicious. The veal meatballs are super tender. Add fresh vegetables and serve it with parsley or other species at will.

Ingredients (8 servings):

Ground veal	1 lb
almond flour	1/2 c
Worcestershire sauce	1 tbsp
Egg	1 pcs
garlic	2 cloves
tomato sauce	½ cup
chili sauce	1/2 cup
vinegar	2 tbsp
pepper and salt to taste	

Directions:
1. Peel the garlic and minced it.
2. Take a large bowl, mix ground veal, cracked egg, minced garlic, Worcestershire sauce.
3. Stir everything well. Add pepper and salt to taste.

4.   Roll ground veal into meatballs. Cover them with almond flour.
5.   Add to the Crock Pot tomato sauce, chili sauce, vinegar and stir everything.
6.   Place the prepared meatballs to the mixture. Cover the Crock Pot and put on LOW for 5 hours. The meatballs must be fully ready.
7.   Toss the meatballs before serving in the sauce.
8.   Serve hot and garnish with parsley at will.
9.   Bon Appetite!

191.Crock Pot veal goulash

This variation of the veal goulash is delicious and amazing. It is not a traditional version of goulash but it is also as tender as beef or chicken. It is usually served in the restaurants with noodles, but following the keto rules, I prefer to eat it with fresh veggies. Add sour cream and red bell pepper at the end of the cooking time.

Ingredients (12 servings):

olive oil divided	2 tbsp
veal	2 lbs
onions	2 pcs
garlic	4 cloves
caraway seeds	1 tsp
black peppercorns	½ tsp
almond flour	2 tbsp
diced tomatoes	1 can (14 oz)
chicken broth	1 cup
paprika	1 tbsp
red bell peppers	2 pcs
chopped dill	½ cup (125 ml)

Sour cream at will

Directions:

1. Wash the veal, dry with a paper towel, trim fat, cut into 1-inch (2.5 cm) cubes.
2. Peel an onion and chop finely.
3. Peel garlic and mince.
4. Crack the black peppercorns.
5. Wash the red pepper, take off the seeds and slice finely.
6. Chop the dill finely.
7. Dissolve paprika in water or chicken broth (2 tbsp).
8. Open the Crock Pot and put the veal cubes on the bottom of it. Add chopped onions to the Crock Pot, add garlic, dissolved peppercorns, caraway seeds.
9. Add flour and stirring everything well.

10. Add tomatoes with juice, add broth.
11. Toss everything thoroughly.
12. Cover the lid of the Crock Pot and put on LOW for 7 hours.
13. Check if the veal is tender once the cooking time is over.
14. At the end of cooking time add red sliced peppers and toss everything well. Put on WARM for half an hour.
15. Remove the dish to a plate, serve with black pepper and dill and sour cream if desired.
16. Bon Appetite!

192.Crock Pot roast lamb leg

Juicy, easy, flavor and tender lamb leg roast are today on your plate! To cook this amazing dish you need to wait 9 hours (yes, I agree – it is rather long, but, believe me, it is worth it!) until your Crock Pot is working hard, but be sure the taste is great! This recipe doesn't need any additions like veggies, noodles, eggs, bread or something like this. It is amazing as it is! Be patient and spend a little bit more your free time as usual. Don't you want to surprise your family or old friends with a new dish and a delicious taste?! I will help you with pleasure! Just follow my instructions and you will see the result!

Ingredients (10 servings):

lamb leg, bone in	4 lb
salt	1 Tsp
Black pepper at will	
garlic	2 large cloves
dried thyme	1 1/2 Tsp
olive oil	1 tbsp
beef stock	2 cups
Gravy:	
Butter	3 tbsp
Almond flour	3 tbsp
liquid from Crock Pot	2 cups
Salt and pepper	

Directions:

1. Wash the lamb and put it into the Crock Pot. Peel the garlic and mince.
2. Season it with salt, pepper, minced garlic and thyme. Spray the oil over it.
3. Add the beef stock to the Crock Pot.
4. Cover the lid and put on LOE for 9 hours. Check from time to time. The lamb must be tender and golden brown.
5. Cook the gravy: take off the liquid from the Crock Pot into a medium-sized bowl. It is approximately 2-3 cups.
6. Melt the butter in a small skillet, add flour. Continue cooking 1 minute. Toss all the time.

7. Add a liquid from the Crock Pot, whisk everything.
8. Pour the ready-made lamb with the gravy.
9. Serve hot!
10. Bon Appetite!

193.Keto Pork Tenderloin Florentine

I came to this recipe when I had a pork tenderloin at home and didn't know what to do with it!? I couldn't even imagine that a simple combination of pork, feta cheese, spinach leaves, ricotta cheese and broth is so delicious! I switched on my Crock Pot and the cooking process began. It didn't take too many skills and preparations to get the pork done after some hours. Sometimes, I like to brown the pork tenderloin before putting to the Crock Pot but this part of the cooking process isn't necessary.

Ingredients (11 servings):

pork tenderloin	about 1¼ pounds
ricotta cheese	½ cup
garlic	2 cloves
salt	½ teaspoon
pepper	¼ teaspoon
red peppers	½ cup
feta cheese	¼ cup
baby spinach leaves	1 cup
olive oil	2 tablespoons
chicken broth	1 cup
white wine	½ cup

Directions:

1. Peel the garlic and mince it finely.
2. Chop the roasted red peppers.
3. Prepare the pork – slice it thinly, remove the unnecessary fat.
4. Take a medium-sized bowl, mix there minced garlic, ricotta, pepper, salt. Spread the mixture over the pork. Put the pork pieces into the Crock Pot, add there chopped roasted peppers, feta cheese, put spinach leaves on the top of the pork.
5. Spread this with olive oil, add optional salt and pepper. Add both wine and broth to the Crock Pot.
6. Cover and put on LOW for 6 hours.
7. Remove the readily prepared pork to the plate, slice into 1-inch slices.
8. Bon Appetite!

194.Keto Pork Meatballs in Marinara Sauce

These easy and delicious Crock Pot meatballs in marinara sauce are simple to prepare. I prefer to add shredded Parmesan cheese to the meatballs, you may add the other cheese or exclude it. The marinara sauce is a perfectly well combination of tomato paste, sauce, tomatoes, rosemary and oregano. It is super delicious and flavor!

Ingredients (17 servings):

Marinara

crushed tomatoes	28 ounces
tomato sauce	8 ounces
tomato paste	6 ounces
fresh oregano	2 sprigs
fresh rosemary	1 sprig
garlic powder	1 teaspoon
sweetener	1 teaspoon
salt	1 teaspoon

Meatballs

ground pork	1 pound
yellow onion	½ medium pcs
garlic	2 cloves
almond flour	⅔ cup
egg	1 pcs
grated Parmesan cheese	3 tablespoons
dried oregano	1 teaspoon
salt	½ teaspoon
ground black pepper	¼ teaspoon

Directions:

1. For marinara sauce: crush the tomatoes from a can, mix them in a small bowl with tomato sauce and paste, fresh rosemary and oregano, sweetener, salt and garlic powder. Stir everything together in the Crock Pot.
2. For meatballs: Peel the onion and dice it. Mince the peeled garlic; grate the Parmesan cheese.
3. In a large bowl mix ground pork, minced garlic, almond flour, cracked egg, grated Parmesan, salt, pepper, and oregano. Make little meatballs using your hands, pour them into sauce in the Crock Pot.
4. Cover and cook on LOW for 5-6 hours, meat must be cooked well.

5. Serve warm. Bon Appetite!

195.Crock Pot Island Jerk Pulled Pork

You can find a plenty of Jerk recipes on the Internet, but not so many recipes that are cooked in the Crock Pot. If you haven't tried my Island Jerk pulled pork yet, you must pay attention to this tasty recipe right now. My recipe is really mouth-watering, I don't know somebody who is indifferent after tasting my Jerk pulled pork. If you would like to surprise your friends or relatives follow the instructions and directions given below.

Ingredients (16 servings):

onion powder	1 tablespoon
garlic powder	1 tablespoon
grated fresh ginger	2 teaspoons
ground cloves	1½ teaspoons
ground allspice	1½ teaspoons
thyme	1½ teaspoons
dry mustard	1½ teaspoons
coarse salt	1½ teaspoons
sweet or hot paprika	1 teaspoon
cumin	½ teaspoon
sweetener	½ teaspoon
black pepper	¼ teaspoon
cayenne pepper	¼ teaspoon
boneless pork	3 pound
balsamic	1 cup
bay leaf	1 pcs

optional - BBQ sauce and chopped fresh cilantro

Directions:

1. Grate fresh ginger.
2. Take a medium pan and mix their garlic and onion powder, grated ginger, thyme, allspice, salt, dry mustard, sweetener, cumin, cayenne, pepper. Stir the mixture. You may stir with hands to let the grated ginger be fully coated.
3. Place the pork to the bottom of the Crock Pot, add the dry mixture over the meat. Pour the vinegar over meat, add the bay leaf.
4. Cover and put on LOW for 8 hours or on HIGH for 4 hours.
5. Serve warm with chopped fresh cilantro and BBQ sauce.
6. Bon Appetite!

196.Thai Pork Crock Pot

If you are a real fan of Thai food, this recipe must be at your dinner today. The classic Thai dish is usually prepared with ground pork, but this recipe is adapted to any type of pork actually. I used here pork loin that I cut into small pieces or strips. The whole my family likes this Thai Pork dish, that's why for me it is also a great pleasure to cook it both for dinner as for supper. There no questions more like «what Thai restaurant should I visit next? » You don't need to go there; you may cook it right in your kitchen.

Ingredients:

dried chilies	2 pcs
hot sauce	tablespoons
red Thai curry paste	3 tablespoon
coconut milk	8 ounces
lemongrass paste	2 tablespoons
sweetener	2 teaspoons
shallots	3 pcs
yellow pepper	1 pcs
red pepper	1 pcs
cumin	2 teaspoons
soy sauce	2 tablespoons
ginger	2 tablespoons
garlic	3 cloves
chili sauce	2 tablespoons
water	½ cup
cubed pork	1 pound

For serving:

mint and cilantro	¼ cup
toasted almonds	½ cup
chopped red pepper	1 cup

pepper and salt at will

Directions:

1. Peel and halve the shallots. Peel the garlic and mince it. Wash and dry with a paper towel the peppers (both of them). Chop the fresh ginger.
2. Cut the pork into cubes.

3. Take a medium bowl, mix there curry paste, sauce, lemongrass, coconut milk, sweetener, shallots, pepper (half of each one), cumin, grated ginger, garlic, chili sauce. Combine thoroughly.
4. Add this mixture to the Crock Pot. Add there pork.
5. Cover and put on LOW for 7 hours or on HIGH for 4-5 hours. Once the cooking time is over, put the rest peppers in the Crock Pot, cover and put on WARM for another half an hour.
6. Serve this dish warm, season with chopped cilantro, mint, chopped red pepper and, of course, roasted tomatoes.
7. Bon Appetite!

197.Crock Pot keto pork roast

Many people prefer to cook simple recipes that don't need actually too many steps and ingredients to be mixed, roasted or boiled. This recipe of keto pork roast is the easiest I can only imagine. This recipe could be coked as a separate dish or as an addition to your favorite vegetables, veggie noodles, cauliflower rice etc. This recipe is awesome that is worth cooking in your Crock Pot.

Ingredients:

pork roast	4 pounds
Worcestershire sauce	1/4 cup
seasoned salt	1 teaspoon
pepper to taste	

Directions:
1. Add a half of the Worcestershire sauce to the Crock Pot.
2. Put the washed pork roast in the Crock Pot, toss with sauce.
3. Season the pork roast with salt and pepper.
4. Cover and put on LOW for 8 hours or on HIGH for 5 hours.
5. Once the pork is done, remove it to the plate, shred with fork and knife into smaller pieces.
6. Serve with vegetables or cauliflower rice.
7. Bon Appetite!

198.Crock Pot Pulled Pork with Fried Shallots and Chiles

The recipe of the pulled pork with chilies and fried shallots is the best variant for the crowd parties! When I have a crowd of guests I'm always quiet because I know definitely what I'll cook. To prepare this pulled pork in the Crock Pot is super easy. As for me, I like to taste the shallots when they are caramelized and dress the pork with them. It's delicious! It will take you a little bit more time, but it worth it, be sure!

Ingredients (17 servings):
Pulled Pork

pork shoulder	3 lb(s)
barbecue sauce	1 cup

sweetener	3 Tbsp
chili powder	2 Tsp
chipotle powder	1 Tsp
vinegar	3 Tbsp
Kosher salt	
onion	1 medium
scallions	3 pcs

Fried Shallots and Chiles

Vegetable oil	1 tbsp
egg whites	2 pcs
almond flour	1 ½ cups
chili powder	1 Tsp
ground cumin	1 tsp
Kosher salt and black pepper to taste	
Fresno chilies	4 pcs
shallots	4 pcs
Celery salt (optional)	

Directions:

Pulled Pork

Slice the pork shoulder into small bites (approximately 2-inch pieces).

1. Peel shallots and chop it, peel the onions, slice thinly.
2. Take a large dish, join together sauce, pork shoulder, sweetener, chipotle and chili powder, vinegar, salt, chopped onions. Toss everything well.
3. Place these components into the bottom of the Crock Pot that you have covered with cooking spray before and put on LOW for 7 hours.
4. Take off the pork to a cutting board once the cooking time is over, shred into pieces using knife and fork. Place the pork in a larger bowl, tack the fluid from the Crock Pot and spread additionally with pepper to taste and salt.

Fried Shallots with Chiles

1. Peel the shallots, cut into rings.
2. Take a fryer, add vegetable oil. At this time, crack the eggs to a little plate and whisk a little. The consistency must be frothy. In the other little plate join together chili powder, flour, pepper, cumin, salt, chilies. Slice onions, pour them into the mixture of the flour (pour all the sides), and after this put the slices into the heated skillet. Fry them until a little bit golden (it takes usually 2 minutes), take them off after this to a paper and add celery salt.

3. Dress the ready-made pork with fried shallots and chilies.
4. Bon Appetite!

199.Crock Pot Sunday gravy

This recipe of Sunday gravy includes three variations of tomatoes. No, it is not too much – tomato paste, sun-dried tomatoes, and tomatoes from a can. As a result, you get a flavor and colorful plate where you can taste all the varieties of tomatoes. The crushed tomatoes will almost melt down into sauce filling the pork ribs with their juice. Mmm... I can't wait for... Let's go cooking together!

Ingredients (10 servings):

olive oil	2 Tbsp
hot Italian sausage	1 ½ lb(s)
tomato paste	2 Tbsp
pork short ribs	4 pcs (about 2 lbs)
Italian herb mix	2 Tsp
Garlic	6 cloves
sun-dried tomatoes	6 pcs
tomatoes	2 (28-oz) cans
large onion	1 pcs
bay leaf	1 pcs

Kosher salt and black pepper

grated Parmesan

Directions:
1. Peel the garlic and mince; crush the tomatoes. Peel the onion, chop it finely. Grate the Parmesan cheese into a small plate.
2. Take a large frypan, add there two tablespoons, heat it and cook the sausages. Turn them from time to time. They must be almost brown, it takes usually 5 to 7 minutes. Place the cooked sausages in the Crock Pot, add tomato paste, stir together. Add there a half of a cup of water, put on LOW for an hour.
3. Add to the Crock Pot pork ribs, minced garlic, Italian herbs, tomatoes (sun-dried), chopped onions, pepper, salt, bay leaf, crushed tomatoes. Toss everything well.
4. Cover the Crock Pot and set on LOW for 6 hours.
5. Once the dish is ready, take it off to a plate, dress with grated Parmesan and black pepper.
6. Serve warm and enjoy!
7. Bon Appetite!

200.Crock Pot Chile Verde

The Crock Pot-chili Verde is special for those who have a rather busy daily life. The pork gets its tenderness through being tossed and cooked for 5 hours at the Crock Pot together with spicy salsa. I like cilantro and red pepper flakes, but if you don't like the same ingredients, you may use basil leaves or green onions.

Ingredients (9 servings):

Coconut oil	2 tbsp
pork shoulder	2-3 lbs
garlic	2 heads
yellow onion	1 pcs
chicken broth	½ cup
tomatillos	2 pounds
jalapenos	4 pcs
cilantro	1 bunch
limes	2 pcs

Cumin (optional)

red pepper flakes, and salt and pepper at will

Directions:

1. Pell the garlic, mince it and split. Peel the onion, slice it finely.
2. Wash and clean the tomatoes, cut into quarters.
3. Prepare the jalapenos - dice them finely too. Take off the stems from cilantro, cut the leaves. Squeeze juice from 2 limes.
4. Cover the bottom of the Crock Pot with coconut oil. Place the garlic and onion on the bottom of the Crock Pot, place the tomatoes, diced jalapenos, broth, squeezed juice, additional species, pepper, salt to taste. You may use a blender to make a smooth consistency or leave so as it is. Place the pork over the mixture, cover and cook on HIGH for 4 hours.
5. Serve hot, add pepper flakes and cilantro.
6. Bon Appetite!

201.Keto ginger pork with broccoli

The main components of this dish are coconut aminos, ginger powder, and species. The combination of the sauce is amazing, it provides the pork with special taste and flavor. Broccoli makes special additions, the whole meal that will satisfy your taste. If you don't like broccoli you may change it with cauliflower.

Ingredients (12 servings):

grass-fed butter	2 tablespoons
pork chops	1 pound

sea salt	1 teaspoon
ground black pepper	¼ teaspoon
garlic powder	1 teaspoon
ginger powder	1 teaspoon
coconut aminos	1 cup
lime juice	¼ cup (2 limes)
fish sauce	¼ teaspoon
broccoli	2 heads (about 4 cups)
cilantro (optional)	¼ cup
red pepper flakes	1 teaspoon

Directions:

1. Slice the pork into 1/3-inch strips.
2. Trim the broccoli florets from the stem. Roughly chop fresh cilantro leaves. Squeeze the lime juice.
3. Melt the butter in a medium fryer. Put the pork slices, season them with a little bit pepper and salt, ginger, and garlic powder.
4. Cook them just 3-4 minutes, they must be brown a little.
5. Place the browned pork into the Crock Pot.
6. Prepare the sauce: in a medium skillet add coconut aminos, juice of limes, fish sauce, whisk everything. Let the sauce simmer 10-12 minutes.
7. Pour it into the Crock Pot.
8. Cover the Crock Pot and put on LOW for 6 hours. Once the time is over, add broccoli florets to the dish for a little and cover. Put on WARM.
9. Serve with cilantro and red pepper flakes.
10. Bon Appetite!

202.Crock Pot keto lamb

There is a traditional dish for Easter in my family – we cook a delicious lamb in the Crock Pot! Instead of preparing it in the oven, I prefer my Crock Pot, I try to escape the stress and finish all my other deals. As a result, I get the super tender meat, flavor enough, with thyme, mint. But if somebody doesn't like it, I don't add it at all. I use also the maple syrup to rich the wished taste of the lamb.

Ingredients (8 servings):

leg of lamb	2 pounds
olive oil	¼ cup
whole grain mustard	2 tablespoons
maple syrup	1 tablespoon
thyme	4 sprigs

mint	6-7 leaves
dried rosemary	¾ teaspoon
garlic	¾ teaspoon

Salt and pepper at will

Directions:

1. Prepare the lamb leg – cover the bottom of the Crock Pot with cooking spray. Place the lamb there, make three snips along the surface of the lamb. The slits have to be approximately 1 inch deep.
2. Spread the lamb with mustard, syrup, pepper, salt.
3. Insert with fingers dried garlic, dried rosemary into the slits.
4. Cover and cook on LOW 9 hours. Once the time is over (the juice must be at the bottom of the Crock Pot), add some sprigs of thyme and mint. Cover again and put on WARM for an additional hour.
5. Remove the lamb from the Crock Pot and slice it.
6. Bon Appetite!

203.Keto lamb with black garlic

I always enjoy meat when I follow my keto diet. It is very comfortable because you can keep it in the fridge for some days. It means you don't need to cook every day something new. This recipe is appetizing when served with lettuce leaves and fresh rosemary. You may also add to the lamb eggs or other favorite veggies. You may find black garlic in big stores. It is rather sweet and is like a balsamic vinegar. When you can't find it at your nearest store, just use the white one.

Ingredients (8 servings):

lamb, whole	(4.4 lb / 70 oz) 1 leg
balsamic vinegar	¼ cup (2 fl oz)
strawberry vinegar	¼ cup
black aged garlic	4 cloves
fresh rosemary	1-2 sprigs
small lettuce	4 heads (14.2 oz)
salt or to taste	½ tsp
water	2-3 cups
pepper	

Directions:

1. Peel the garlic, slice finely.
2. Place the lamb leg into the Crock Pot, add the strawberry and balsamic vinegar, rosemary, sliced garlic. Dress with pepper and salt, pour water.
3. Cover and cook for 5 hours on LOW.
4. After 2 times, open the Crock Pot, turn the lamb leg and cover again.

5. Once the time is over, open the Crock Pot, remove the lamb to the plate and let it cool for a while.
6. Shred the meat with a fork, pour the juice from the Crock Pot over the meat.
7. Wash and separate lettuce leaves. Put the shredded meat into the leaves, roll them.
8. Dress with black pepper and fresh rosemary leaves.
9. Bon Appetite!

204.Keto coconut lamb curry

This incredible curry lamb was a real finding for me. It has a magnificent creamy texture that is cooked regularly in my family. Such species like garam masala is an Indian flavoring that contains cardamom, clove, fennel, coriander seed, pepper, cumin, nutmeg. It may also contain caraway or cinnamon seeds. It could be found in almost all the supermarkets. You may prepare this in the oven but the result will not be so perfectly well as while cooking in the Crock Pot. You can change the red chili when the kids are at home too)

Ingredients (15 servings):

coconut oil	1 tablespoon
diced lamb	1.5 lb
brown onion	1 large
long red chili	½
celery sticks	2 medium
garlic	3 cloves
garam masala	2½ teaspoons
turmeric powder	1¼ teaspoons
fennel seeds	1 teaspoon
ghee	1½ teaspoons
coconut milk	1 can or 1½ cups
tomato paste	1½ tablespoons
water	1 cup
sea salt	1⅓ teaspoon
A squeeze of lime or lemon juice	1 pcs
parsley to garnish	

Directions:

1. Peel the onion and slice it finely. Peel the garlic and dice. Finely dice long chili. Be careful. Dice the celery sticks.
2. Cover the bottom of the Crock Pot with coconut oil. Put there onion, celery, chili, stir everything.

3. Add there diced garlic, masala, turmeric powder, ghee, fennel seeds.
4. Pour coconut milk, water, salt and tomato paste. Stir all the ingredients together. The mixture must be of smooth consistency.
5. Put the diced lamb to the mixture, toss it to coat. Cover and cook for 5 hours on LOW.
6. Chop fresh parsley. Remove the dish to the plate and garnish with chopped parsley.
7. Serve with vegetables, avocado slices, cauliflower rice.
8. Bon Appetite!

205.Crock Pot Lamb Shanks

The lamb shanks prepared on this recipe are perfectly well, tender and flavor. I think, the main ingredient for me is... cream! Yes, it is really the king of this recipe. And do you know why? Because the final texture of lamb is tender definitely because of this cream. You may add so many creams as you want. It wouldn't be worse. Serve this dish with cauliflower mash or other vegetables.

Ingredients (9 servings):

Lamb shanks	4 pcs
Red wine	½ cup
Garlic	6 cloves
Tomatoes	1 can
Italian Herbs	1 tbsp
Onion	1 pcs
Shallots	4 pcs
Zucchini	1 small pcs
Cream	½ cup

Salt and pepper at will

Directions:
1. Prepare the lamb shanks – put them on the bottom of the Crock Pot (that is already spread with the cooking spray).
2. Peel the onion, shallots and slice, peel garlic, mince it finely. Wash, dry with a paper towel zucchini and slice them.
3. Add to the Crock Pot onions and minced garlic, crushed tomatoes from a can.
4. Cover and put on LOW for 7 hours.
5. Once the time is over, add zucchini, shallots, and cover once more. Put on LOW for an hour.
6. Before serving, add pepper, cream, and salt. Let it cool a little bit.
7. Serve with cauliflower at will.
8. Bon Appetite!

206. Keto pork roast with creamy gravy

One of the main benefits of the Crock Pot – is cooking the dishes in its own juice. This flavor, spicy juice may become a constituent of your dish. When you mix together whipping cream (or another one you prefer) with juice, it could be a great supplement to the main dish.

Ingredients (12 servings):

pork shoulder or pork roast	2 lbs
salt	½ tablespoon
bay leaf	2 pcs
black peppercorns	5 pcs
water	2½ cups
dried thyme or dried rosemary	2 teaspoons
garlic	2 cloves
fresh ginger	1½ oz.
olive oil or coconut oil	1 tablespoon
paprika powder	1 tablespoon
ground black pepper	½ teaspoon

Creamy gravy

heavy whipping cream	1½ cups
juices from the roast	

Directions:

1. Place the pork shoulder to the bottom of the Crock Pot and water (the meat must be covered with it).
2. Add bay leaf, thyme, and peppercorns.
3. Cover the Crock Pot and put on HIGH for 5 hours.
4. Once the time is over, take off the meat, pour the juice of the meat in a large bowl.
5. Peel garlic, grate it and grate the ginger in a little frypan. Add there pepper, herbs, oil and stir everything.
6. Pour this mixture over the meat.
7. Return the meat (with a mixture) to the Crock Pot, and put on LOW for 1 hour. The pork must get a golden color.
8. Remove it from the Crock Pot, slice and serve with whipping cream and a little bit juice from a large bowl.
9. Enjoy with keto bread or vegetables.
10. Bon Appetite!

SEAFOOD

207.Shrimp and onion zucchini pasta

Onion and shrimp zucchini pasta is a light and delicious recipe. I also like marinara sauce, added basil, oregano and other wished species. But you also may use another species if you like. Parmesan cheese is great for this dish, but Swiss cheese one is also perfect here.

Ingredients (9 servings):

Olive oil	2 tbsp
White onions	½ lb
Butter	2 tbsp
Shrimp	12 oz.
Zucchini	1 Large
Marinara sauce	½ cup
Salt at will	
Pepper if desired	
Red Pepper Flakes	
Basil	1 tbsp
Oregano	1 tbsp
Parmesan Cheese	½ cup

Directions:

1. Peel the shrimp.
2. Peel the onion and chop it finely.
3. Take a middle saucepan, heat olive oil over medium heat. Fry the onion until they are softened.
4. Add two tablespoons of butter to the softened onions.
5. Open the Crock Pot and pour the onions into the bottom.
6. Add shrimp and season them with salt.
7. Add oregano, red pepper flakes, marinara sauce.
8. Cover the Crock Pot and put on LOW for 2-3 hours.
9. While the shrimp are cooking, make noodles using a spiralizer.
10. Once the shrimp are cooked (they must get pink color), toss the noodles with cooked shrimp in the Crock Pot. Let it stay for some minutes.
11. Finally season with salt and pepper.
12. Toss it all together and sprinkle with Parmesan cheese!
13. Bon Appetite!

208.Easy Lobster Bisque Crock Pot

Lobster bisque prepared in the Crock Pot is an amazing option for anybody who loves lobster and who prefer to cook seafood at all. In my lobster bisque recipe, you can easily count fat, adding a rather good amount of cream, use a low sugar tomato paste and enjoy high carb vegetables. Don't hesitate to prepare it today!

Ingredients (16 servings):

lobster chunks	24 oz
garlic	4 cloves
red onion	1/2 pcs
celery	4 stalks
tomato paste	1/2 cup
seafood broth	1 quart
white wine	2 cups
olive oil	1 tbsp
heavy cream	1 cup
bay leaves	3 pcs
salt	1 tbsp
peppercorns	1 tsp
paprika	1 tsp
thyme	1 tsp
xanthan gum	1 tsp
fresh lemon juice	1 tbsp
Parsley	

Directions:

1. Peel and chop the garlic.
2. Slice the celery and onion finely.
3. Take a medium-sized pan, add olive oil, place the onions and cook for some minutes. The onions must get fragrant.
4. Add garlic and cook until tender.
5. Add the white wine to the pan, deglaze everything a little and add sliced celery.
6. Open the Crock Pot, pour the mixture into it.
7.   Add broth, tomato paste and stir well.
8. Don't forget to add salt, pepper, and species. Add the bay leaves.
9. Cover and cook on LOW for 2 hours.
10. Once the soup is almost cooked, remove and take off the bay leaves.

11. Add the cream and let it be covered for some time.
12. After this add a small amount of xanthan gum while stirring the soup. It must start to thicken.
13. Pour the ready-made soup in a food processor and blend. It must get a creamy consistency.
14. Cut lobster into chunks and saute it in olive oil or in butter in a small pan.
15. Pour your bisque into a deep bowl and add the lobster chunks, stir until combined.
16. Dress with lemon juice, chives, green onion or parsley and enjoy!
17. Bon Appetite!

209.Keto halibut in the Crock Pot

Some types of meat, as well as fish, are great without adding something special. I think I have made the right choice when I decided to cook halibut without some specialties. Adding hot species, a little bit lemon, fennel or celery or both is enough to get juicy and tasty fish. Sometimes, I don't even need something for garnish. I eat it as it is or with some fresh vegetables.

Ingredients (4 servings):

skin-on halibut	1 to 2 pounds
fish broth	1 to 1 1/2 cups
Fennel	½ cup
Celery	½ cup

Spices hot (optional)

Salt and black pepper at will

Lemon slices at will for garnish

Directions:

1. Wash the halibut, take off the skin. Rinse well once more. Cut them into pieces or use the whole one.
2. Wash the celery and fennel, chop them finely.
3. Spread the bottom of the Crock Pot with cooking spray.
4. Put the halibut on the bottom. Sprinkle it with black pepper and salt.
5. Add fish broth.
6. Add your favorite species on the top of the halibut.
7. Cover and cook on LOW for 3 hours.
8. Open and remove the fish to a plate.
9. Serve with chopped fennel and celery, add lemon slices at will.
10. Bon Appetite!

210.Crock Pot keto juicy cod

Keto juicy cod cooked in the Crock Pot is a rather good alternative to fish we have usually prepared on a rack. Sometimes you get not the result you have waited before, have no time to check the dish and to control the cooking process. Cooking your delicious dishes in the Crock Pot is everything you need in a busy world.

Ingredients (5 servings):

Cod	5 slices (fresh)
Sour-cream sauce	1/2 cup
lime juice	1/8 cup
soy sauce	1/4 cup
garlic	2 tsp.

pepper and salt at will

Directions:

1. Peel the garlic and crush it finely.
2. Squeeze the juice of one lime.
3. Spread the bottom of the Crock Pot with cooking spray.
4. Place the cod slices into a Crock Pot.
5. Take a little bowl and mix there sour-sauce, lime juice, soy sauce, garlic, and pepper.
6. Pour the mixture into the Crock Pot. Cover and cook on LOW for 4 hours.
7. This dish tastes pretty well both cold and hot.
8. Bon Appetite!

211.Seafood soup Crock Pot

Today we have a great variety of seafood in the store – fresh, frozen, half done etc. I decided to throw this amazing marine life into a one delicious and flavorful seafood soup that you'll like it for sure. This soup is absolutely great to cook for some days and keep it in the fridge. My family thinks it tastes even better after some days. Don't worry if your fish is frozen, it will take you a little more time but it will be also so delicious as with fresh one. Here you have a recipe with frozen wild caught cod!

Ingredients (22 servings):

Soup

wild caught cod	10 oz
calamari	8 oz
shrimp	8 oz
coconut oil	1/4 cup
tomato sauce	1.5 cup
coconut cream	1/2 cup
seafood broth	1 quart
water	2 cups
celery	4 stalks
green onion	4 stalks

garlic	4 cloves
onion	1 medium pcs
lime	1 pcs
lemon	1 pcs

Spices

Salt	1 Tbsp
Pepper	2 Tsp
red pepper flakes	2 tsp
thyme	1 Tsp
dill	1 Tsp
bay leaves	3 whole
basil	2 Tsp
oregano	2 tsp

fresh parsley

Directions:

1. Take a medium-sized saucepan, heat two tablespoons of coconut oil on a medium flame.
2. Peel the onion, chop it finely.
3. Peel the garlic and crush.
4. Add onions and crushed garlic to the saucepan and cook until softened.
5. Peel the celery and add to the mix also.
6. Open the Crock Pot, pour the fish broth, water and tomato sauce.
7. Add the mixture of onions, garlic, and celery in the Crock Pot.
8. Cover and cook on LOW for two hours. The liquid must simmer slowly. Add salt and pepper at will.
9. While the liquid is cooking, peel the shrimp, if unpeeled.
10. Rinse well and cut the calamari tubes into about 1/2 inch pieces. Place them in a bowl with lemon juice. This will help to prevent calamari turning rubbery if you cook them too long.
11. Open the Crock Pot and add coconut cream. Cover the Crock Pot and put it on WARM, the soup must not be cooled.
12. Rinse the wild cod. Slice if it is not sliced yet.
13. After 10-15 minutes open the Crock Pot again and add the wild caught cod and Take a wooden spoon and carefully break the fish down in the Crock Pot into smaller pieces. Cover the Crock Pot. Put it on LOW for 1 hour more.
14. While this is cooking, prepare the shrimp: take a medium-sized bowl, let the water simmer over a medium heat. Add the shrimp in the simmering water and let them cook for about 4 minutes.
15. After this, add in the calamari and shrimp to the soup and set on WARM. Don't let it cook longer, the calamari may become rubbery and the shrimp hard.
16. Once the cooking time is over, add the juice of one lime, or more if you like.
17. Garnish with chopped green onion and fresh parsley.

18. Remove the bay leaves.
19. Bon Appetite!

212. Crock Pot keto salmon pie

My lovely combination of fresh chopped dill and smoked salmon. This cheesy and hearty keto pie prepared in the Crock Pot is amazing! I don't n know words that can express my feelings when I taste this salmon pie. You must cook it at once!

Ingredients (17 servings):

Pie crust

almond flour	¾ cup
sesame seeds	4 tablespoons
coconut flour	4 tablespoons
ground psyllium husk powder	1 tablespoon
baking soda	1 teaspoon
salt	1 pinch
olive oil or coconut oil	3 tablespoons
egg	1 pcs
water	4 tablespoons

Filling

smoked salmon	8 oz.
mayonnaise	1 cup
eggs	3 pcs
fresh dill, finely chopped	2 tablespoons
onion powder	½ teaspoon
ground black pepper	¼ teaspoon
cream cheese	4¼ oz.
shredded cheese	1¼ cups

Directions:

1. In a large bowl combine sesame seeds, almond flour, ground flour, ground psyllium husk powder, salt, baking soda, coconut or olive oil, cracked fresh egg and water at room temperature.
2. Using a food processor blend until mixture forms a ball. If you don't have a food processor, use your hands.
3. Open the Crock Pot and spray the bottom and walls with cooking spray thoroughly.

4. Oil your fingers or a spatula, and gently press the dough into the bottom and sides of the Crock Pot.
5. Cover the Crock Pot and put on HIGH for 2 hours. Pre-bake the pie until lightly browned.
6. While the pie is cooking prepare the filling: take a medium-sized bowl, mix mayo, eggs, onion powder, ground black pepper, cream cheese and stir everything well.
7. Wash and chop the fresh dill and add it to the mixture also.
8. Shred the Cheddar or Swiss cheese (at will) and add to the mix too. Combine everything well.
9. Open the Crock Pot and pour these ingredients into the pie crust.
10. Add the salmon, cover the Crock Pot and set on HIGH for 2 hours more until the pie is golden brown.
11. Let cool for a few minutes and serve with a salad or other vegetables.
12. Bon Appetite!

213.Sesame keto scallops with wasabi mayonnaise

Exotic and elegant. What do you need more?? Sesame keto scallops are fresh and fun, simply light and tangy. These scallops are going to become a dinner party. Keto fast food at its finest!

Ingredients (9 servings):

Scallops	8 pcs
sesame seeds	4 tablespoons
coconut oil or olive oil	1 tablespoon
wasabi paste	½ tablespoon
lime juice	1 tablespoon
mayonnaise	5 1⁄3 tablespoons
sesame oil	1 tablespoon
bok choy	4 oz.
scallions	2 pcs

Directions:

1. In a medium-sized bowl combine the lime juice and wasabi paste with mayo. Dress with salt to taste. Set aside.
2. Open the Crock Pot and spray thoroughly the bottom and the sides of it with cooking spray. Add coconut oil.
3. Rinse the scallops, roll the scallops in sesame seeds and put to the Crock Pot. Be attentive! Put on HIGH for half an hour, after this turn on the other side quickly. Check they must get brown quickly. Keep hot.
4. Wash and peel scallions, wash the bok choy.
5. Take off the scallops on a plate and put the chopped scallions and bok choy in the same liquid (after the scallops), add sesame oil if necessary.
6. Place the scallops directly on a plate. Add lime juice at will.
7. Serve immediately with wasabi mayo.
8. Eat hot!

9. Bon Appetite!

214.Keto salmon meatballs with lemon béchamel

Fishballs? Never tried? Really? Whatever you can call them, these amazing salmon meatballs are perfect when eaten with lemon bechamel sauce. If you don't like lemon bechamel, prepare another hot sauce you like!

Ingredients (15 servings):

Salmon	2 lbs
egg yolks	2 pcs
heavy whipping cream	¾ cup
salt	1 teaspoon
dried dill (optional)	1 tablespoon
ground black pepper	½ teaspoon
butter	2 oz.
cauliflower	1½ lbs

Lemon béchamel sauce

heavy whipping cream	1¾ cups
cream cheese	7 oz.
lemon juice	2 tablespoons
salt	½ teaspoon
ground black pepper	¼ teaspoon
ground nutmeg (optional)	¼ teaspoon
lemon, zest	2 teaspoons

Directions:
1. Rinse and cut the fish into small pieces, put everything into a food processor.
2. Take a medium-sized bowl, mix egg yolks, cream, and some spices. Dress with salt and pepper. Using a blender, mix everything into a smooth batter.
3. Using your wet hands, make little rolls they must be approximately size of 2 tablespoons each.
4. Open the Crock Pot and add cooking spray or olive oil or butter on the bottom.
5. Put the rolls in butter, cover the Crock Pot and set on HIGH for two hours until the rolls get golden brown. Turn them from one side to another from time to time.
6. While the rolls are cooking, wash and cut the cauliflower into big wedges and place in a large pot. Cover with water. Let it boil over medium heat and dress with a pinch of salt until the cauliflower fork-tender but not mushy. Drain well.
7. Once the rolls are done, serve them with cauliflower and a lemon béchamel.

Lemon béchamel

1. Take a medium-sized saucepan, place whipping cream, salt, lemon juice, cream cheese, pepper, nutmeg and lemon zest. Bring it to a boil while stirring continuously.
2. Lower the heat and let it simmer for a few minutes. The sauce must reach a smooth consistency.
3. Finally, add the lemon zest.
4. Season with salt and pepper.
5. Bon Appetite!

215.Cajun crab keto Crock Pot

A tasty and quick keto cajun crab dish with delicious seasoning is perfect for both breakfast, dinner and even supper. If you don't prefer celery stalks you may don't use them at all or add other veggies – onions, basil leaves etc. Enjoy warm!

Ingredients (11 servings):

Butter	1 oz.
yellow onion	1 pcs
celery stalks	5 1⁄3 oz.
mayonnaise	1¼ cups
eggs	4 pcs freshly
shredded cheese	2⁄3 lb
crab meat (120 g/can be drained)	1 lb canned
paprika powder	2 teaspoons
cayenne pepper	¼ teaspoon
salt and pepper	

For serving

leafy greens	3 oz.
olive oil	2 tablespoons

Directions:

1. Peel and chop the onion and celery finely.
2. Take a medium-sized saucepan, add butter and roast a little onion and celery until translucent. Dress with salt and pepper at will.
3. Shred the cheese and set aside.
4. Take another deep bowl, add mayo, freshly cracked eggs, crab meat, seasonings and ⅔ of the shredded cheese.
5. Add the fried onion and celery. Mix everything well and season at will.
6. Open the Crock Pot and spray with the cooking spray finely. Pour the mix into the Crock Pot.
7. Add the remaining cheese on top and on LOW for 3 hours until golden brown.

8. Serve with salad and black pepper!
9. Bon Appetite!

216.Keto smoked mussels Crock Pot

Have a busy weekend but still want to cook some delicious? Canned seafood to the rescue! Take a bowl and combine smoked mussels with cheese and cauliflower, and have a perfect keto dinner on the table in half an hour.

Ingredients (9 servings):

Cauliflower	1 lb
yellow onion	½ pcs
Dijon mustard	2 tablespoons
Mayonnaise	1 cup
shredded cheddar cheese	7 oz.
fresh chives (optional)	2 tablespoons
mussels	10 oz. canned
salt and pepper	

Serving

Lettuce	4¼ oz.
olive oil	4 tablespoons

Directions:

1. Wash and cut the cauliflower into small florets and put them in a pot.
2. Add water, it must cover the florets.
3. Add salt and bring to a boil. Let the cauliflower boil for a couple of minutes.
4. Drain the cauliflower and discard the water.
5. Peel the onion and chop the onion finely.
6. Shred the cheddar cheese. Set aside.
7. Take a deep bowl, put the onion, mustard, mayo and ⅔ parts of the cheese in a bowl and mix everything well.
8. Open the Crock Pot, pour the mixture, add cauliflower and mussels.
9. Cover and put on LOW for 3 hours.
10. Once the dish is ready, sprinkle the remaining grated cheese on top and set on WARM.
11. Serve with lettuce.
12. Bon Appetite!

217.Broiled Sea Bass with Chili Basil Glaze

Seabass with basil-chili glaze tastes super tender and amazing. You may serve this dish with cauliflower rice or noodles, fresh veggies or anything you like but that correspond the ketogenic diet. You don't need to much time, just to wash the filets, sprinkle with species. The other part of work will do the Crock Pot.

Ingredients (7 servings):

Vinegar	2 tablespoons
chopped basil	1 teaspoon
red pepper	1/8 teaspoon
garlic	1 clove
salt, divided	3/4 teaspoon
sea bass fillet	4 (6-ounce)
black pepper	1/4 teaspoon

Cooking spray

Directions:

1. Wash the fish fillet and dry it with a paper towel.
2. Peel the garlic and mince.
3. Wash fresh basil, chop finely.
4. Crush the red pepper. Set aside.
5. Open the Crock Pot, spray with cooking spray the bottom and sides of it.
6. Take a medium bowl, conjoin vinegar, basil, red pepper, garlic, salt.
7. Season the fillets with salt and black pepper at will.
8. Place the sea bass fillets on a bottom of the Crock Pot, sprinkle with species.
9. Cover the lid and put on HIGH for 4 hours or until the fillets are tender when tested with a fork.
10. Bon Appetite!

218.Crock Pot keto sea bass

Cooking of the sea bass in a traditional way is of high importance to check the time. The sea bass must not be overcooked or undercooked, otherwise, the taste and the fish will be damaged. The time that is suggested at the recipe is the optimal period for cooking the fish tender but stay juicy.

Ingredients (5 servings):

sea bass	1 whole fish
sea salt	1 tsp
fresh dill	3 sprigs
fresh parsley	2 sprigs
lemon zest	
pepper at will	

Seasoning: 1 tsp sea salt + 2 tsp olive oil

Directions:

1. Shred the lemon zest in a plate. Set aside. Wash fresh parsley and dill.

2. Wash the fish thoroughly, rinse well. Take off the scales, wipe dry.
3. Season with sea salt from both sides - inside and outside of the sea bass.
4. Open the Crock Pot, spray with cooking spray the bottom and sides of it.
5. Put the whole fish on the bottom of the Crock Pot.
6. Dress the fish with sprigs of dill and parsley. Put the lemon zest over the fish. Drizzle a little with olive oil.
7. Cover the lid and put on HIGH for 3 hours, the sea bass must get tender when tested with a fork.
8. Remove the fish carefully from the Crock Pot once the cooking time is over and serve on a plate.
9. Serve hot.

219.Sea bass with fennel and tomatoes in Crock Pot

The tender taste of sea bass is combined with flavor tomatoes and fennel in this recipe... How delicious is it! You can't imagine. Check the tenderness of sea bass all the time while cooking it in the Crock Pot, it is of high importance cooking the fish in a right way. It is a super tasty combination of the Mediterranean classic ingredients.

Ingredients (11 servings):

Cooking the sea bass:

fillets of sea bass	6 oz
olive oil	1 tbsp
salt and ground black pepper at will	

Cooking tomatoes and fennel:

fennel	4 bulbs
extra virgin olive oil	6 fl oz
tomatoes	1 big can
garlic	1 head
boiling water	5 fl oz
dry white wine	120ml/4fl oz
chopped fresh oregano leaves	2 tbsp
balsamic vinegar	2 tbsp
basil leaves	12 pcs

Directions:

1. Wash the fish thoroughly, rinse well. Take off the scales, wipe dry. Take off the skin. Place the pieces in the fridge.
2. Peel the garlic and mince. Wash the fresh leaves of oregano and chop.
3. Remove leaves from fennel.
4. Cut the fennel lengthways into quarters.

5. Heat the oil in a medium-sized saucepan and put the fennel. Cook the fennel turning frequently, for 15 minutes. Fennel must be of brown color.
6. Add the chopped tomatoes, minced garlic, boiling water, wine, oregano and black pepper at will.
7. Let the mixture boil, cover the lid of the saucepan and cook for 20 minutes.
8. Once the ingredients are almost cooked, add balsamic vinegar and basil leaves. Cover with lid again.
9. Take the sea bass from the refrigerator, season with salt and pepper.
10. Open the Crock Pot, spray with cooking spray the bottom and sides of it.
11. Place the sea bass on a bottom of the Crock Pot.
12. Cover the lid and put on HIGH for 4 hours or until the fish is tender when tested with a fork.
13. Remove the fish carefully from the Crock Pot once the cooking time is over and serve on a plate.
14. Place with a spoonful of the tomatoes and fennel into the center of each piece of fish.
15. Enjoy warm!

220.Keto sea bass Cuban style

This recipe of the sea bass fish fillets is easy to cook and sure to please! This one is great for parties, guests, friends and you don't need special time (if you don't have it at all) to be present all the day long at the kitchen.

Ingredients (9 servings):

olive oil	2 tsp
white onions	1 1/2 cups
minced garlic	2 tsp
fresh tomatoes	4 cups
dry white wine	1 1/2 cups
red pepper flakes	1/8 tsp
fillets sea bass	4 (6 ounces)
butter	2 tsp
fresh cilantro	1/4 cup

Pepper and salt at will

Directions:

1. Peel the onion and chop. Peel the garlic and mince finely. Wash and chop fresh cilantro. Set aside.
2. Wash the tomatoes, dry with paper towel, take off the seeds, chop them.
3. Heat olive oil in a medium saucepan over high heat. Sautee onions for some time until it gets brown color. Add garlic, and saute for minutes.
4. Add tomatoes. They must begin to soften.
5. Add wine, toss and add red pepper flakes. Let everything boil a little bit. Add butter. The sauce must thicken.

6. Open the Crock Pot, spray with cooking spray the bottom and sides of it.
7. Place the sea bass fillets on a bottom of the Crock Pot. Pour the sauce over the fillets.
8. Cover the lid and put on LOW for 6 hours or until the fish is tender when tested with a fork. But check the tenderness of fish fillets from time to time they must not be overcooked.
9. Remove the fish carefully from the Crock Pot once the cooking time is over and serve on a plate together with sauce from the Crock Pot.
10. Serve with fresh dill or cilantro at will.
11. Bon Appetite!

221.Keto Sticky Asian Sea Bass

I like this recipe for Asian sea bass very much. Delicate and a little bit soft, but it is still totally versatile. It tastes delicious. Take off the skin from the fillets, prepare the sweet-soy sauce that is a perfect adding to your fish and wait until the Crock Pot will cook the fish fillets for you. Add to the fish chili and coriander. It is perfectly well!

Ingredients (9 servings):

sesame oil	1 tbsp.
red chili	½ pcs
sweetener	3 tbsp.
dark soy sauce replaces with tamari	1 tbsp.
ground ginger	1/4 tsp
garlic	1 clove
Juice of lime	¼ of a lime
Sea Bass fillets - skin on	2 fillets
Almond flour	1/2 tsp
fresh coriander torn	
pepper and salt at will	

Directions:

1. Peel the garlic and mince finely.
2. Take off the skin of the sea bass fillets.
3. Take a medium-sized bowl, mix the oil, chili, sweetener, soy sauce, ginger, minced garlic.
4. Squeeze the juice of a lime and add to the mixture.
5. Open the Crock Pot, spray with cooking spray the bottom and sides of it.
6. Place the sea bass fillets on a bottom of the Crock Pot.
7. Sprinkle with the flour.
8. Sprinkle with sweet-soy sauce mix.
9. Cover the lid and put on LOW for 6 hours or until the fish is tender when tested with a fork.
10. Once the cooking time is over, remove the fillets from the Crock Pot on a plate and sprinkle with remained sauce, season with coriander and chili slices.
11. Enjoy warm.

222.Healthy Crock Pot fish fillet

I think every person is going to eat only healthy organic food. What could be healthier than to consume fish that is full of microelements and vitamins? To prepare the fish fillets following this recipe you may choose almost any fish you prefer most and mix with favorite species. Add lemon slices to get the tender taste of the fish and to avoid the smell.

Ingredients (5 servings):

salt, or to taste	1 tsp
fresh ground black pepper	1/2 tsp
white fish (cod, sea bass or catfish)	2-3 lb
fresh herbs (mix of parsley, basil, savory, tarragon)	
lemons	2-3 pcs

Directions:

1. Wash and dry with paper towel lemons. Slice thinly. Set aside.
2. Wash the fish thoroughly, rinse well. Take off the scales, wipe dry. Take off the skin.
3. Sprinkle all the sides of the fish with pepper and salt.
4. Open the Crock Pot, spray with cooking spray the bottom and sides of it.
5. Place the fillets on a bottom of the Crock Pot.
6. Place the lemon slices and herbs on top of the fish.
7. Cover the Crock Pot and put on HIGH for 4-5 hours (depending on the fish) until the fish is cooked through fully.
8. Once the cooking time is over, remove the lemon slices and serve the fish fillet with your favorite species.
9. Bon appetite!

223.Crock Pot Tuna Mornay

This tuna Mornay is super easy and tender. Everything you need is to buy a can of tuna, add your favorite cheese (Parmesan or Cheddar, as for me), add sour cream and celery soup and wait for tasty dinner!

Ingredients (6 servings):

condensed cream of celery soup	1 can
tuna, with brine (with liquid)	1 425g can
sour cream	½ cup
shallots	3 pcs
water	1/3 cup
Parmesan or cheddar cheese	1 cup
salt and pepper at will	

Directions:

1. Pell and chop the shallots.
2. Take a medium-sized bowl, join the condensed cream of celery soup, tuna, sour cream, water, shallots. Add also the rest liquid from the tuna.
3. Open the Crock Pot, put all the mixture, cover the lid of the Crock Pot and put on LOW for 4 hours.
4. Once the cooking time is over, open the lid, add shredded cheese and cover for 30 minutes.
5. Serve hot.
6. Bon Appetite!

224.Crock Pot Fillet of Sole with Pesto

This amazing recipe needs only three main ingredients! Could you imagine this?! You need only fish fillets, pesto, and shredded cheese. I don't recommend to add the water as the fish fillets could be overcooked. When the fillets are done they are of white color and tender, check this using a fork.

Ingredients (3 servings):

white fish (sole)   1 to 2 pounds

bottled pesto   1 bottle

shredded Parmesan cheese   ½ cups

salt and pepper at will

mint for dressing

Directions:

1. Shred the Parmesan cheese. Set aside.
2. Wash the fish thoroughly, rinse well. Take off the scales, wipe dry. Take off the skin.
3. Open the Crock Pot, spray with cooking spray the bottom and sides of it.
4. Place the fillets on a bottom of the Crock Pot.
5. Cover the sole fillets with pesto (1-2 spoons on each fillet).
6. Sprinkle with shredded Parmesan each piece of sole.
7. Cover the lid and put on LOW for 4 hours.
8. Once the cooking time is over, open the Crock Pot and remove the ready-made fish fillets on a plate.
9. You may serve the fish fillets with veggies like spinach, zucchini, asparagus etc.
10. Eat warm. Serve with fresh mint.
11. Bon Appetite!

225.Sole in herbed butter Crock Pot

This recipe was advised me many years ago by my old friend. Since that time I have prepared this dish many times as it is simple and quick. Dill and lemon is the best mix of herbed butter and sole. Don't hesitate to cook it today!

Ingredients (7 servings):

Butter	4 tsp
dill weed	1 tsp
onion powder	1/2 tsp
garlic powder	1/2 tsp
salt	1/2 tsp
white pepper	1/4 tsp
sole fillets	2 pounds

Fresh dill and lemon wedges for dressing

Directions:

1. Wash the fish thoroughly, rinse well. Take off the scales, wipe dry. Take off the skin.
2. Take a medium-sized bowl, conjoin the butter, onion powder, dill, garlic powder, salt at will and pepper if desired.
3. Open the Crock Pot, spray with cooking spray the bottom and sides of it.
4. Add the sole on a bottom of the Crock Pot and put the herbed mixture over each fish fillet.
5. Garnish with lemon and dill if desired.
6. Cover the lid and put on LOW for 5 hours.
7. Once the cooking time is over, open the Crock Pot and take off the fish fillets on a serving plate.
8. Bon Appetite!

226.Jamaican salmon Crock Pot recipe

Preparing the salmon according to this recipe you may mix all the species that are mentioned below or just buy the mix of species in a store. As for me, I Like to use my handmade species because I know what I want to mix and the ingredients are always fresh. I advise you to follow strictly my instructions. Don't open the foil packet during the cooking time, otherwise, the juice from fish will flow out.

Ingredients (11 servings):

Cloves	1/8 teaspoon
Ginger	1/8 teaspoon
Nutmeg	1/8 teaspoon
kosher salt	1 teaspoon
onion powder	1 teaspoon
sweetener	2 teaspoons
chipotle chili powder	1/4 teaspoon
cayenne pepper	1/2 teaspoon

black pepper	1/4 teaspoon
thyme	1/8 teaspoon
cinnamon	1/2 teaspoon

Directions:

1. Peel the garlic and mince finely.
2. Mix in a medium-sized bowl garlic minced, ginger, nutmeg, salt and pepper, onion powder, sweetener, chili powder, cayenne pepper, cinnamon.
3. Open the Crock Pot, spray with cooking spray the bottom and sides of it.
4. Put the fish on of foil in the middle. Season all sides of the fish with mix once more. Make an enclosed packet from the foil, the fish juice must stay inside.
5. Put the foil into the Crock Pot. Be attentive! Do not add water.
6. Cover the lid and cook on LOW for 3 hours. Don't open the foil until the finish of the cooking time.
7. Serve hot on a large plate (without foil) with fresh veggies!
8. Bon Appetite!

227.Clam chowder Crock Pot

This is the recipe for the clam chowder from England! This amazing dish with a creamy texture is perfect and light for sunny days. I usually serve it with salad or keto bread. My family likes seafood prepared in the Crock Pot very much. You may serve the clam chowder with chopped fresh parsley or bacon slices. I'm sure the seafood fans would like this creamy soup very much!

Ingredients (11 servings):

Onion	1 pcs large
clams	3 cans (ca. 6.5 ounces each)
clam juice	8 ounces
dried thyme	1/2 teaspoon
salt or at will	1/4 teaspoon
pepper or at will	1/4 teaspoon
butter	2 tablespoons
almond flour	3 tablespoons
half and half	1 cup
whole milk	1 cup
bacon	2 slices chopped
parsley for garnish	

Directions:

1. Peel one large onion and dice it. Set aside.

2. Chop the clams finely. Slice the bacon.
3. Spread the bottom of the Crock Pot with cooking spray, add there diced onion.
4. After this, add there two full cans of clams (with juice) and also one without it.
5. Pour one bottle of clam juice, add pepper, dried thyme, salt in the Crock Pot. Mix everything well.
6. Cover the Crock Pot and cook on HIGH for 3-4 hours.
7. Take a large bowl, place it on high heat and melt the butter there. Add almond flour.
8. Toss the mixture until the smooth consistency. Pour slowly half and half and milk. Continue to stir until thickened.
9. Pour this mixture into the Crock Pot, cover and continue to cook for an hour on LOW.
10. Serve warm, add sliced bacon strips and parsley.
11. Bon Appetite!

228.Keto shrimp Crock Pot

Have you already cooked the shrimps in the Crock Pot? Not yet!? It takes only an hour but it is divine! The BBQ sauce adds a special taste to the shrimp minced garlic and melted butter do their best. This dish is very simple but I think it has definitely a leading place in your keto cookbook. I usually serve shrimps with vegetable salad, cauliflower rice. Enjoy it right now!

Ingredients (5 servings):

shrimp	2 lbs.
butter	3 Tbsp
Worcestershire sauce	3 Tbsp
minced garlic	2 Tsp
BBQ sauce	1 cup

Salt and pepper to taste

Directions:

1. Peel and devein the shrimps into a medium bowl. Wash them and place in the Crock Pot.
2. Peel and mince the garlic cloves.
3. Place the butter in the Crock Pot, dress with salt, add Worcestershire sauce, pepper, and minced garlic. Mix everything well. Add BBQ sauce and stir once more.
4. Cover and cook on LOW for an hour.
5. Serve with fresh veggies or keto bread.
6. Dress in a lemon wedge.
7. Bon Appetite!

229.Crock Pot Indian fish curry

This dish is of bright yellow color and has a delicious flavor of mixed species in it. The fish fillets are cooked very fast, they get tender, melt in your mouth and don't let you apathetic. You may also add the other species that you or your family prefers more. Serve this Indian fish curry over the cauliflower rice! Enjoy warm.

Ingredients (14 servings):

canola oil	1/3 cup (3 fl. oz./80 ml)
yellow onion	1 pcs large
garlic	2 cloves
hot green chilies	2 small
fresh ginger	1-inch (2.5-cm) piece
ground cumin	1 Tbs.
ground coriander	2 tsp.
brown mustard seeds	2 tsp.
ground turmeric	2 tsp.
tomatoes	2 pcs
sweetener	1 Tbs.
Kosher salt	
fish fillets (such as tilapia, cod or halibut)	2 lb.
cilantro	3 Tbs.

Directions:
1. Peel and chop finely yellow onion. Peel the garlic and mince.
2. Peel and grate the fresh ginger. Chop fresh cilantro. Wash hot chilies, take off the seeds and mince them.
3. Wash tomatoes, take off the seeds and chop them finely.
4. Wash the fish fillets, cut them into 1-inch pieces.
5. Cover the bottom of the Crock Pot with oil, add there chopped onion and stir.
6. Add minced garlic, minced chilies, coriander, cumin, ginger, turmeric, mustard, and toss.
7. Add the tomatoes, sweetener, pepper, salt and stir everything in the Crock Pot. Toss until tomatoes begin to release the juice (ca. 1 minute).
8. Cover and cook on LOW for 1-2 hours.
9. Once the time is over, open the Crock Pot, add fish fillets. Filets must be coated with sauce fully.
10. Recover and continue cooking for about 1 hour on LOW. The sauce must be of thick consistency.
11. Serve with black pepper and salt at will.
12. Remove the filet with sauce to a plate.
13. Bon Appetite!

230.Keto salmon in the Crock Pot

I always say that sometimes it is better to cook something simple than to buy 15-17 ingredients, spend a lot of time in the kitchen and don't astonish your friends finally. Keto salmon in the Crock Pot is the easiest dish I could imagine. It is the best way to get extremely tender salmon full of your favorite species dressed with lemon slices. You may place the salmon in the Crock Pot in two layers. In this case, you have to add a little bit more liquid (broth or water). I also don't recommend cooking salmon by using more than two layers, your fillets could be overcooked.

Ingredients (2 servings):

skin-on salmon fillets	1 to 2 pounds
liquid (water or broth)	1 to 1 1/2 cups

Salt and black pepper at will

Lemon slices at will for garnish

Fennel or celery (optional)

Spices (optional)

Sliced lemon (optional)

Directions:

1. Wash the salmon filets. Cut them into pieces. Wash the celery or fennel (depending on what you choose), chop them finely.
2. Spread the bottom of the Crock Pot with cooking spray.
3. Put the salmon fillets on the bottom. Sprinkle the salmon pieces with black pepper and salt.
4. Add broth or water.
5. Add your favorite species on the top of the salmon pieces.
6. Cover and cook on LOW for 2 or 3 hours (it depends on the thickness of the fillets).
7. Open and remove the fillets to a plate.
8. Serve with chopped fennel or celery, add lemon slices.
9. Bon Appetite!

231.Shrimp Scampi Crock Pot

This recipe is special for those who like shrimp scampi. I serve this dish usually with keto bread or fresh green. When I add the shrimps to the bottom of the Crock Pot, be sure that you leave the tail on. You also may put the Crock Pot on High, this time you'll cook the shrimps for an hour. But anytime this is the quickest and easiest way to cook the shrimps for dinner. You may also cook the shrimps as an appetizer!

Ingredients (7 servings):

chicken broth	1/4 cup
olive oil	2 tablespoons
butter	2 tablespoons
garlic	1 tablespoon
parsley (dried could be also used)	2 tablespoons
freshly squeezed	1/2 lemon
raw shrimp	1 pound

salt and pepper at will

Directions:
1. Peel the garlic and mince it.
2. Wash and cut the fresh parsley. Wash the lemon and squeeze a juice from it to a cup. Set aside.
3. Wash, peel and devein shrimps.
4. Spread the Crock Pot with cooking spray. Put there butter, olive oil, add chicken broth, chopped parsley, minced garlic, juice from a lemon, add pepper and salt to taste.
5. Add shrimps.
6. Cover and cook on LOW for 2 hours.
7. Once the time is over, remove to a plate, serve with fresh green.
8. Bon Appetite!

232.Crock Pot crab and shrimp bisque

Instead of many ingredients of this dish, they are all simple to find in the store. Lump crab costs pretty much but I suspect it is worth to cook this dish one time a month. This ingredient makes the dish something special. All the steps that could be seen as a little bit complicated at the first gaze. But be sure, following the steps you'll achieve the best result that could be only imagined!

Instructions (24 servings):
Preparing the bisque:

avocado oil	1 tbsp
butter	2 tbsp
leek	3 pcs
garlic	4 cloves
red pepper	a pinch of flakes
tomato paste	2 tbsp
fish stock	4 cups
water	2 cups
tomatoes (diced)	1 (15-oz) can
seasoning	1 tbsp
Sweetener	1 tbsp
salt	2 tbsp
black pepper	1 tbsp
almond flour	¼ cup
heavy cream	1 cup

shrimp	1 lb
jumbo lump crab	1 cup
parsley	2 tbsp.

For the Crab Topping:

lemon juice	½ a lemon
Mayo	2 tbsp.
Dijon mustard	1 teaspoon
Mustard grains	1 teaspoon
parsley	1 tbsp
jumbo lump crab	1 cup

Salt and pepper at will

Directions:

Preparing bisque:

1. Wash, dry with a paper towel, slice the leeks.
2. Peel garlic, mince it.
3. Wash, peel and devein shrimps.
4. Wash, chop finely fresh parsley.
5. Place butter and avocado oil in the Crock Pot, add sliced leeks, garlic, red pepper. Mix everything together.
6. Add also tomato paste, broth, diced tomatoes, water, seasoning, sweetener, stir well.
7. Dress in white or black pepper, salt.
8. Add flour and combine everything well. Cover the Crock Pot and put on LOW for 3 hours or on HIGH for ca. 2 hours.
9. Once the time is over, add heavy cream, shrimps, crab, chopped parsley. Covert and go on cooking for 1 hour more. The shrimps must be of pink color.

Preparing topping:

1. While the bisque is preparing, take a medium bowl and mix the lemon juice, mustard, mayo, chopped parsley. Fold in the crab meat gently.
2. Dress with salt and pepper.
3. Add parsley (chopped previously).
4. Eat warm.
5. Bon Appetite!

233.Crock Pot spicy barbecue shrimp recipe

This dish is also named as New Orleans spicy barbecue shrimp. It contains a mix of species such as Cajun seasoning, shrimp, hot sauce (you may choose anyone you like), juice of lemon, large juicy shrimps, garlic, green onions for serving and… and nothing more! Take patience until the shrimps will be cooked in the Crock Pot.

Ingredients (8 servings):

Garlic	2 cloves
Cajun seasoning	1 tbsp
unsalted butter	1/2 cup
Worcestershire Sauce	1/4 cup
hot pepper sauce	1 tbsp
juice	1 lemon
large shrimp, unpeeled	1 1/2 pounds
green onion	1 pcs large
salt and pepper at will	

Directions:

1. Peel the garlic and mince it finely. Wash and chop the green onions. Set aside.
2. Cut butter into pieces.
3. Squeeze the juice of one lemon into a cup.
4. Peel the onion and chop it finely.
5. Take a medium bowl and combine there butter, Cajun seasoning, Worcestershire Sauce, pepper, hot sauce, salt, minced garlic.
6. Place this in the Crock Pot, cover and cook on LOW for half an hour on LOW until hot.
7. While the sauce is cooking, rinse the shrimp and drain.
8. Place the shrimp into the Crock Pot and toss with already-cooked sauce. Shrimps must be coated.
9. Cover and continue cooking another 30 minutes.
10. Once the time is over put on WARM until serving.
11. Dress with chopped green onions.
12. Eat warm.

234.Crock Pot keto maple salmon

Maple salmon could be cooked from fresh or frozen salmon both are rather well to cook in the Crock Pot. To mince the ginger root I keep it a little bit frozen (I put it in the freezer) and then grate the frozen ginger root. It is rather convenient I must say. Be sure that that chosen soy sauce doesn't contain sugar.

Ingredients (5 servings):

Salmon	6 fillets (fresh or frozen)
maple syrup	1/2 cup
lime juice	1/8 cup
soy sauce	1/4 cup
garlic	2 tsp.
minced ginger root	1 tsp.

Directions:

1. Peel the garlic and crush it finely.
2. Squeeze the juice of one lime.
3. Peel the ginger root and mince carefully.
4. Spread the bottom of the Crock Pot with cooking spray.
5. Place the salmon pieces into a Crock Pot.
6. Take a little bowl and mix the maple syrup, lime juice, sauce, garlic and ginger root.
7. Pour the mixture into the Crock Pot. Cover and cook on LOW for 2 hours.
8. This dish tastes pretty well both cold and hot.
9. Serve with cauliflower rice or broccoli.
10. Bon Appetite!

235.Crock Pot salmon curry

Creamy, astonishing, appetizing, flavor salmon curry prepared in the Crock Pot is rather comfort food for me at any time of the day. I hope you'll like it too. The salmon curry is aromatic and tender it melts like butter in your mouth. I grew up on this recipe it is one of my favorite ones. It doesn't need other additions like rice (cauliflower rice) or other veggies. Just cook right now and eat!

Ingredients (15 servings):

Salmon	6 pieces
onion	1 pcs
garlic	6 cloves
ginger	2 teaspoons
celery	3 stalks
coconut milk	2 cans
vegetable stock	½ cup
tomato paste	1 12 ounces can
coriander	1 ½ teaspoons
cumin	1 ½ teaspoons
chili powder	1 teaspoon
smoked paprika	2 teaspoons
turmeric	1 teaspoon
pepper	½ teaspoon
salt	¼ teaspoon

parsley or chili flakes to garnish (optional)

Directions:

1. Take off the skin from the salmon pieces. Set aside.
2. Peel onions, garlic, crush them finely.
3. Peel and grate the fresh ginger.
4. Chop the celery stalks finely.
5. Chop parsley for garnish (optional).
6. Pour cans of coconut milk into the Crock Pot.
7. Add tomato paste there also, vegetable stock, cumin, coriander, paprika, turmeric, chili.
8. Season with salt and pepper.
9. Stir well all the ingredients.
10. Place the salmon pieces into the mixture in the Crock Pot.
11. Add garlic, onion, grated ginger, celery.
12. Cover and cook on LOW for 3 hours.
13. Garnish with chili flakes or parsley.
14. Bon Appetite!

236.Crock Pot lemon dill halibut

Why have I chosen the lemon dill halibut for my cookbook? It is a light, tasty and flaky dish cooked in the Crock Pot. Preparing the fish in the Crock Pot doesn't smell bad in the whole house you don't need to clean too many dishes, skillets or saucepans. I like to add dill (both dried or freshly chopped) to fish fillets. I like also to add extra lemon slices on the top of the fish or add some more black pepper and fresh dill.

Ingredients (4 servings):

seafood halibut (fresh or frozen)	12 oz
lemon juice	1 Tbsp
olive oil	1 Tbsp
dried dill (1 Tbsp fresh dill)	1 1/2 Tsp

Salt and pepper at will

Directions:

1. Wash, peel the fresh halibut (or use the frozen one).
2. Squeeze the juice of one lemon.
3. Spray the bottom of the Crock Pot with olive oil.
4. Place the halibut to the bottom of the Crock Pot.
5. Dress with pepper, salt to taste.
6. Take a small bowl, whisk the lemon juice, dill, and olive oil together.
7. Pour this mixture over the halibut.
8. Cover and cook on LOW 2 hours.
9. Once the time is over, check if the fish is tender and ready.
10. Serve halibut with an extra one lemon slice or fresh dill.
11. Bon Appetite!

237.Crock Pot cod with red curry

The keto cod cooked in the Crock Pot is rather simple, tender dish in a tasty red curry sauce. This dish is great if you change the cod fillets with chicken or pork if you are not a fish fan. But, still, I recommend to cook and to taste this amazing one! If you don't like cod you may change this fish with salmon or another one preferred. Sometimes I add to the Crock Pot the whole fish, sometimes only pieces (fillet) of it. But both variants are great!

Ingredients (8 servings):

coconut milk	2 – 15 oz. cans
red curry paste	3 Tbsp
curry powder	1 Tbsp
ground ginger	1 Tsp
garlic powder	1 Tsp
bell pepper	1 pcs
codfish fillet	1 lb.

Salt and pepper at will

Fresh basil or green onion, garnish

Directions:
1. Wash and slice the bell pepper, take off the seeds and slice.
2. Wash the fish fillet, dry it with a paper towel.
3. Wash and cut the green onions or basil (optional).
4. Open the Crock Pot, add the coconut milk, add curry paste, ginger, curry powder, garlic powder and whisk together.
5. Put into the sauce the sliced peppers and fish fillet.
6. Cover and cook on LOW for 2-3 hours.
7. Once the fish is ready, put it on a plate and cut into pieces.
8. Serve with fresh basil leaves or chopped green onions.
9. Bon Appetite!

238.Coconut cilantro curry shrimp

This dish needs only 6 simple ingredients. The junction of shrimp and milk tastes great it is one among my lovely combinations of tastes. Coconut cilantro curry shrimp is served in the Thai restaurants as usual. To stress the relish you may add the grated ginger, lemongrass or lime juice. But I don't recommend putting all of them in one Crock Pot at once. If you can't find seasoning (lemon-garlic) at the store, make it your own!

Ingredients (6 servings):

Shrimp	1 lb
coconut milk	30 ounces
water	15 ounces

red curry paste	1-2 tbsp
seasoning	2½ tsp
cilantro	¼ cup

Directions:

1. Take a medium bowl, mix water, curry paste, coconut milk, seasoning, cilantro.
2. Add this mixture to the Crock Pot and put on LOW for an hour.
3. Place shrimp in the sauce, continue cooking for half an hour more. Shrimp must be done fully.
4. Serve with cilantro.
5. Bon Appetite!

239. Crock Pot Cilantro-Lime Fish Tacos

The keto recipes cooked in the Crock Pot are always easy and great for large companies and holidays. This dish goes usually over well. The cooking process is rather easy, you just need to buy the fillets at the nearest store (I prefer tilapia, but you may also use salmon or cod), add on the top of the fillets some flavor species, garlic, cilantro, lime juice. The fillets couldn't be overcooked or raw.

Ingredients (5 servings):

fish fillets (frozen)	6 pcs
Rotel	1 large can
garlic	1/2 tsp.
dried cilantro	1 1/2 Tbsp
lime juice	2 Tbsp
salt to taste	
taco shells (for garnish, optional)	

Directions:

1. Peel the garlic and mince.
2. Wash the cilantro and cut it (if you use the fresh one).
3. Squeeze the juice from one lime into a cup.
4. Put the fillets into the Crock Pot.
5. Cover the fillets with minced garlic, drained can of Rotel, squeezed juice, cilantro, pepper.
6. Cover and put on HIGH for 1 hour. Check the readiness with a fork.
7. Serve the dish in taco shells.
8. Bon Appetite!

240. Roasted keto shrimps Crock Pot

I have gathered many recipes how to prepare the shrimp tastily and quick. But I think cooking shrimp in the Crock Pot is without a rival! This time you don't need to roast the shrimp using a large skillet, bottles of oil, many dishes and so on. Cooking the roasted shrimp in the Crock

Pot saves time, useful residues, electricity and your energy and free time. My family likes to consume the roasted keto shrimp with avocado slices or feta cheese.

Ingredients (9 servings):

raw shrimp	11 oz
fire roasted stewed tomatoes	14.5 oz can
spicy salsa	2 tbsp
bell pepper	5 oz or 1/2 cup
cumin	1/2 tsp
cayenne pepper	1/4 to 1/2 Tsp
garlic	1/2 Tsp
cilantro	3-4 tbsp
olive oil	1-2 tbsp

sea salt and black pepper

optional feta cheese, slices of avocado.

Directions:

1. Peel the shrimp lay them on the bottom of the Crock Pot.
2. Spread the shrimp with olive oil.
3. Wash the bell pepper, dry it with a paper towel, take off the seeds and slice.
4. Peel the garlic and mince. Wash the fresh cilantro and mince finely.
5. Dress the shrimp with pepper and salt. Add tomatoes (if using frozen shrimp – drain the liquid from tomatoes), add pepper slices, cumin, cayenne pepper, a half of all cilantro, garlic.
6. Toss everything well.
7. Cover and put on LOW for 3 hours.
8. Once the dish is ready, dress with remained cilantro, slices of avocado, feta cheese.
9. Eat warm!

241.Crock Pot Ginger Steamed Pompano

Yesterday I found a fresh Pompano at the store near my house. I remembered about this tasty, delicious dish at once and decided to cook it today for supper. Sometimes, it is a real trial for me to cook fish – I don't like the smell during the cooking process, too many dishes need to be cleaned after preparation process. But when you cook in the Crock Pot it changes all my prejudices. All you need here just to take off the inside and gills from the fish, prepare the sauce and pour your fish. That's all! For those who don't like pompano, I advise using halibut, seabass, tilapia, grouper.

Ingredients (9 servings):

Pompano	1 Whole pcs
Soy Sauce	1/4 Cup

Sesame Oil	1/4 Cup
Chinese Cooking Wine	1/4 Cup
Sweetener	2 Tablespoons
Ginger	1 2" Piece
garlic	6 Cloves
Leeks	1 Bunch
Cilantro	1 Bunch

Directions:

1. Wash the fish, take off the inside, scale, make the slits (diagonal) on both sides.
2. Pell the ginger and grate it. Set aside. Wash and chop the cilantro for garnish. Peel the garlic and mince.
3. Take a medium bowl, mix there sesame oil, sauce, wine, sweetener, grated ginger and whisk everything. Add pepper and salt at will.
4. Cut the leeks and put them into the bottom of the Crock Pot.
5. Place the fish over the leeks, pour the mixture over the fish.
6. Cover the Crock Pot and cook on LOW 2 hours.
7. Serve hot with fresh cilantro and minced garlic.
8. Bon Appetite!

242.Razor Clams in Spicy Sauce

Razor claims is a product that doesn't eat by all. Once you have decided to cook the clams in the Crock Pot, I can recommend using this recipe. After you have bought the clams at the store, let them rinse in a cold or a little bit warm water or just leave them in a bowl with water for some minutes. If some shells are opened, don't use them at all! Put the clams into the Crock Pot very carefully don't disturb the bottom of the Crock Pot. As soon as the shells are opened, it means they are ready. Once the clams are ready, take them off and pour the liquid into a large bowl and prepare a flavor mixture. If you wish you may add some more chili or other hot sauce.

Ingredients (11 servings):

Razor Clams	1 lb
Garlic	1 Tablespoon
Shallots	1 Tablespoon
Ginger	1 Tablespoons
Red Chili	2-3 Pieces
Oyster Sauce	1/4 Cup
Soy Sauce	2 Tablespoons
Sweetener	2 Tablespoons
Water	1/4 Cup

Cilantro   2 Tablespoons

Flour (almond)   2 Tablespoons

Salt, pepper at will

Directions:
1. Peel the garlic and shallots and mince both finely.
2. Peel the ginger and mince it. Chop the red chili carefully. Wash and chop the fresh cilantro.
3. Take a large bowl, combine water, sweetener, both sauces, salt, chili, ginger, garlic, shallot, razor clams.
4. Cover and cook on HIGH for an hour until the shells open.
5. Once the cooking time is over, pour the liquid into a large bowl, add a little bit water an flour. Stir everything well. The consistency must be smooth.
6. Serve the clams in shells with the smooth mixture.
7. Bon Appetite!

243.Crock Pot Vietnamese Braised Catfish

This is one of the best recipes for cooking the catfish. I cooked the catfish for my friends recently and they have appraised worthy this one. I'm sure this dish will be definitely included in the list of your favorite seafood recipes! Your catfish mustn't «swim» in the sauce in the Crock Pot. It must reach at least the half of the height of fish. I cook usually this dish for 5-6 hours because the catfish is firm enough and all the flavors must «enter» the fish meat. Enjoy it with me!

Ingredients (7 servings):
Catfish   1 Piece

Sweetener   1/2 Cup

Fish Sauce   1/4 Cup

Shallot   1 Piece

Red Chilies   2-3 Pieces

Ginger   1 2" Piece

Vietnamese Coriander Leaves

Pepper and salt to taste

Directions:
1. Wash the catfish, remove the inside, cut into steaks. Set aside.
2. Peel shallot and slice thinly.
3. Chop red chilies finely.
4. Peel and cut ginger into thin strips.
5. Take a large bowl, add a little bit water, salt, shallots, ginger, black pepper, chili. Stir well.
6. Take another little saucepan, add the sweetener and melt it a little. Pour to the mixture in a large bowl.
7. Pour the sauce into the Crock Pot, place the fish stakes, cover and cook on LOW for 5-6 hours.
8. Garnish with coriander leaves.

9. Bon Appetite!

244.Keto Crock Pot Chili Prawns

This keto chili prawn is one of the recipes that stress not only the heat of chili but also its flavor. All you need to prepare this recipe is to buy prawns and chili) it leaves you a little bit choice to add to the dish your favorite ingredients (species). I think, the catsup corresponds to the hot base of chili and creates here an interesting substitute. You may also try coconut cream if you prefer it more. Don't hesitate to create new tastes! In most supermarkets, you may find Sambal Oelek as an Asian condiment, combine it also with jalapenos, habaneros, etc.

Ingredients (12 servings):

Prawns shell-on	500 lb
Ginger	1 thumb-sized Piece
Shallot	1 Pieces
Garlic	1 clove
Scallions	1/2 Cup
Sambal Oelek	2 Tablespoons
Sweetener	1 Tablespoons
Cider Vinegar	2 Tablespoons
Catsup (sugar-free)	1/2 Cup
Sesame Oil	2 Tablespoons
Fish Sauce	1 Tablespoons
Egg	1 Piece

Pepper and salt at will

Directions:

1. Peel the ginger and mince it finely.
2. Peel the shallot and mince too. Peel the garlic, mince or press it.
3. Slice thinly the peeled shallots.
4. Take a medium bowl, mix there shallots, ginger, sambal oelek, scallions, sweetener, garlic, vinegar, catsup. Whisk all together.
5. Pour the mixture into a Crock Pot, cover and cook on HIGH for an hour.
6. Once the time is over, open the Crock Pot, add the prawns. Continue cooking half an hour more.
7. Once a half an hour is over, open the Crock Pot and add there cracked egg and sesame oil. Keep under cover for 15 minutes.
8. Season with fish sauce at will.
9. Bon Appetite!

245.Crock Pot Tuna Salpicao

I can't remember how many times I have exactly cooked this delicious tuna in Crock Pot for my husband and kids! I really enjoyed the results all the time, so this variant of dinner is sure-fire. I usually choose the freshest fish I could only find. In the nearest supermarkets, tuna could be found all year-long. The frozen tuna is also well as the fresh one. Fresh tuna must be a little bit firm and of pink color. Cut tuna into slices larger or small as you prefer and follow my instructions.

Ingredients (7 servings):

Tuna	1/2 lb
olive oil	1 Cup
garlic	1 Clove
Jalapeno Peppers	4 Pieces
Red Chili	3-5 Pieces
Black Peppercorns	2 Teaspoons
Salt	1 Teaspoon

Directions:

1. Wash the tuna fish, remove the inside, cut into 1-inch cubes.
2. Peel and chop finely the garlic.
3. Wash, take off the seeds, slice the jalapeno peppers.
4. Finely chop the red chili (be careful!)
5. Take a medium bowl, combine there olive oil, jalapenos, garlic, red chili, peppercorns, salt. Whisk everything well.
6. Pour the mixture into the Crock Pot.
7. Cover and cook on LOW for an hour.
8. Once the time is over, open the Crock Pot, put the tuna there and close the cover.
9. Cook on LOW for an hour more.
10. Serve with salt and black pepper.
11. Bon Appetite!

246.Crock Pot Miso-Poached Salmon

The miso-poached salmon prepared in the Crock Pot is delicious, amazing, flavor…. All the dishes cooked with salmon are simple but appetizing. It is the most delicious fish I know! The base of this dish is miso, it could be found in any Asian or Japanese section at the supermarket. You may choose any color of the miso pasta – yellow, red or white variant.

Ingredients (6 servings):

Salmon Fillet	2 Pieces
Miso Paste	1/2 Cup
Fish Stock	3 Cups
Scallions	1/2 Cup
Ginger	1 2" Piece

Salt   2 Teaspoons

Black pepper at will

Directions:

1. Wash the salmon fillets. Set them aside.
2. Thinly slice the washed scallions.
3. Peel the ginger and thinly slice it too.
4. Take a medium bowl and combine there miso paste, fish stock, scallions, ginger, whisk everything.
5. Cover and put on LOW for 3 hours.
6. Once 3 hours are over, open the Crock Pot and put the salmon fillets there.
7. Put on HIGH and cook for half an hour, turn to WARM after this time.
8. Season with fish salt, black pepper, salt at will.
9. Bon Appetite!

247.Crock Pot Soy-Ginger Braised Squid

You may ask me why I cook squid so long. Most people cook squid for a couple of minutes, it mustn't be too rubbery or tough. Yes, but there is one exception. Squid are full of natural collagen, the cooking process that I have chosen – is braising. It is the best way of squid preparation. Braising lets collagen fibers be hydrolyzed and as a result, they get extremely tender (while cooking squid slowly on LOW). They will absorb as much species as you add to the braising liquid. Surprise your family today!

Ingredients (10 servings):

Squid   1 lb

Ginger   1 2-inch Piece

garlic   1 clove

Sweetener   1/2 Cup

Soy Sauce   1/4 Cup

Oyster Sauce   1/4 Cup

Chinese Cooking Wine   1/4 Cup

Leeks   2 Stalks

Bay Leaves   2 Pieces

Red Thai Chili (optional)

Directions:

1. Wash and cut squid into rings.
2. Peel and finely chop the ginger.
3. Peel and crush the garlic clove.
4. Thinly slice the leeks.
5. Take a large bowl, combine squid pieces, chopped ginger, garlic, sweetener, sauce (Oyster and soy), cooking wine. Mix everything well.

6. Pour the mixture into the Crock Pot, add bay leaves, salt, and pepper to taste, Thai chili (at will).
7. Cover the Crock Pot and put on LOW for 7 hours.
8. Check if the squid is tender.
9. Bon Appetite!

248.Crock Pot Seabass in Coconut Cream Sauce

I must recognize that my love for coconut cream and seabass is unlimited. My taste receptors are too excited with amazing and rich flavors of fish and tender texture of the coconut cream. This delicious dish doesn't need other ingredients except those listed below. I enjoy it always in the evenings after long busy days, when I sit in the kitchen and delight seabass. This recipe is also well for other fish like halibut or salmon.

Ingredients (7 servings):

Seabass	2-3 lb
Ginger	1 2" Piece
Scallions	2 Stalks
Coconut Cream	2 Cups
Fish Sauce	1 Tablespoon
Bok Choy	4 Stalks
Jalapeno Peppers	3-5 Pieces

Salt, pepper at will

Directions:

1. Peel and cut ginger into strips.
2. Wash seabass, take off the inside, make two-three snips on seabass.
3. Slice scallions thinly. Wash the jalapeno peppers, wash the Bok Choy.
4. Take a medium bowl, combine ginger, coconut cream, scallions, peppers, pepper, salt, fish sauce.
5. Pour the mixture into the Crock Pot, put the fish on it. Put the Bok Choy over the fish.
6. Cover and cook on LOW 2 hours.
7. Remove seabass to a plate, dress with jalapenos and Bok Choy.
8. Bon Appetite!

249.Crock Pot seafood cioppino

The basic component of this dish is salted cod. Before cooking the seafood cioppino I soaked the cod in 5 cups of water for a day. I also changed the water 2 times. The cod wasn't salty at all. In my recipe, I used a combination of shrimp, mussels, scallops with cod. But you may combine also other ingredients that you prefer – crab meat, clams etc. You may also use the homemade fish stock or buy it at the store.

Ingredients (16 servings):

Cristobal salted cod	1 lb

Shrimp	½ lb
Scallops	½ lb
Mussels	½ lb

Stew:

diced tomatoes	28 ounces
tomato sauce	6 ounces
onion	1 medium
celery	2 stalks
bell pepper	1 pcs
fish stock	2 cups
garlic	4 cloves, minced
Italian Seasoning	2 tsp
Salt	½ tsp
red pepper flakes	½ tsp
laurel leaf	1 pcs
olive oil	1 tbsp

Fresh parsley (optional)

Pepper and salt at will

Directions:

1. Peel and dice the onions.
2. Wash the sweet pepper, take off the seeds, slice. Wash and dice celery stalks.
3. Wash and chop the parsley finely.
4. Take a large bowl, combine diced tomatoes, tomato sauce, fish stock, onion, celery, sliced bell pepper, garlic, salt, seasoning, pepper flakes, olive oil. Stir well everything.
5. Pour this compound into the Crock Pot, add the laurel leaf.
6. Cover and cook on HIGH for 3 hours.
7. Once the preparation time is over, open the Crock Pot, add cod, scallops, mussels, and shrimp.
8. Cover and continue cooking for 30 minutes on LOW.
9. Take off the laurel leaf before eating.
10. Season with chopped parsley, black pepper at will.
11. Bon Appetite!

250. Pepper lemon tilapia with asparagus

This recipe contains only 5 simple ingredients. It is one of the easiest and tastiest recipes for seafood products. You may use also lime juice instead of lemon one and another seasoning you prefer. I think this is the best combination of tilapia, asparagus, lemon and butter you could only think!

Ingredients (5 servings):

Asparagus	1 bundle
Tilapia fillets	4-6 pcs
lemon juice	8-12 tablespoons
pepper lemon seasoning	1/2 tablespoon
butter	1/2 tablespoon

salt and pepper at will

Directions:
1. Wash and divine the asparagus bundle by the number of fillets.
2. Spread the bottom of the Crock Pot with cooking spray, put the fillets on the bottom, sprinkle fillets with seasoning.
3. Squeeze the juice of a lemon and add to fillets.
4. Add butter on the top of each fillet.
5. Dress with salt and pepper, top the fillets with asparagus.
6. Cover and put on LOW for 3 hours.
7. Enjoy warm.
8. Bon Appetite!

251.Crock Pot keto mackerel

This recipe is rather simple and pretty tasty for those who are lazy or are busy all day long during the whole weekend. I don't know what could be easier than to prepare the mackerels using only water, a fish sauce that could be bought at the store, Asian species and ginger. It is appetizing. Try to cook it today!

Ingredients (6 servings):

Mackerels	2 pcs
Water	3 cups
Fish sauce	1 cup
Ground ginger	2 tbsp
Parsley	3/4 cup
Asian 5 spice, to taste	½ tablespoon

Pepper and salt at will

Directions:
1. Wash, clean the mackerels, take off the inside, cut into slices.
2. Peel the ground ginger and slice.
3. Spread the cooking spray over the bottom of the Crock Pot.

4. Put there mackerels slices, add water and fish sauce, ginger, chopped parsley, species, salt at will.
5. Cover and cook 4 hours on LOW.
6. Serve warm.
7. Bon Appetite!

252.Crock Pot seafood gumbo

Frankly speaking, I have never cooked the seafood gumbo before I visited my old friend. This amazing dish could be served both for lunch, dinner or supper. It contains both main dish and stews or soups. It is perfectly well in a cold time of the year when you are dreaming about sunny summer and sea…

Ingredients (7 servings):

Mussels	2 lb
medium shrimp	2 bags
head of cabbage	1 half
clams	4 can
onion	1 pcs medium
tomato paste	1 small can
water	½ cup

salt and pepper to taste

Directions:

1. Peel the onion and mince finely. Chop the cabbage into pieces.
2. Take the Crock Pot, put shrimps, clams, chopped cabbage, minced onion, mussels.
3. Take a little bowl, combine water with tomato paste, whisk all together. Pour the mixture into the Crock Pot over the mussels.
4. Cover and cook on LOW for 5 hours.
5. Once the time is over, season the dish with salt and pepper.
6. Eat warm.
7. Bon Appetite!

253.Crock Pot sole in onion sauce

Among the usual dishes in Spain sole is the most expanded dish. But it is usually roasted and eaten with rice. I decided to cook this tender fish in the Crock Pot and I must say I have chosen the right route! If you would like to eat the sauce of the smooth consistency with this fish I advise you to add a little bit flour and stir the sauce.

Ingredients (7 servings):

Sole	4 medium pcs
Brown onion sauce	½ cup
red onions	4 medium pcs

garlic	5 cloves
cooking wine	1 glass
water	2 glasses
salt at will	
olive oil	2 tablespoons
fresh parsley (optional)	

Directions:

1. Peel red onions and slice. Peel the garlic, mince it finely.
2. Wash fresh parsley and chop.
3. Take a medium skillet. Add olive oil, garlic minced, dry a little bit and take them out into a large bowl.
4. Add at the same skillet sliced onions, roast until golden. Add water, after some minutes add wine and steam it. Season with pepper and salt, add chopped parsley. Stir everything a little bit.
5. Add to the Crock Pot a mixture from the skillet and a bowl. Toss everything. Add onion sauce.
6. Put the sole into the sauce.
7. Cover and cook on LOW for 2 hours.
8. Once the time is over, take the fish out and let the sauce simmer some minutes more. It must get a smooth consistency.
9. Serve warm with keto bread.
10. Bon Appetite!

254.Crock Pot keto stuffed squid

Many people don't like to cook squid because of its smell. As for me, I like the result more than cooking process. For me it's not a problem to cook them and breathe their smell, I think more about their tender meat and delicious taste that I will get in some hours. I usually fill the squids and sale them with a toothpick when they are hot. Pour the ready-made squids with the rest of the liquid and enjoy!

Ingredients (6 servings):

Squids	8 large pcs
red onions	10 medium pcs
prawns	16 pcs
garlic	3 tsp
parsley	3 tsp
olive oil	2 tbsp
salt and pepper to taste	

Directions

1. Peel red onions and slice. Peel the garlic.
2. Wash squids finely. Rinse them, chop tentacles, remove the fins.
3. Add to the bottom of the Crock Pot olive oil and the sliced onions. Put on HIGH, onions must get a golden color.
4. Take a medium bowl, add water and boil prawns for 1 minute. They mustn't be cooked through! Once the minute is over, remove them and put in the cold water. Peel them finely and chop.
5. Once the onions are golden, add squid. After some minutes add prawns. Dress with pepper and salt.
6. Cover and cook on LOW for 2 hours.
7. Once the time is over, remove the squid to a plate and stuff them with cooked prawns, garlic, parsley, onions.
8. Seal the filled squids with a toothpick.
9. Serve hot, season with fresh parsley optional.
10. Bon Appetite!

255.Mediterranean octopus casserole

Everything I could say about this dish – delicious! This simple, light and flavor casserole is a full swallow of the sea foods. Red and yellow pepper let your dish be full of color and taste. You may add also more or less spicy paprika to stress the taste or to reduce it (without using paprika at all).

Ingredients (10 servings):

boiled octopus	1 lb
onion	1 1/2 large pcs
yellow peppers	2 medium pcs
red pepper	1 1/2 large
garlic	6 cloves
salt	1 Tsp
spicy paprika	1 tsp
parsley	2 Tsp
olive oil	2 tbsp
water	½ cup

pepper to taste

Directions:

1. Peel the onion and dice. Peel the garlic, mince.
2. Wash and chop finely parsley. Set aside.
3. Wash the peppers, take off the seeds, cut julienne style.
4. Wash and cut octopus, slice 1-inch or less, let them boil in a medium bowl for 4-5 minutes.

5. On the bottom of the Crock Pot, add olive oil, minced garlic, diced onions, salt, sliced peppers, black pepper (optional), paprika, water. Stir everything well.
6. Add octopus to the mixture in the Crock Pot. Cover and cook on LOW for half an hour.
7. Serve right away.
8. Season with fresh parsley.
9. Bon Appetite!

256.Crock Pot tuna casserole

I prepare this tuna casserole as an addition to cauliflower rice or keto bread that I cook in the Crock Pot for my family also. It has a creamy texture, is light and is the best variant for supper actually. If you or your family doesn't like celery soup, use another one. Don't be afraid. The taste will be also well. What about the mayo, homemade or bought in the store are also possible.

Ingredients (9 servings):

canned tuna	2 (12 ounces) cans
hard-boiled eggs	6 pcs
condensed cream	1 (10 3/4 ounce) can
condensed cream of celery soup	1 (10 3/4 ounce) can
mayonnaise	1 cup
onion powder	1/2 tsp
garlic powder	1/2 tsp
black pepper	1 tsp
diced celery	3 cup
salt to taste	

Directions:

1. Drain the liquid of tuna and add it into the Crock Pot.
2. Peel the eggs and chop them. Add to the Crock Pot too.
3. Wash and dice the celery.
4. Add to the Crock Pot also condensed cream, celery soup, onion powder, mayo, garlic powder, salt and black pepper. Stir everything well.
5. Cover and cook on LOW for 4 hours.
6. Serve warm with keto bread.
7. Bon Appetite!

257.Crock Pot squid stew

This time I recommend you to cook squid stew Spanish style. Cooking the squids slowly in the Crock Pot they totally change their natural structure. The collagen in the squid melts and turns into gelatin. I think the taste of squid is something like silken Tofu. I don't recommend you to season the stew too much because chorizo is salty enough. Just taste your dish all the time. Enjoy the delicious flavor of the fresh seafood.

Ingredients (12 servings):

Squid Tubes	1 lb
Shallot	1 large pcs
Spring Onions	2-3 cloves
Fresh Tomatoes	3-4 pcs
White wine	1 cup
Butternut Pumpkin	1 pcs
Chorizo Sliced	1 cup
Chili Pepper	1 pcs
Paprika	1 pinch
Bay leaves	2 pcs
Lemon Thyme	1 sprig
Butter	2 tbsp

Pepper and salt to taste

Directions:

1. Clean the squids, score the tubes of the squids with a knife, make criss-cross scores on the squids.
2. Peel shallots and onions and cut them. Chop finely the chili pepper.
3. Wash and dice the butternut pumpkin (10 mm cubes).
4. Wash fresh tomatoes, cut into halves.
5. Take a medium saucepan, add butter, melt and add chorizo. Fry 5 minutes until golden, take off to a plate.
6. To the same saucepan add shallots, roast a little bit, remove. Add the thyme, paprika, onions, let it soften 3-4 minutes.
7. Add wine and steam alcohol fully. Add tomatoes and simmer 8-9 minutes. Tomatoes must be collapsed fully. Season with pepper.
8. Pour the mixture into the Crock Pot, add chorizo, shallots, toss the squid. Be sure the squid is covered with liquid fully.
9. Add bay leaves, cubes of butternut pumpkin, chilies.
10. Cover and put on LOW for 1 hour.
11. Season with a little bit paprika.
12. Bon Appetite!

258.Crock Pot Indian-style fish curry

What is the best way to cook your keto fish? No, not roasting at the skillet! But to cook in the Crock Pot! Let it simmer 2 hours on HIGH and your favorite fish fillet will be mild and will take all flavors of species. I used halibut for this recipe, but it could be also another fish you prefer – sole, cod, seabass, etc.

Ingredients (11 servings):

serrano chilies	2 pcs
coriander seeds	1 teaspoon whole
onion	½ pcs
fresh turmeric	1 inch
fresh ginger	1 inch
garlic	2 cloves
tamarind paste	2 tablespoons
ground cumin	1 teaspoon
mild curry powder	1 tablespoon
unsweetened coconut milk	2 cans (13.5 ounces each)
firm white-fish fillets (halibut)	2 pounds
Fresh cilantro (optional)	
Kosher salt	

Directions:

1. Peel and finely chop the onion.
2. Peel and grate ginger.
3. Peel the garlic, slice thinly.
4. Wash and chop fresh cilantro (optional).
5. Remove the seeds from chilies and slice.
6. Wash the fish fillets and cut into 2-3-inch pieces.
7. Add to the blender (or food processor) chilies, coriander seeds, turmeric, onion, garlic, ginger, curry powder, cumin, a little bit salt, blend everything until smooth form.
8. Put this mixture in a skillet and add coconut milk, let it boil.
9. Pour the mixture into the Crock Pot, place fish fillets into it.
10. Cover and cook on HIGH 2 hours.
11. Season with black pepper, fresh cilantro.
12. Bon Appetite!

259.Crock Pot Brazilian Fish Stew

It seems that every nation has its own version of seafood stew. The Brazilian fish stew is also called *moqueca*, it is cooked of fish fillets, onion, garlic, tomato sauce, coconut milk. I tried to cook this Brazilian stew with many various fish fillets, like salmon, tilapia, sole. My best choice is for the sole. The recipe is very simple, it is exotic, flavor and delicious.

Ingredients (6 servings):

Fish Fillet (sole)	2 lb
Tomatoes	2-3 large pcs

Onions	2 pcs medium
tomato sauce	1 cup
coconut milk	2 cups
olive oil	1 teaspoon

Parsley and cilantro for garnish

Salt, pepper at will

Directions:

1. Wash the fish fillets, take all the bones if necessary.
2. Cut fillets into smaller pieces.
3. Peel onion, slice.
4. Peel the garlic and mince.
5. Wash tomatoes, cut into large pieces and put into the bottom of the Crock Pot.
6. Add onion, fish, garlic, tomato sauce, coconut milk, olive oil.
7. Cover and cook on HIGH 3 hours.
8. Season with cilantro or fresh parsley.
9. Serve with vegetable salad or cauliflower rice!
10. Bon Appetite!

260.Squid puttanesca recipe

As you have already understood cooking in the Crock Pot is my favorite technique. My Crock Pot cooks squids very tender after some hours. They get the soft texture soak the flavor and species I add. Serve this appetizing dish for dinner or supper with friends. Surprise them with unforgettable taste!

Ingredients (9 servings):

Squid	1 large
olive oil	1 tablespoon
onion	1 large
garlic	2 cloves
tomatoes	1 can (400 grams)
fish stock	150 ml
thyme	2 to 3 sprigs
fennel seeds	1 teaspoon
sweetener	1 teaspoon

Salt and pepper to taste

Directions:

Wash and clean the squid, remove tentacles. Rinse inside the squid well.

1. Slice squid into thin pieces (rings).
2. Peel and chop the onion. Peel garlic, mince finely.
3. Chop tomatoes from a can. Crush the fennel seeds.
4. Take a medium saucepan, add olive oil, toast onion, garlic and soft ca. 2 minutes.
5. Add chopped tomatoes, stock, salt, thyme, pepper, seeds, sweetener. Stir everything well.
6. Let the sauce boil for some minutes.
7. Pour it into the Crock Pot, add squid rings. Toss everything.
8. Cover and put on LOW for 3 hours.
9. Enjoy warm!
10. Bon Appetite!

261.Crock Pot creamy garlic king prawns

The creamy garlic king prawns are the best appetizing, side dish both for crowd party or family dinner. I think the combination of prawns and creamy sauce is the best compound one could only imagine. Be sure, you can't spoil the products anyway.

Ingredients (7 servings):

green king prawns	2 lb
butter	½ cup
cream	1/2 cup
garlic	2 cloves
chicken stock	1 cup
mustard powder	1/2 tsp
almond flour	1 tbsp

Salt & Pepper at will

Fresh parsley to garnish if desired

Directions:
1. Peel garlic and crush.
2. Peel and devein king prawns.
3. Take a medium pan, heat the butter with garlic until butter is melted.
4. Add flour and stir.
5. Add stock slowly, add cream and continue to stir everything well.
6. Pour the mixture into the Crock Pot, cover and put on HIGH for 30 minutes.
7. Once the time is over, add mustard, pepper, salt to taste.
8. Add king prawns and continue cooking on HIGH for 20minutes.
9. Check the prawns. They must be tender.
10. Bon Appetite!

VEGETARIAN AND VEGAN

262.Crock Pot vegetable soup

This recipe of vegetable soup is excellent for calming the nervous system. You may also add the other herbs according to your own tastes or tastes of your family. Blend the mixture until smooth once the cooking time is over.

Ingredients (11 servings):

Cauliflower	1 head
Watercress	½ cup
olive oil	2 tablespoons
sweet onion	1 medium
leek	1pcs
celery 1 stalk	
water (or vegetable stock)	6 cups
bay leaf	1 pcs
thyme	1 branch
sea salt	2 pinches
dill	1/4 cup

black pepper at will

Directions:

1. Peel and chop the onion. Set aside.
2. Chop the leek, celery, dill.
3. Chop finely the cauliflower.
4. Take a medium-sized skillet, heat the olive oil over medium heat.
5. Add onion, leeks, celery into the skillet and cauliflower florets. Cook about 5 minutes, the onions must be translucent.
6. Add water thyme, and salt at will, bay leaf to the Crock Pot, pour the ready-made veggies from the skillet.
7. Cover the Crock Pot and set on HIGH for 3 hours.
8. Using a blender blend the soup until smooth mix.
9. Add black pepper or cilantro and serve.
10. Dress with watercress.
11. Bon Appetite!

263.Crock Pot broccoli Tofu soup

This easy Crock Pot recipe is great if you need a healthy meal but you don't have time to prepare this meal. It is quick, healthy, full of minerals and vitamins, keto-friendly and tasty! Add Tofu cheese for garnish or fresh basil leaves!

Ingredients (9 servings):

broccoli florets	5 cups (about 16 ounces)
yellow onion	1 medium
garlic	3 cloves
dried oregano	1 teaspoon
freshly grated nutmeg	1/4 teaspoon
vegetable broth	2 1/2 cups
kosher salt	1/2 teaspoon
black pepper	1/4 teaspoon
Tofu cheese low-carb	1 (8-ounce) block

Directions:

1. Peel the onion and slice finely.
2. Peel the garlic and mince.
3. Chop the broccoli florets.
4. Open the Crock Pot and put the broccoli, onion, and garlic in the bottom of the Crock Pot. Add oregano, nutmeg, and vegetable broth.
5. Add Tofu. Cover the Crock Pot and set on HIGH for 2 hours.
6. Once the cooking time is over, use the blender and puree the soup, it must be of smooth consistency.
7. Serve warm. Season with fresh parsley or grated Tofu.
8. Bon Appetite!

264.Easy Vegetarian Roasted Chestnut Soup

I know that not everybody likes chestnuts, but if you still like, you will definitely cook this soup recipe! This vegan chestnut soup is delicious and light. I advise you to check the soymilk when you will buy it at the store as some kinds of them contain sugar.

Ingredients (9 servings):

olive oil	3 tbsp. vegan
celery	1 rib
onion	1 pcs
strong vegetable broth	6 cups
fresh parsley	1/4 cup

ground cloves   1/4 tsp.

bay leaves   2 pcs

chestnuts (roasted and peeled)   12 oz.

unsweetened soymilk   1/4 cup

Salt and pepper at will

Directions:
1. Mince celery. Peel the onion and mince.
2. Wash the parsley and chop.
3. Peel and the cloves and mince finely.
4. Peel and roast the chestnuts.
5. Take a large saucepan, saute minced garlic, celery, onion with oil until softened, about 7 minutes.
6. Open the Crock Pot, add vegetable broth. Add chopped fresh parsley, cloves, bay leaves and the chestnuts. Put the mixture in the skillet. Add soymilk.
7. Toss everything well. Put the Crock Pot on HIGH for 3 hours.
8. Once the cooking time is over, take off the bay leaves, using a blender make a puree.
9. Dress with salt and pepper before serving.
10. Bon Appetite!

265.Crock Pot keto aubergines

An easy vegetarian Crock Pot recipe, full of summer flavors is great for hot sunny days. Simply easy put the ingredients in the morning to the Crock Pot and this one will be ready for dinner, supper or lunch. Enjoy!

Ingredients (14 servings):
olive oil   4 tbsp

red onion   1 pcs

garlic   2 cloves

aubergines   1 lb

ripe tomatoes   6-7 pcs

fennel bulb   1 small

sundried tomatoes   3-4 pcs

coriander seeds   1 tsp

Dressing:

flat leaf parsley   ¼ cup

basil   ¼ cup

chives   2 Tsp

| olive oil | 2 tbsp |
| juice of lemon | 1 pcs |

Topping

| toasted flaked almonds | ½ cup |

keto bread for serving

Directions:

1. Peel the red onion and slice. Peel the garlic and crush it.
2. Slice the bulb.
3. Wash the tomatoes and cut.
4. Wash parsley and chop, wash the basil leaves, chop the chives.
5. Squeeze the juice of a lemon.
6. Open the Crock Pot, pour a little bit olive oil into the Crock Pot, put the onions into the bottom, add crushed garlic.
7. Wash and slice the aubergines into thick slices and salt. Put them into the Crock Pot on top of the mix from onions and tomatoes, fennel and sundried tomatoes.
8. Spread the coriander seeds, season well with salt and pepper.
9. Cover and cook on LOW for 7 hours, the aubergines must be softened.
10. Prepare the dressing – mix together parsley and basil, olive oil, juice of lemon, chives.
11. Transfer the ready dish to a serving plate and drizzle with the dressing.
12. Top with flaked almonds and serve with keto bread.
13. Bon Appetite!

266.Italian vegetable keto bake

An Italian vegetable dish prepared in the Crock Pot, full with sunny courgettes, tomatoes, herbs, and aubergine is irresistible! You may cook this keto dish for parties as an addition to the main dish or eat it without anything.

Ingredients (7 servings):

garlic	3 cloves
tomato	1 can
bunch oregano	
pinch chili flakes	
baby aubergines	11oz
Courgettes	2 pcs
roasted red peppers	½ large jar
beef tomatoes	3 pcs
bunch basil if desired	
green salad at will	

Directions:

1. Peel the garlic and mince.
2. Chop tomatoes from the can
3. Wash the courgettes and slice, chop baby aubergines. Slice beef tomatoes.
4. Open the Crock Pot, put the garlic, chopped tomatoes, oregano leaves, chili and some seasoning, add olive oil if necessary.
5. Add chopped aubergines, tomatoes, courgettes, red peppers, basil and remaining oregano. Repeat vegetable layer, herb, and tomatoes. Push down well to compress, set on HIGH for 5 hours.
6. Serve with the basil leaves and the green salad.
7. Bon Appetite!

267.Vegetarian Korma Crock Pot keto

Today I would like to present you an exotic Indian dish, extremely flavorful and spiced. I usually serve this keto dish with cooked cauliflower rice and keto bread. Enjoy the real Indian food full of tasty veggies and an unreal mix of species.

Ingredients:

vegetable oil	1 1/2 tablespoons
onion	1 small pcs
fresh ginger root	1 teaspoon
garlic	4 cloves
fresh jalapeno pepper	1 pcs
ground unsalted cashews	3 tablespoons
tomato sauce	1 (4 ounces) can
salt	2 teaspoons
curry powder	1 1/2 tablespoons
frozen onions	1 cup
green bell pepper	1/2 pcs
red bell pepper	½ pcs
fresh cilantro for garnish	1 bunch

Directions:

1. Peel the onion and slice.
2. Mince fresh ginger.
3. Take off the seeds from jalapeno pepper.
4. Peel the onion and mince.
5. Chop the previously wash pepper, remove the seeds and chop finely.
6. Take a medium-sized skillet, heat the oil over medium heat. Add the onion, cook until tender. Add ginger and garlic, continue cooking 3 minutes.

7. Open the Crock Pot, add pre-cooked mix, put jalapeno, toasted cashews, tomato sauce. Add frozen onions.
8. Place into the Crock Pot bell peppers, add curry powder, cover and put on LOW for 3 hours.
9. Garnish with cilantro.
10. Enjoy!

268.Crock Pot easy keto soup

You know, something happens to fresh vegetables usually when they are cooked slowly for a long time in the Crock Pot. Your kitchen is full of aromas and the veggie soup is super tender and light!

Ingredients (5 servings):

Leeks	8 oz (225 g)
spinach	8 oz
onion	1 pcs small
vegetable stock	2½ pints
bay leaves	2 pcs

salt and black pepper at will

fresh chives for garnish

Directions:

1. Trim and wash the leeks, cut into 2-inch pieces.
2. Peel chop finely the onions.
3. Wash and cut the spinach.
4. Open the Crock Pot and put the leeks, onion, bay leaves, dressed with pepper and salt. Add vegetable stock.
5. Cover the lid and put on LOW for 3 hours.
6. When the time is almost finished, open the lid and put spinach.
7. Serve warm fresh chives, dress with pepper and salt.
8. Bon Appetite!

269.Crock Pot vegetarian stew keto recipe

One of my favorite flavor vegetarian stews is this one. If you want to get the creamy texture of it, use the blender or the food processor you have at home and blend the stew at the end of the cooking.

Ingredients (11 servings):

Onion	1 medium pcs
Celery	1 stalk
Kale	4 cup
garlic	4 clove

Italian Seasoning   1 tsp

diced tomatoes   1 can

pumpkin   2 cups canned

chicken broth   4 cup

chicken breast   2 breast

sea salt   1/8 tsp

black pepper, ground 1/8 tsp

Directions:
1. Peel the onions, chop finely.
2. Chop the leek. Chop the kale.
3. Peel the garlic and mince.
4. Open the Crock Pot and put everything into the Crock Pot, cover the lid and set on LOW for 7 hours.
5. Once the time is over, serve the dish tor and season additionally with black pepper.
6. Bon Appetite!

270.Crock Pot pumpkin chili recipe

Have you ever tried pumpkin chili recipe? Not yet!? Poor you! It is amazing, flavor, delicious recipe. Smooth texture and tender veggies are perfect! You may also add other variations of veggies if you don't like tomatoes, onion or something else.

Ingredients (11 servings):
diced tomatoes   2 (14.5-ounce) cans

pumpkin pureed   1 cup

diced yellow onion   2 cups

yellow bell pepper   1 medium pcs

chili powder   1 Tsp

cinnamon   1 tsp

cumin   1 tsp

nutmeg   1/4 tsp

ground cloves   1/8 tsp

kosher salt   1/2 tsp

ground black pepper 1/2 Tsp

Directions:
1. Peel the onion and dice finely.
2. Wash the pepper and slice finely.

3. Open the Crock Pot, put diced tomatoes, pumpkin puree, onion, pepper, a little bit chili powder, cinnamon, cumin, nutmeg, ground cloves, pepper and salt at will.
4. Toss everything together. Add water if needed.
5. Cover the lid and put on LOW for 4 hours.
6. Serve hot!
7. Bon Appetite!

271.Crock Pot tomato soup recipe

Crock Pot tomato soup is perfectly well on hot summer days. Do you know my keto bread recipe? Not yet? Search quickly for this recipe and enjoy with colorful tomato soup during hot days. Serve with fresh parsley, dill or basil leaves.

Ingredients (10 servings):

Diced Tomatoes Canned	56 ounces
Vegetable Broth/Stock	2 cups
yellow onion	½ pcs
dried thyme	1 teaspoon
oregano	1 teaspoon
garlic	½ teaspoon
salt	½ teaspoon
black pepper	¼ teaspoon
Bay Leaf	1 whole
Butter	4 tablespoons

Parsley or dill for garnish

Directions:
1. Peel the onion and cut finely. Peel the garlic and mince it.
2. Open the Crock Pot, put diced tomatoes, vegetable stock, onion, dried thyme, oregano, minced garlic, salt at will, bay leaf, black pepper, butter. Toss everything well.
3. Cover the lid and put on LOW for 3 hours.
4. Once the cooking time is over, serve the ready-made tomato soup to the deep plates. Eat with keto bread.
5. Bon Appetite!

272.Crock Pot spaghetti squash

This vegan spaghetti squash is the best one among vegan recipes. You may it this with various dressings, fish, vegetables, sauces. To cook spaghetti squash in the Crock Pot is so easy! No efforts, no troubles, you don't need to wash a huge number of dishes! Simplicity is a virtue!

Ingredients (2 servings):

squash	1 pcs large

water   1-2 cups

salt at will

Directions:
1. Take squash that corresponds to the size of a Crock Pot.
2. Wash it and make some holes with fork Pierce 4-5 times.
3. Put the squash in the Crock Pot, add water.
4. Cover and put on HIGH (4 hours).
5. Take off the squash to a plate, let it cool 25 minutes.
6. Cut the squash in half lengthwise, separate the strands by pulling a fork along the flesh.
7. Bon Appetite!

273.Crock Pot Mediterranean eggplant salad

You may eat Mediterranean eggplant salad both hot and cold – anyway it is delicious! I tried two ways of its cooking – roasting the onions with peppers or adding them to the Crock Pot at once. You may also add other species to get the dish more flavor.

Ingredients (6 servings):

red onion   1 pcs large

bell peppers   2 pcs

eggplant   1 large

whole tomatoes   1 24 ounces can

smoked paprika   1 tablespoon

cumin   2 teaspoons

salt   1 teaspoon

black pepper to taste

juice lemon   1 pcs

Directions:
1. Peel and slice the onion.
2. Wash, take off the seeds and slice sweet peppers. Set aside.
3. Wash and quarter the eggplant.
4. Squeeze the juice of a lemon into a cup.
5. Open the Crock Pot, add the juice of lemon, pepper, cumin, paprika, onion, tomatoes, eggplant, peppers, salt. Stir everything well.
6. Cover and put on LOW for 6 hours.
7. Enjoy hot with keto bread!
8. Bon Appetite!

274.Keto Vindaloo vegetables

This dish is great for those who like one-pot meals. It could be eaten as an addition to the main dish or as a separate dish. You may add here also other veggies you prefer. Don't cook the veggies more than mentioned time, otherwise, your veggies would be mushed.

Ingredients (14 servings):

garlic   3 cloves

ginger   1 tablespoon

ground coriander   1 1/2 teaspoon

ground cumin   1 1/4 teaspoon

dry mustard   1/2 teaspoon

cayenne pepper   1/2 teaspoon

turmeric   1/2 teaspoon

cardamom   1/4 teaspoon

vinegar   1 tablespoon

yellow onion   1 large

cauliflower florets   4 cups

tomato paste   6 ounces (one small can)

zucchini   2 small

bell pepper   1 small

Salt and freshly ground black pepper to taste

Directions:

1. Peel the garlic and mince.
2. Peel the ginger and chop.
3. Peel the onion and chop.
4. Wash and cut zucchini into 1/3-inch pieces.
5. Wash and take off the seeds from the bell pepper, slice.
6. Mix garlic, ginger, coriander, vinegar, cardamom, turmeric, mustard, cayenne pepper in a blender. Mix until smooth. Set aside.
7. Add to the Crock Pot smooth mixture, cauliflower florets, zucchini, peppers, tomato paste, salt at will.
8. Cover and cook on LOW for 25 minutes.
9. Serve hot!
10. Bon Appetite!

275.Crock Pot cauliflower Bolognese with zucchini noodles

Nothing is so flavor as this vegan cauliflower Bolognese made in the Crock Pot! The cauliflower is engrained with tomato sauce, species, pepper. It is like hearty pasta but without meat. The consistency of cauliflower Bolognese is like a real meat sauce! I'm sure, even those who are not vegan will like this dish.

Ingredients (9 servings):
Preparing for bolognese:

Cauliflower	1 head
red onion	3/4 cup
garlic	2 small cloves
dried oregano flakes	2 tsp
dried basil flakes	1 tsp
tomatoes	2 14oz Cans
vegetable broth	1/2 cup
red pepper flakes	1/4 tsp
salt and pepper, to taste	

Preparing pasta:

Zucchinis	5 large

Directions:
1. Cut cauliflower into florets.
2. Peel onions and dice. Peel the garlic and mince.
3. Wash zucchini. Make zucchini noodles.
4. Place the cauliflower florets, garlic, onion, oregano, basil, tomatoes, broth, pepper flakes, salt into the Crock Pot.
5. Cover and put on HIGH for 3 hours.
6. Once the Bolognese is done, mash cauliflower with a fork, put over the noodles.
7. Bon Appetite!

276. Red Thai veggie curry

This Thai curry is easy while cooking in the Crock Pot. It could be also cooked with coconut cream, for me, it is better when I use coconut milk. Coconut cream gets the dish creamy and smooth texture, as for me I like the light variant of it. You may also change the soy sauce with a hot one. But don't forget to choose the sauces without sugar.

Ingredients (10 servings):

Cauliflower	1/2 head
Onion	1 small
coconut milk	1 (14 oz.) can
soy sauce	3 tbsp

sriracha sauce	1-2 tsp.
salt	1/2 tsp.
red curry paste	3 tbsp
sweetener	1 tbsp
toasted cashews (optional)	1/2 cup
fresh cilantro (optional)	1/4 cup
fresh basil leaves at will	

Directions:

1. Wash and cut cauliflower into florets.
2. Wash cilantro and chop. Set aside.
3. Peel the onion and chop finely.
4. Take a medium bowl, mix coconut milk, both sauces, curry paste, sweetener, pepper, and salt.
5. Pour the mixture into the Crock Pot, add cauliflower and onion. Toss everything together. The veggies must be coated.
6. Cover and put on LOW for 2 hours.
7. Once the dish is done, serve with toasted cashews, chopped cilantro, basil.
8. Bon Appetite!

277.Spicy Maple Meatballs

The natural Canadian maple syrup together with allspice allows the meatballs be spicy and flavorful. These vegan meatballs are incredible! If you would like to get the one-pot meal you may add a little (1-2 cups) of vegetable broth or water and get delicious meatball soup.

Ingredients (11 servings):

olive oil	1 tbsp.
white onion	½ pcs
red bell pepper	1 pcs
green bell pepper	1 pcs
jalapeno peppers	2 pcs
plain tomato sauce	1 1/2 cups
maple syrup	1 cup
almond flour	2 tbsp.
ground allspice	2 tsp.
liquid smoke (optional)	1/8 tsp.
frozen vegan meatballs	1 bag

Directions:

1. Peel the onion, chop it finely.
2. Wash and take off the seeds from the peppers, slice them. Set aside.
3. Add olive oil to the Crock Pot, add onion and peppers.
4. Take a medium bowl add flour, maple syrup, tomato sauce, allspice, liquid smoke. Mix all together until smooth consistency. Pour into the Crock Pot.
5. Add frozen meatballs. Cover and cook on LOW for 5 hours.
6. The sauce should be thick and cover the meatballs.
7. Serve warm over cauliflower rice.
8. Bon Appetite!

278.Crock Pot spiced cauliflower

It is a classic Indian cauliflower dish. This hot, flavor dish tingle my taste buds. I can't say I am a fan of cauliflower, but this combination is amazing! You just forget you eat simple cauliflower dish! I think you must also give this dish go. Add your favorite species to this one.

Ingredients (13 servings):

cauliflower	1 large
onion	1 medium pcs
tomato	1 medium
ginger root	1 2-inch piece
garlic	2 cloves
jalapeño peppers	2 pcs
cumin seeds	1 Tbsp
cayenne pepper	1 pinch
garam masala	1 Tbsp
kosher salt	1 Tbsp
turmeric	1 tsp
vegetable oil	3 Tbsp
fresh cilantro	1 Tbsp

Directions:

1. Rinse cauliflower, cut into 1-inch pieces.
2. Peel and dice onion.
3. Wash tomato, dry with paper towel, dice.
4. Peel and grate ginger root.
5. Peel and grate the garlic.
6. Remove the seeds from jalapenos, slice.
7. Wash fresh cilantro, chop finely.

8. Put in the Crock Pot cauliflower florets, onion, tomato, ginger, garlic, peppers, masala, salt, turmeric, oil. Stir everything well.
9. Cover and put on LOW for 2 hours.
10. Serve with fresh cilantro.
11. Bon Appetite!

279.Crock Pot flavor Brussels sprouts

This simple dish is appetizing and flavor. This dish includes only 4 simple ingredients (and pine nuts optional. You may also use other nuts you prefer.) All steps you need to do – just to wash the sprouts, put them to the machine and wait. Pour the flavor mixture and that's all!

Ingredients (4 servings):

Brussels sprouts	2 pounds
olive oil	2 tablespoons
salt at will	
pepper optional	
pine nuts at will	
balsamic vinegar	½ cup
sweetener	1-2 tablespoons

Directions:

1. Rinse the sprouts, halve them.
2. Pour olive oil and place sprouts, season them with salt.
3. Cover the Crock Pot, put on LOW for 2 hours.
4. Take a bowl and mix balsamic vinegar with sweetener (like Splenda).
5. Once the veggies are almost done, remove them to a plate and drizzle with the mixture.
6. Dress with toasted pine nuts.
7. Enjoy warm!
8. Bon Appetite!

280.Crock Pot keto ratatouille

I think everyone has eaten ratatouille or has heard about this famous dish at least. This recipe isn't new to you but this is the keto version prepared in the Crock Pot. As for me, I think, it is easier than to cook it in the oven. Just put the ingredients in the Crock Pot and do your business!

Ingredients (7 servings):

sauce

tomato	4 medium
Red sweet pepper	2 small
Garlic	1 clove
Water	1/4 cup

black pepper

ratatouille

zucchini	1 medium
eggplant	1/2 lb
Green pepper	1 oz

Directions:
1. Prepare the sauce – wash the sweet pepper, take off the seeds, slice.
2. Peel the garlic, chop finely.
3. Wash and crush tomatoes.
4. Blend tomatoes, pepper, salt, garlic, water in a blender. Set aside.
5. Wash and slice zucchini and eggplant.
6. Place veggies into the Crock Pot, pour the sauce.
7. Cover and put on LOW for 2 hours.
8. Bon Appetite!

281.Crock Pot Butternut Dhal

I'm always happy when the dish is simple to cook and it satisfies my taste buds! This dish is perfect for all my family, it comes on our weekly meal plan. One may prepare this in the morning and leave (on WARM) till supper. You may also keep it in the fridge for some days.

Ingredients (10 servings):

red onion	1 pcs
avocado oil	2 tbsp
garlic purée	1 tsp
ginger purée	1 tsp
red chili	1 pcs
curry powder	4 Tsp
coconut milk	3 cups
vegetable stock	1 Tsp
butternut squash	1 lb
green chili	1 pcs

fresh coriander at will

Directions:
1. Peel and chop the onion. Take off the seeds from chili, slice.
2. Take a medium saucepan, add oil, fry onions, add garlic and ginger puree, curry and chili. Stir everything well. It takes ca. 5 minutes. Set aside.
3. Wash, peel the butternut squash. Cut it into cubes.

4. Pour this in the Crock Pot, add coconut milk, vegetable stock. Add squash. Season with salt and pepper.
5. Cover and cook on HIGH 3 hours. The consistency must be creamy.
6. Wash the coriander and chop finely.
7. Dress the ready-made dish with fresh coriander.
8. Bon Appetite!

282.Crock Pot keto aubergines

This simple vegan recipe is ideal for busy mornings. You may dress this dish with additional species you prefer, roasted almonds or cashews. One may also use avocado oil or vegetable oil at will. Eat this flavor one warm!

Ingredients (12 servings):

olive oil	4 tbsp
red onion	1 pcs
garlic	2 cloves
aubergines	1 lb
ripe tomatoes	2 cups
fennel bulb	1 small
sundried tomatoes	½ cup
coriander seeds	1 tsp
For the dressing:	
Parsley	1/4 cup
Basil	¼ cup
olive oil	2 tbsp
lemon juice	1 lemon

Directions:

1. Peel the onion and slice.
2. Wash and quarter the tomatoes. Slice fennel.
3. Wash and chop finely the parsley and basil leaves.
4. Squeeze the juice of a lemon.
5. Peel the garlic and crush.
6. Wash the aubergines, slice thinly.
7. Pour the olive oil into the Crock Pot (a half), put onions, garlic, sliced aubergines. Pour the rest of olive oil.
8. Put on the top of the tomatoes, fennel, sundried tomatoes, season with pepper, coriander seeds, salt.
9. Cover and cook on LOW for 5 hours.
10. Combine in a little bowl parsley, basil, olive oil and lemon juice. Whisk everything well.

11. Remove the ready dish to a plate and pour the dressing.
12. Bon Appetite!

283.Crock Pot cabbage soup

If you have some cabbage in the refrigerator, you must definitely cook this cabbage soup. It is very easy and is great for dinner! Simple ingredients that cost not so much and could be found at any store. This keto soup is cooked in the Crock Pot, it means it could be cooked even when you are not at home!

Ingredients (8 servings):

cabbage	1/2 small (4-5 cups)
onion	1 pcs
garlic	4-5 cloves
diced tomatoes	3 1/2 cups
tomato sauce	1 1/2 cups
vegetable broth	4-5 cups
dried parsley	1 tbsp
oregano	1 tsp
salt at will	

Directions:

1. Peel and chop the onion.
2. Peel the garlic and mince.
3. Shred the cabbage.
4. Put cabbage, onion, garlic, sauce, diced tomatoes, broth, oregano, and parsley.
5. Cover and cook on HIGH 3 hours.
6. Serve hot.
7. Bon Appetite!

284.Keto creamy cauliflower soup

The keto cauliflower soup is definitely easy to cook. The coconut milk adds the creamy texture, it gets light and silk. Serve this soup with fresh basil leaves or chopped parsley, veggie salad or keto bread.

Ingredients (9 servings):

Cauliflower	1 large head
red pepper	3/4 cup (1 medium)
onion	1/2 cup
curry powder	3 tsp
fresh ginger	2 tsp

salt	1/2 tsp
red pepper	1/8 tsp
vegetable broth	4 cups
coconut milk	1 14 oz can

Directions:

1. Rinse the cauliflower, cut into about 1 1/2" pieces.
2. Wash and chop the red peppers.
3. Peel the onion, chop finely. Peel the ginger and grate it.
4. Mix florets, pepper, onion, curry, ginger, salt, broth in the Crock Pot. Stir everything well.
5. Cover and put on LOW for 3 hours. The veggies must be tender.
6. Pour the coconut milk and continue cooking 2 hours more.
7. Once the time is over, blend the mixture until smooth.
8. Serve warm.
9. Bon Appetite!

285.Creamy Roasted Red Pepper Soup

I like this vegan red pepper soup for its color! Bright, sunny, happy soup will make your day today! It is full of the flavor of roasted pepper, coconut milk make its consistency tender. A combination of shallots, kale, peppers creates a velvety smooth soup.

Ingredients (11 servings):

organic coconut oil	2tablespoons
red pepper	1/2cup
shallot	1large
celery salt	1teaspoon
organic paprika	1teaspoon
red pepper flakes	1pinch
kale	4 to 5 cups
vegetable stock	4cups
cider vinegar	1splash
fresh thyme	1pinch
coconut milk (canned)	1cup

Directions:

1. Peel the shallots, chop finely. Chop the kale.
2. Crush the pepper flakes. Wash and remove the seeds from the peppers. Slice them
3. Take a medium saucepan, add oil and put on a high heat.
4. Sautee shallots ca. 2-3 minutes. Add there sliced peppers. Season them well. Roast them ca.3-4 minutes.

5. Add to the Crock Pot the mixture from the saucepan, salt, paprika, pepper flakes, kale, stock, vinegar. Stir everything well.
6. Cover and put on LOW for 2 hours.
7. Add coconut milk, thyme, vinegar and blend everything.
8. Cook another half an hour.
9. Bon Appetite!

SIDE DISHES

286.Mashed Cauliflower with Chives and Parmesan cheese

Cauliflower is a healthy ingredient and great substitute for potatoes and other vegetables full of carbohydrates. Firstly, this new recipe doesn't appear so delicious, tender and creamy. But if you follow my instructions, you'll get the tender texture of cauliflower with chicken broth (you may also use vegetable one), joined with grated cheese and also chives. Remember, that potato isn't as healthy as you think. Just say «hello» to your new friend – cauliflower!

Ingredients (4 servings):

Cauliflower   2 small heads

chicken broth   2 cups

Parmesan cheese   ¼ cup

fresh chives   ¼ cup

Kosher salt

ground black pepper at will

Directions:
1. Wash the cauliflower, remove the leaves and core, cut it into small pieces (florets).
2. Grate the Parmesan cheese on a plate. Set aside.
3. Wash and chop the fresh chives.
4. Take a bowl medium-size, combine the cauliflower florets and two cups of chicken broth.
5. Pour it into the Crock Pot, cover and set on LOW for 1 hour, until the cauliflower florets get tender It must not fall apart. Be attentive!
6. Once the time is over, use a long spoon and take off the cauliflower to a blender if you have in a food processor. Puree cauliflower until smooth texture.
7. Transfer mashed cauliflower into a small bowl and stir in the grated Parmesan and fresh chives.
8. Season with salt at will and ground pepper.
9. Serve warm.

287.Rosemary garlic cauliflower Crock Pot

You may ask me, what do we prepare this side dish for? The mashed cauliflower recipe is frequently compared with mashed potatoes. It has a similar texture, consistency and conjoined with similar foods. But wait, it tastes quite different! Cauliflower isn't the same product as a potato. Both taste amazing, but don't forget about your ketogenic diet! I hope you give this recipe a try.

Ingredients (5 servings):

Cauliflower   1 large

fat cream cheese   3 ounces

unsalted butter	2 tablespoons
minced garlic	1 1/2 teaspoon
fresh rosemary	1 tablespoon

salt and pepper at will

Directions:

1. Wash the cauliflower, remove the leaves and core, cut it into small pieces (florets).
2. Peel the garlic and mince it. You may saute it if you prefer.
3. Wash the rosemary and chop into small pieces.
4. Open the Crock Pot and put the cauliflower florets into, add a little bit water (1/2 cup), cover and put on LOW for 1 hour.
5. Once the time is ready (the cauliflower florets must be tender), remove them from the Crock Pot and let them cool a little.
6. Put the cooked cauliflower in a food processor or a blender, add fat cream cheese, unsalted butter, minced garlic, chopped rosemary and salt if desired. Blend until smooth texture.
7. Serve cool.
8. Bon Appetite!

288.Cauliflower casserole with tomato and Goat cheese

I like to cook the dishes that don't need to much time especially if I'm tired after a hard working day! So, today I cook the cauliflower casserole with crumbled Goat cheese and canned tomatoes. It is a perfect casserole, full of vegetables and tastes. Tomatoes, Goat cheese, and cauliflower – what could be easier?

Ingredients (12 servings):

cauliflower florets	6 cups
olive oil	4 Tsp
dried oregano	1 tsp
salt	1/2 Tsp
ground pepper	1/2 Tsp
goat cheese crumbled	2 oz.

The Sauce:

olive oil	1 tsp
garlic	3 cloves
crushed tomatoes	1 (28 oz.) can
bay leaves	2 pcs

| salt | 1/4 tsp |
| minced flat-leaf parsley | 1/4 cup |

Directions:

1. Wash the cauliflower, remove the leaves and core, cut it into small pieces (florets).
2. Spray the bottom of the Crock Pot with cooking spray, put the cauliflower florets on the bottom of it, add olive oil, oregano, and pepper. Salt if desired.
3. Cover and cook on LOW for 2 hours until the cauliflower florets get tender and a little bit brown color.
4. While the cauliflower is cooking prepare the sauce: peel the garlic cloves and mince it. Take a medium-sized skillet, heat the olive oil, add garlic and cook 1 minute, stir it thoroughly all the time.
5. Add the crushed tomatoes and bay leaves, let it simmer for some minutes. Remove the bay leaves, dress with pepper and salt. You may also add parsley if you want.
6. Pour the sauce over the cauliflower florets in the Crock Pot once the time is over.
7. Spread the Goat cheese over the dish, cover the Crock Pot and continue cooking for 1 hour on LOW until the cheese is melted.
8. Serve warm!
9. Bon Appetite!

289.Cauliflower with celery puree and garlicky greens

I would like to present you one of my precious purée. It has a creamy combining of tender cauliflower and delicious celery root. This is a quiet combination that is rather tender and delicious when seasoned with a pile of garlicky greens. This time I get excited about this keto side recipe.

Ingredients (8 servings):

For Purée:

celery root	1 medium
cauliflower head	1 small head
salt	1/2 teaspoon
butter	3 Tablespoons

For the preparation of Chard:

Swiss chard	2 bunches
Butter	1Tablespoon
garlic cloves	2 small pcs
red pepper flakes	one pinch or 1/8 tsp

sea salt at will

Directions:

Prepare the purée:

1. Wash the cauliflower head, remove all green leaves and core, cut it into medium-sized pieces (florets).
2. Peel the celery, cut in little or cubes.
3. Open the Crock Pot, put the celery, cauliflower, put the lid and cook on LOW for 2 hours.
4. Take off the vegetables and place them in the saucepan, conjoin butter, salt and blend thoroughly until puree texture.
5. Dress with salt or pepper if desired. Cover while preparing the garlicky greens and set it aside.

Make the Chard:

1. Stack the leaves of Swiss chard, wash, braid them and slice into 1/3-inch strips. Cut the stems very thinly.
2. Take a skillet, heat the butter in it.
3. Peel the garlic and mince it.
4. Add garlic, pepper flakes. Toss everything for 40 seconds just wait until the garlic is tender.
5. Stir in the leaves of chard, toss it in the butter, garlic for 2-4 minutes.
6. Cover the lid of the skillet and let it cook for 4 minutes until the mixture is tender.
7. Dress with sea salt.
8. Dress the puree with the garlicky greens.
9. Bon Appetite!

290.Squeak and Bubble Crock Pot

This English side dish I cooked firstly because I simply liked the name. This traditional recipe is cooked of cauliflower puree, cabbage, roasted and chopped bacon, scallions and Cheddar cheese. So easy and so perfect!

Ingredients (5 servings) :

cauliflower puree	2 cups
cabbage	1 cup
scallion, green only	1/4 cup
salt & pepper to taste	
cooked bacon	1/4 cup
Cheddar cheese	2 oz

Directions:

Prepare the cauliflower puree:

1. Wash the cauliflower, remove the leaves and core, cut it into small pieces (florets).
2. Open the Crock Pot and put the cauliflower florets into, add a little bit water (1/2 cup), cover and put on LOW for 1 hour.
3. Once the time is ready (the cauliflower florets must be tender), remove them from the Crock Pot and let them cool a little.
4. Put the cooked cauliflower in a food processor and blend until smooth texture.

5. Shred the cabbage and steam it for some minutes until softened.
6. Chop the washed scallions.
7. Join the cabbage with the cauliflower puree and scallions, dress with salt and pepper.
8. Shred the Cheddar cheese and chop the bacon.
9. Put in the Crock Pot, season with shredded cheese and put on LOW for 1 hour.
10. Serve with chopped bacon on top.
11. Bon Appetite!

291.Cheddar cauliflower bacon bites Crock Pot

Thinking about more recipes for the side dishes? Here you are! A light mix of cauliflower florets, Cheddar cheese, flour and bacon strips! Light, easy, quick and tasty! I think it is the best way to follow your keto diet and prepare in the Crock Pot. And what about you?

Ingredients (8 servings):

cauliflower florets	4 cups
bacon crisps	6 ounces
egg	1 pcs
baking soda	1 teaspoon
salt	1/4 teaspoon
scallions	1/3 cup
coconut flour	1/2 cup
Cheddar cheese	1 cup

Salt at will

Directions:

1. Wash the cauliflower, remove the leaves and core, cut it into large pieces (florets).
2. Open the Crock Pot and put the cauliflower florets into, add a little bit water (1/2 cup), cover and put on LOW for 1 hour.
3. Once the time is ready (the cauliflower florets must be tender), remove them from the Crock Pot and let them cool a little.
4. Put the cooked cauliflower in a food processor and blend until smooth texture.
5. Wash and chop the scallions. Shred the Cheddar cheese and set aside.
6. Take a large bowl, mix the cauliflower with salt, add cracked egg, chopped scallions, coconut flour, baking soda. Mix everything well.
7. Spray the bottom and sides of the Crock Pot with cooking spray and put the mixture into it.
8. Cover the Crock Pot and put on HIGH for 1 hour.
9. Once the time is over, put the bacon crisps on the top and spread the shredded Cheddar cheese. Cover and put on WARM for one additional hour.
10. Serve warm and enjoy immediately!
11. Bon Appetite!

292.Keto cheese pancetta cauliflower

More variations with cauliflower puree and other vegetables like scallions, adding butter a lot of cheese and pancetta!? Not a problem! Here the recipe for the keto side dish you have looked for! Don't hesitate to cook it!

Ingredients (10 servings):

cauliflower	2 pounds
butter	1/4 cup
salt	1/4 tsp
pepper	1/4 tsp
garlic powder	1/2 tsp
pancetta diced	8 ounces
smoked gruyere	8 ounces
Monterey Jack cheese	8 ounces
cheddar cheese	8 ounces
scallions	1/2 cup

pepper and salt at will

Directions:

1. Wash the cauliflower, remove the leaves and core, cut it into large pieces (florets), you have to cut off all the stems.
2. Open the Crock Pot and put the cauliflower florets into, add a little bit water (1/2 cup), cover and put on LOW for 1 hour.
3. Once the time is ready (the cauliflower florets must be tender), remove them from the Crock Pot and let them cool a little.
4. Put the cooked cauliflower in a food processor and blend until smooth texture.
5. Wash and chop the scallions. Shred the cheese, divide into small portions and set aside.
6. Dice the pancetta. Cook it in a skillet over medium-high heat until crisp. Drain it with the paper towel.
7. Mix in a large bowl butter, salt, pepper, shredded cheese (half), cauliflower, scallions, garlic powder.
8. Add pancetta and save a few pieces for topping.
9. Spread the bottom of the Crock Pot with cooking spray. Pour the mixture, sprinkle the rest of the cheese over the top of the mixture.
10. Cover and put on LOW for 2 hours.
11. Remove the dish from the Crock Pot and let it cool for about 10 minutes.
12. Season with extra pancetta, scallions before eating.
13. Enjoy!

293.Creamy Greek zucchini Crock Pot

This creamy Greek zucchini side dish is flavor and tender. This recipe is a set of health, spring, color, and taste. I advise you to use only the organic eggs, fresh herbs that you may buy at the farmers' shops and fresh feta cheese. You may also change Feta with the other cheese you prefer more.

Ingredients (9 servings):

zucchini	2 lbs (about 7 large)
organic eggs	2 large
fresh herbs	1 cup
almond meal (or keto breadcrumbs)	1 cup
feta cheese	1 cup
ground cumin	1 teaspoon
fine grain sea salt	1 teaspoon
Ground black pepper at will	
olive oil	3 tablespoons

Directions:

1. Wash zucchini, take off the ends.
2. Put them in a blender and grate.
3. Put the grated zucchini in a medium bowl and season with salt. Leave them to drain for 30 minutes.
4. Take handfuls of the grated zucchini, squeeze all of the moisture. Set aside.
5. Take a medium bowl, beat eggs, add zucchini, cumin, herbs, meal. Mix everything. Add salt, feta, and pepper. Stir well.
6. Place the ready mixture in the refrigerator for 30 minutes.
7. Open the Crock Pot, spread the cooking spray or olive oil over the bottom and sides.
8. Put the mixture into the Crock Pot and set on HIGH for 1 hour.
9. Remove the side dish once the time is over.
10. Serve!

294.Garlicky zucchini noodles with Buratta and tomatoes

This recipe of the keto side dish is perfectly well for summer and spring when you have a lot of fresh tomatoes, basil, and zucchini. First time I enjoyed Buratta was a really delicious opening for me! Such a great taste of it. I will not recommend you to change Buratta with the Goat cheese because in this way you wouldn't taste this flavor and taste!

Ingredients (7 servings):

Zucchini	3 medium 9 – 10 inches long each
cherry or grape tomatoes	1 1/2 cup
olive oil	2 Tbsp

garlic	2-3 large cloves
Italian Herb Blend	1 tsp.
Burrata cheese	3 balls

fresh basil for garnish at will

salt and pepper

Directions:

1. Wash the zucchini and take off the ends.
2. Then make the noodles using a julienne cutter.
3. Wash the basil leaves, chop. Set aside.
4. Wash and cut the cherry tomatoes in half.
5. Cut each ball of Burrata cheese into fourths (you may also or crumble it). Heat the oil in a skillet over medium heat.
6. Peel the garlic and mince. Add the garlic cloves, cook until fragrant. It takes you about a minute.
7. Remove garlic from the skillet, add the tomatoes and cook about 3 minutes.
8. Open the Crock Pot, put the noodles, top with tomatoes, cheese add species.
9. Cover and cook on LOW for 1 hour.
10. Serve immediately once the cooking time is over.
11. Bon Appetite!

295.Zucchini noodles in a creamy tomato sauce

Try these delicious and flavor zoodles for a keto dinner as a side dish. Zoodles are quickly covered with the creamy tomato sauce full of brown onion and garlic. A rich pinch of fresh thyme, black pepper, and shredded Parmesan add a special taste to this dish.

Ingredients (10 servings):

olive oil	2 tablespoons
zucchini	3 pcs
onion	1 small
garlic	4 cloves
canned tomatoes	2 cup
water	1/4 cup
vegetable bouillon	1/2 cube
fresh thyme	1/4 teaspoon
heavy cream	1/2 cup
Parmesan cheese	½ cup
Red pepper flakes	

Paprika at will

Salt at will

black pepper if desired

Directions:
1. Wash the zucchini and take off the ends.
2. Then make the noodles by mean of a julienne cutter.
3. Heat a medium-sized skillet over high heat adding a little bit olive oil.
4. Peel the onion, chop finely. Peel the garlic and mince.
5. Sautee the chopped onions, add garlic. It takes you approximately a minute of time. Check the onion it must be softened but not dark brown.
6. Dress with pepper, paprika, salt. Continue cooking for about 3 minutes, onions must be softened.
7. Grate the Parmesan into a bowl. Set aside.
8. Add the crushed tomatoes, solve the bouillon cube in 1/3 cup of water in a large bowl.
9. Pour this mix into the Crock Pot and add thyme. Cover and cook on LOW for 1 hour.
10. Dress with red pepper and salt at will. Once the cooking time is over, add heavy cream, cover and set on WARM for half an hour.
11. Add zucchini noodles and toss. Put on LOW for half an hour.
12. Serve warm.
13. Sprinkle the dish with grated cheese, thyme.
14. Bon Appetite!

296.Crock Pot Keto Cheesy zucchini

Speaking about keto side dishes, I must say, I like light vegetable variations in creamy-cheesy combinations. This recipe recommended as a side dish, prepared in the Crock Pot is a really creative combination of cheese (you may also choose Swiss or parmesan cheese) milk, butter and zucchini noodles. Let's try to cook!

Ingredients (6 servings):

Zucchini	1 pcs
Water	1/2 cup
Salt	1 Tsp
Butter	1 tbsp
Milk	2 tbsp
Cheddar cheese	2/3 - 1 cup

black pepper at will

Directions:
1. Wash the zucchini, dry with a paper towel. Cut the ends of it and with a help of spiralizer make „noodles".
2. Take a saucepan medium-sized, put the noodles into a saucepan, add water, season with salt and let them boil. Noodles must get soft.

3. Shred the Cheddar cheese.
4. Remove the noodles from the Crock Pot, butter, milk, pepper and shredded cheese.
5. Cover and cook on LOW for 30 minutes.
6. Serve warm, add if desired black pepper!
7. Bon Appetite!

297.Keto easy cheesy zucchini gratin

It is a perfect low carb recipe prepared in the Crock Pot! This tasty and flavorful veggie side dish would be a great addition to a roasted chicken or good steak for dinner! I must say, I eat this easy cheesy late in the evenings even without steaks or chickens. It is delicious!

Ingredients (7 servings):

zucchini	4 cups
onion	1 small pcs
pepper Jack cheese	1 1/2 cups
butter	2 Tbsp
garlic powder	1/2 tsp
heavy whipping cream	1/2 cup
salt and pepper to taste	

Directions:

1. Wash and dry with a paper towel zucchini. Slice them. Set aside.
2. Peel the onion, slice thinly.
3. Shred the Jack cheese.
4. Spray the bottom of the Crock Pot with cooking spray. Put the zucchini slices, onion, sprinkle with salt and shredded cheese. Repeat this layer two or three times.
5. Take a little bowl, combine butter, garlic powder, heavy cream, whisk together.
6. Pour the mixture over the zucchini-onion layers. Cover and cook on LOW for 1 hours. The liquid must be thickened; the top must be of brown color.
7. Eat warm.

298.Crock Pot French onion-zucchini

If you would like to inspire a little bit France today, I advise you to prepare this French dish in the Crock Pot. When it comes to healthy and easy food I always remember this recipe. It is my second favorite French recipe after the most famous one French soup.

Ingredients (8 servings):

Zucchinis	2 pcs small
yellow onion	1 small
Splenda	1 teaspoon
fresh thyme	1 teaspoon

unsalted butter	2 tablespoons
beef broth	1/4 cup
Worcestershire sauce	1/4 cup
fontina cheese	1 cup

salt and pepper to taste

Directions:
1. Peel the onion, slice it thinly.
2. Wash and chop fresh thyme. Set aside.
3. Grate fontina cheese.
4. Prepare the French mixture – take a medium skillet, melt butter. Put the sliced onion, season with salt, Splenda, pepper, thyme, Worcestershire sauce. It takes a couple of minutes to let the onion be golden.
5. Wash and dry with a paper towel zucchini. Slice them thinly.
6. Spray the bottom of the Crock Pot with cooking spray, put sliced zucchinis, add broth, pour the French mixture over them, add grated cheese.
7. Cover and cook on LOW for 1 hour.
8. Once the time is over, remove from the oven and cool them a little bit.
9. Garnish with a rest fresh thyme and black pepper.
10. Enjoy!

299.Keto spaghetti-squash with Ricotta

This spaghetti-squash Ricotta will definitely help to keep your keto diet and let you forget about boring spaghetti from flour. When you really want to enjoy your meal, spend a little bit more time than usual preparing spaghetti-squash. It is worth it! I'm pretty sure, you'll be surprised at the result! I try to be creative with the side dishes all the time!

Ingredients (9 servings):
Squash	1 pcs medium sized
olive oil	1 tbsp.
Ricotta cheese	1 3/4 cup
Parmesan cheese	¾ cup
Greek yogurt	1 cup
egg	1 pcs
garlic powder	1/2 tsp.
oregano	1 tsp.

fresh parsley

salt & pepper to taste

Directions:

1. Wash and dry with a paper towel squash.
2. Cut squash in half (lengthwise), remove the seeds.
3. Pour a little bit water into the Crock Pot, put the squash, cover and cook on HIGH for 1 hour. Check the readiness with a fork. Let it cool.
4. Remove the squash, make spaghetti squash. Put them on a plate and add olive oil.
5. Grate the Parmesan and Ricotta cheese into a medium bowl, crack an egg, add Greek yogurt, garlic powder, oregano, black pepper, salt. Mix everything well.
6. Put the spaghetti squash into the Crock Pot again, add the mixture, cover and cook on LOW 1 hour.
7. Wash fresh parsley and garnish the ready dish with it.
8. Bon Appetite!

300.Keto spaghetti-squash with pesto

Spaghetti-squash with pesto is a perfect side dish for weekends! Using a basil pesto makes this dish flavor and appetizing. The dish could be also eaten with marinara sauce instead. Don't forget to add basil pesto after removing the spaghetti-squash to a plate, otherwise (when you add pesto to the Crock Pot) you'll get completely another taste and unappetizing grey color of your dish.

Ingredients (4 servings):

cooked spaghetti squash	2 cups
olive oil	1 Tbsp
fresh mozzarella cheese	4 oz
basil pesto	1/4 cup

Salt and pepper to taste

Directions:

1. Wash the squash.
2. Cut it in half (lengthwise), remove the seeds. Pour a little bit water into the Crock Pot, put the squash, cover and cook on HIGH for 1 hour. Check the readiness with a fork. Let it cool.
3. Remove the squash, make spaghetti squash using a fork. Put them on a plate.
4. Cube the mozzarella cheese.
5. Put the spaghetti-squash into the Crock Pot again, sprinkle with olive oil, add pepper and salt. Put the cubes of mozzarella over spaghetti, cover and cook on LOW 30 minutes.
6. Remove spaghetti to a plate, let it cool about 7 minutes.
7. Drizzle with pesto and black pepper.
8. Bon Appetite!

301.Broccoli Gratin with Parmesan and Swiss cheese

The combination of Parmesan, Swiss cheese, mayo, and broccoli is the best recipe for the keto diet side dish! Once the dish is on the table you see a golden-white color of its covering. Just take a fork and deep into the middle – you'll see a green, bright color of broccoli. A rainbow of tastes and colors in one plate!

Ingredients (7 servings):

bite-size broccoli flowerets	8 cups
Swiss cheese	1 1/2 cups
mayo	8 Tsp
lemon juice	1 1/2 Tbsp
Dijon mustard	3/4 Tsp
green onions	3 Tbsp
Parmesan cheese	1/4 cup

black pepper and salt to taste

Directions:

1. Wash broccoli and cut into small florets.
2. Grate both parmesan and Swiss cheese into a bowl. Set aside.
3. Squeeze juice of a lemon into a cup.
4. Wash and chop the green onions.
5. Spread the cooking spray or olive oil (optional) over the bottom of the Crock Pot.
6. Put broccoli florets in a single layer.
7. Mix in a separate bowl lemon juice, mustard, mayo, black pepper, add to the mixture green onion and grated cheese.
8. Put the mixture over the broccoli, cover and cook on LOW 1 hour.
9. Serve hot.

302. Keto Garlic-Parmesan broccoli

Are you looking for the best recipe for baked broccoli? Here you are! This veggie-cheese combination is everything you need. It will be the best side dish that will fully complete your meal. It is the easiest and quickest way to prepare delicious broccoli. If the main dish doesn't have enough to be a full meal, the garlic-Parmesan broccoli will definitely solve this problem.

Ingredients (5 servings):

broccoli florets (not frozen)	24 ounces
olive oil	3 tbsp
garlic minced	3 Tsp
salt to taste	1 pinch
Parmesan cheese	1/4 cup

Directions:

1. Peel the garlic and mince it. Set aside.
2. Wash the broccoli florets, put them in the bottom of the Crock Pot.

3. Spread the olive oil over the florets, add minced garlic, pepper, and salt to taste. Toss everything well.
4. Cover and cook on LOW for 0.5-1 hour until broccoli is cooked through.
5. Shred the Parmesan cheese.
6. Once the broccoli is done, sprinkle with shredded cheese and serve.
7. Bon Appetite!

303.Keto asparagus casserole recipe

Asparagus casserole is creamy, a cheesy side dish that could be served both for holidays and as a daily meal. You may use here another homemade sauce or the sauce you prefer instead of soy sauce. This light variation of veggie side dish will be a great addition to pork or chicken.

Ingredients (6 servings):

Asparagus	2 cups
heavy cream	1/4 cup
cream cheese	2 ounces
dried onions	1-1/2 teaspoons
gluten-free soy sauce	1 tablespoon
mild Cheddar	1-1/2 ounces

ground pepper and salt at will

Directions:

1. Shred the Cheddar cheese into a little bowl.
2. Take a medium saucepan, mix heavy cream, cream cheese, dried onions, soy sauce. Whisk everything together.
3. Put asparagus on the bottom of the Crock Pot, pour the mixture over it.
4. Season with pepper and salt.
5. Sprinkle with shredded Cheddar cheese.
6. Cover and cook for 30 minutes, the top of the dish must be of golden color.
7. Serve hot!
8. Bon Appetite!

304.Creamed Kale with Bacon and Walnuts

This appetizing and flavor creamed kale with walnuts and crispy bacon strips is a great way to keep your keto diet. The nutmeg gets savor to the Parmesan (Romano)-mascarpone creamy sauce. This creamy sauce, milk, and butter make the texture of this dish silky and delicious. You may add more crispy bacon or walnuts if you like.

Ingredients (9 servings):

raw bacon	4 slices
butter	1 Tbsp
garlic	2 cloves

almond milk	1/2 cup
ground nutmeg	1/4 tsp
raw kale	10 cups
mascarpone cheese	1 cup
Parmesan or Romano cheese	1/3 cup
walnuts	1/4 cup

salt and pepper to taste

Directions:

1. Chop the bacon. Peel and mince the garlic.
2. Chop the raw kale. Grate the Parmesan (or Romano cheese).
3. Chop the walnuts.
4. Cook bacon in a medium saucepan until brown, add garlic and butter. Garlic must be fragrant. Add also the nutmeg and almond milk. Stir well everything.
5. Spray the Crock Pot with cooking spray, add the chopped kale.
6. Blend well the grated Parmesan cheese and mascarpone and pour over the kale.
7. Season with pepper and salt. Add the mixture to the saucepan.
8. Cover and cook on LOW for 1 hour.
9. Remove and serve with walnuts.
10. Eat warm.
11. Bon Appetite!

305.Brussels Sprouts with Lemon and Pine Nuts

This is an easy dish to cook but how flavor is it! You may cook the Brussels with cheese and bacon. Today I decided to cook sprouts with nuts and lemon (or lime if you wish), so a great variation! The lemon zest gets our dish crispy and flavor; the toasted nuts add some sweetness. I really enjoy this recipe and I'm sure you'll do the same.

Ingredients (5 servings):

pine nuts	1/3 cup
olive oil	3 Tbsp
lemon zest	2 Tbsp
Brussels sprouts	6 cups
lemon juice	2 Tbsp

salt and pepper to taste

Directions:

1. Quarter the Brussels sprouts.
2. Squeeze the juice of a lemon into a cup.
3. Toast the nuts in a medium saucepan for about 3-4 minutes. Stir them all the time.

4. Put the Brussels sprouts into the Crock Pot, drizzle with olive oil. Season with lemon zest, add salt and pepper.
5. Cover and cook for about 30 minutes, not more.
6. Season with toasted nuts and sprinkle with lemon juice.
7. Enjoy warm.
8. Bon Appetite!

306.Keto collard with cherry tomatoes

I like easy and light side dishes that are great both for meat and fish. This recipe is the easiest I could only think. It is a fantastic flavor and delicious recipe. It is amazing keto food. You can eat it as much as you want and don't worry about the carb count.

Ingredients:

bacon	3 strips
collard	1 lb
cherry tomatoes	1/4 cup
chicken broth	2 tablespoons
cider vinegar	1 tablespoon

salt and pepper to taste

Directions:
1. Slice bacon strips and roast them a little over high heat in a medium pan until golden.
2. Wash the collard greens and tomatoes.
3. Put the collard in the Crock Pot, pour the chicken broth, vinegar, dress with pepper and salt, add cherry tomatoes. Top with bacon strips.
4. Cover and cook on LOW for 30 minutes.
5. Eat warm.

307.Crock Pot keto creamy spinach

Cheesy, creamy, flavor spinach is eaten almost every week in my family as a side dish. Fantastic veggies are the best addition to your daily healthy food, that allows you to follow the keto diet and taste the best combinations and variations one could only imagine. Add as much species as you like!

Ingredients (11 servings):

Butter	2 tbsp
shallots	1/2 cup
garlic	1 tbsp
Half & Half	1 1/2 cups
Salt	1/2 Tsp
Pepper	1/2 Tsp

smoked paprika	1/2 Tsp
nutmeg	1/8 tsp
cayenne pepper at will	1/8 Tsp
Swiss cheese	8 ounces
spinach	16 ounces

Directions:
1. Peel and chop the shallots.
2. Peel the garlic and mince.
3. Shred the Swiss cheese.
4. Take a medium saucepan, melt butter, add garlic and shallots. Cook them until tender. Set aside.
5. Wash spinach. Put them into the Crock Pot, add golden garlic and shallots.
6. Take a medium bowl, mix Half & Half, pepper, smoked paprika, nutmeg, cayenne pepper, salt, and whisk. Pour the mixture into the Crock Pot.
7. Add shredded cheese, cover and cook until cheese is melted (ca. 30 minutes).
8. Once the time is over, toss everything until spinach is fully covered with cheese.
9. Bon Appetite!

308.Keto artichoke hearts Au Gratin

Keto artichokes Au Gratin is a leading combination among dozens of different variations of cooking artichokes in the Crock Pot. I used Cheddar and Pecorino-Romano cheese, but if you don't have this combination at home, you may use another one and I'm sure it will be delicious too!

Ingredients (12 servings):

frozen artichoke hearts	1 pkg. (12 oz.)
green onions	3-4 pcs
olive oil	2 tsp.
Cheddar cheese	1/3 cup
Pecorino-Romano cheese	1/3 cup
Almond flour	1/3 cup
dried thyme	1/2 tsp.
dried oregano	1/4 tsp.
mayo or light mayo	1/3 cup
juice	1 pcs
lemon zest	1 tsp.
garlic puree	1/2 tsp.
salt and black pepper to taste	

Directions:
1. Cut artichoke hearts lengthwise.
2. Green onions thinly sliced.
3. Grate the cheese. Mix both cheese in a medium bowl, add thyme, oregano.
4. Put the olive oil in the Crock Pot, arrange the artichoke hearts in a single layer, cover them with chopped onions, season with pepper, salt.
5. Take a medium bowl, mix the mayo, zest, almond flour, juice of lemon, garlic puree, whisk everything well. Combine cheese mixture with this one.
6. Spread this mixture over the artichoke hearts.
7. Cover and cook on LOW 4 hours.
8. Enjoy warm!

309.Crock Pot Garlic Artichokes

To cook the artichokes in the Crock Pot doesn't take you too many efforts. Everything you need, to rinse them, cut, peel the garlic and mince and put these ingredients in the Crock Pot. Chose the right regime and wait for flavor side dish!

Ingredients (5 servings):

Artichokes	4 medium pcs
fresh garlic	4 tablespoons
balsamic vinegar	4 tablespoons
chicken broth	1/2 cup
extra virgin olive oil	4 teaspoons

Directions:
1. Peel the garlic and mince.
2. Rinse the artichokes and cut them ½-inch off the top. They must stand flat (trim the stem).
3. Place the artichokes into the Crock Pot, season with black pepper, salt, drizzle ca. 1 tablespoon of the vinegar. Add broth to the Crock Pot (if it is necessary to add water a little bit).
4. Cover and cook on HIGH 3 hours. Check the readiness with a knife (it must insert the stem easily, the leaves have to be pulled away)
5. Remove the artichokes to a plate, sprinkle with the rest of the olive oil.
6. Bon Appetite!

310.Asiago zucchini and sun-dried tomato bread

Today I introduce you my recipe of tender and crusty keto bread prepared at the Crock Pot. This amazing cheesy keto zucchini bread has fluffy and light texture. This bread is served usually with meat, chicken or fish instead of usual roasted or cooked veggies.

Ingredients (15 servings):

butter	3/4 cup
eggs	4 pcs

almond milk	1/2 cup
zucchini	1/2 cup
sun-dried tomatoes	2 Tbsp
almond flour	2 cups
coconut flour	1/4 cup
baking powder	4 Tsp
Swerve	1 Tsp
xanthan gum	1/2 Tsp
kosher salt	1 1/4 Tsp
dried oregano	1/2 Tsp
dried parsley	1/2 Tsp
garlic powder	1/4 Tsp
Asiago cheese	1/2 cup

Directions:

1. Wash zucchini, shred into a plate and squeeze the rest of the liquid.
2. Chop the tomatoes. Melt the butter.
3. Take a large bowl, combine butter, cracked eggs, zucchini, almond milk, chopped tomatoes. Stir until the mixture is smooth.
4. Take another medium bowl, mix coconut and almond flour, sweetener, baking powder, salt, xanthan gum, oregano, garlic powder, parsley. Stir well.
5. Join the ingredients from both bowls in one until dry ingredients are fully absorbed.
6. Shred the cheese.
7. Spread the bottom of the Crock Pot with cooking spray, pour the mixture, spread the cheese on the top.
8. Cover and cook on HIGH 4 hours.
9. Season with the rest of the Asiago cheese.
10. Bon Appetite!

311.Crock Pot keto pumpkin bread

This super awesome French pumpkin bread is finally on the list of the keto side dishes in my cookbook. The original recipe of this bread is really tender and colorful. It is delicious, silky and flavor. It is a rather good addition to veggies, tomatoes, dips and other recipes that you may find in my cookbook.

Ingredients 912 servings):

butter	¾ cup
large eggs	4 pcs
unsweetened almond milk	1/4 cup

canned pumpkin puree	1 cup
almond flour	2 cups
coconut flour	1/3 cup
baking powder	4 Tsp
erythritol sweetener	½ cup
pinch of salt	
ground cinnamon	1 tsp
ground nutmeg	¼ tsp
ground allspice	¼ tsp

Directions:

1. Melt the butter. Combine it with cracked eggs, almond milk, pumpkin puree until smooth texture (use a blender).
2. Take another bowl, mix coconut and almond flour, salt, baking powder, allspice, stir well everything.
3. Combine the dry ingredients with the mixture and stir well once more.
4. Spread the cooking spray on the bottom and sides of the Crock Pot.
5. Pour the mixture into it. Cover and cook for 3 hours on HIGH.
6. Remove the bread, let it cool and slice before serving.
7. Enjoy!

312.Pumpkin bread, sausage, and Feta stuffing

Remember, I have advised you the recipe for the pumpkin bread? (See above) This time I cook the sausage-Feta-pumpkin bread side dish that is quick and substantial. To prepare this recipe you need to have pumpkin bread already cooked. Don't hesitate to follow my instructions.

Ingredients (8 servings):

cubed pumpkin bread	4 cups
pork sausage	16 oz
onion	1/2 cup
chicken or turkey broth	1/3 cup
butter	2 Tbsp
Bell's seasoning	1 Tsp
Feta cheese	3/4 cup
fresh parsley	2 Tbsp

Directions:

1. Cube the pumpkin bread. Toast them a little bit until golden.

2. Peel and chop the onion. Wash and chop the parsley.
3. Cut the sausage, cook them in a little saucepan until cooked, add chopped onions and let them soften.
4. Add the broth, butter, seasoning to the Crock Pot put onions and sausages.
5. Cover and let it cook 30 minutes on LOW.
6. Open the Crock Pot, add Feta cheese, bread cubes, and parsley. Cover and put on HIGH for half an hour.
7. Serve warm.

313.Keto bacon and Goat cheese cauliflower

When there is no time to cook but I must still have something as a side dish, I use this recipe. The cauliflower is like a «superman» among other vegetables. There are a lot of variations of it prepared in the Crock Pot, adding your favorite species and shredded cheese. Anyway, it will not be boring.

Ingredients (6 servings):

Cauliflowers	2 large head (8 cups chopped)
Smoked Bacon	4 strips
Onion	1 cup
Garlic	4 teaspoons
Goat Cheese	10 ounces
Cream Cheese	1/4 cup

Salt and Pepper at will

Green Onion (optional) for garnish

Directions:
1. Rinse and chop the cauliflowers.
2. Peel the onions and garlic. Chop finely. Cut the bacon strips into small pieces.
3. Wash and slice green onions.
4. Spread the cooking spray over the Crock Pot, place the cauliflower. Put the chopped onion and garlic, season with pepper and salt. Add a little bit water (1-2 tablespoon) if needed.
5. Cover and cook on LOW for 2 hours.
6. Remove the cooked cauliflower with garlic and onion in a blender, add Goat cheese, cream cheese and blend everything until totally smooth mixture.
7. Put the ready-made cauliflower with bacon slices to the Crock Pot again, put on HIGH for 30 minutes until the top begins to brown.
8. Serve with pepper and green onion.
9. Bon Appetite!

314.Keto cauliflower gratin Crock Pot

I think each of us doesn't like to cook too long. Especially, as for the side dishes, they must be always quick and easy. I hope, this cauliflower recipe will be a great benefit to you! I haven't even shredded the cheese, just sliced it and that's all. And, you may add so many cheeses as you like!

Ingredients (4 servings):

raw cauliflower florets   4 cups

butter   4 Tbsp

heavy whipping cream   1/3 cup

pepper Jack cheese   6 deli slices

salt and pepper to taste

Directions:
1. Rinse the cauliflower, cut into florets.
2. Slice the pepper Jack cheese.
3. Put the cauliflower florets into the Crock Pot, add butter, salt, cream, and pepper. Mix everything thoroughly.
4. Cover and cook on LOW 2 hours.
5. Remove it from the Crock Pot, mash the cauliflower using a fork, season with more pepper at will.
6. Place the mashed cauliflower again in the Crock Pot, slice the cheese and put on WARM for 1 hour.
7. Serve hot!

315.Jalapeno popper cauliflower casserole

Spicy, creamy and cheese – this all about this recipe! This side dish is almost eaten with keto fish and veggies. This keto recipe is simple, quick and flavorful. You may eat it as much as you will!

Ingredients (11 servings):

Preparing the puree:

cauliflower   1 head

heavy cream   2 Tbsp

butter   1 Tbsp

Sharp Cheddar cheese   1/4 cup

raw jalapenos   1 Tbsp

garlic powder   1/4 tsp

salt and pepper to taste

Preparing the cream layer:

cream cheese   6 oz

Cheddar cheese   1/2 cup

| salsa verde | 1/4 cup |

Preparing the topping:

| Colby Jack cheese | 3/4 cup |

| raw jalapenos | 1/4 cup |

Directions:

Puree:

1. Rinse cauliflower, cut into florets. Put the florets into the Crock Pot, add butter, cream and cook on LOW for 2 hours.
2. Shred the cheese.
3. Wash and remove the seeds from jalapenos. Slice them thinly.
4. Once the time is over, remove the cauliflowers, put them in a blender, add jalapenos and cheese. Blend well everything.
5. Dress with salt at will.

Cream cheese layer:

1. Shred the Cheddar cheese and mix it with salsa verde, stir thoroughly.
2. Put the prepared cauliflower into the Crock Pot again, pour the cream sauce. Shred additionally the Jack cheese and put on the top jalapenos (seeds removed and washed). Cook everything on LOW for an hour.
3. Serve hot!
4. Bon Appetite!

316.Crock Pot Mexican cauliflower rice

Cauliflower is a natural source of useful minerals and vitamins. I know a lot of people who eat cauliflower rice instead of usual one and feel themselves better than ever. A little thing you need to do here – to make the rice from cauliflower florets, it means to use the food processor or a blender.

Ingredients (12 servings):

Cauliflower	1 head
tomato sauce	1 cup
chicken stock	1/2 cup
tomato paste	1 heaping tbsp
white onion	1 medium
bell peppers	2 pcs
jalapeno peppers	2 pcs
garlic powder	1 tbsp
chipotle powder	2 Tsp

ground cumin	2 tsp
dried oregano	1 tsp
black or white pepper	1 Tsp

Salt to taste

Directions:

1. Rinse the cauliflower, remove the stems, cut into florets.
2. Peel and dice the onion.
3. Wash and remove the seeds from bell peppers and jalapenos, dice.
4. Put tomato sauce, stock and tomato paste to the Crock Pot and stir.
5. Add the garlic powder, chipotle powder, cumin, oregano black pepper, salt, and stir.
6. Add peppers and onion to the Crock Pot, add cauliflower florets. Toss everything. Florets must be covered with sauce fully.
7. Cover and cook on LOW 5 hours.
8. Once the time is over, mash the florets until they break up like rice consistency.
9. Drain the remained liquid and serve!
10. Bon Appetite!

317.Southern asparagus Crock Pot

The easiest way of preparing the asparagus is to cook it in the Crock Pot. The package of bacon, chicken broth, chopped fresh onion and a little bit pepper and salt – the best combination for your keto asparagus. You don't need to clean the saucepans after roasting the bacon – use already-prepared one.

Ingredients (6 servings):

fresh asparagus	2 lbs
chicken broth	2 cups
real bacon pieces	1 (2.8-ounce) package
yellow onion	½ pcs
kosher salt	3 teaspoons
black pepper	½ teaspoon

Directions:

1. Peel and dice the onion.
2. Spray the bottom and sides in the Crock Pot with cooking spray.
3. Add the asparagus, broth, pepper, onion, slat.
4. Add a half of all bacon.
5. Cover and cook on HIGH for 3 hours. Asparagus must get its tenderness.
6. Stir them from time to time.
7. Serve with the remained bacon strips.
8. Bon Appetite!

318.Lemon Pepper Asparagus Keto

This delicious and easy recipe is a little bit spicy, crunchy and flavor! The almonds add amazing taste to the dish! You may add to this recipe your favorite species, cayenne pepper at will.

Ingredients (4 servings):

fresh asparagus	1 pound
butter	2 tablespoons
sliced almonds	1/4 cup
lemon pepper	2 teaspoons
salt	

Directions:
1. Rinse well asparagus.
2. Place asparagus in the Crock Pot, add a little bit water.
3. Cover and cook on LOW for 2 hours.
4. Melt the butter in a little skillet, saute almonds until golden.
5. Remove asparagus to a plate, add salt, add almonds.
6. Bon Appetite!

319.Mashed cauliflower with rosemary

For those who prefer potatoes but remember about this keto-forbidden product, the mashed cauliflower with rosemary that is the best choice for the holidays and other days of the year. I hope, this side dish will be your new favorite one.

Ingredients (5 servings):

Cauliflower	1 large
cream cheese	3 ounces
unsalted butter	2 tablespoons
minced garlic	1 1/2 teaspoon
fresh rosemary	1 tablespoon
salt and pepper at will	

Directions:
1. Wash the cauliflower, chop into small florets.
2. Peel the garlic and mince it finely.
3. Wash rosemary and chop into small pieces.
4. Cover the Crock Pot with cooking spray, put the cauliflower florets. Add a little bit water if necessary.
5. Cover and cook on LOW for 2-3 hours until cauliflower is tender.
6. Put the cooked cauliflower in the blender, add cream cheese, butter, garlic and rosemary and blend well.
7. Season with pepper and salt.
8. Bon Appetite!

320.Indian spiced cauliflower rice

I have introduced this cauliflower rice not so many years ago and got in love with it at once. This dish is healthy because it is cooked with vegetables, it IS vegetables! I call it just «rice» without the word «cauliflower» sometimes because it looks like real rice. I substitute with it many dishes, especially those where I'd like to serve my meat or fish over rice. Follow the directions listed below to get the right consistency of cauliflower rice, not like mashed potatoes or cereals. You may also serve this side dish with pork, lamb, chicken, beef or just with other vegetables.

Ingredients (10 servings):

Cauliflower	1 head
Butter	1 tablespoon
olive oil	1 tablespoon
cumin	½ teaspoon
turmeric	¼ teaspoon
ground ginger ¼ teaspoon	
cardamom	1/8 teaspoon
cinnamon	1/8 teaspoon
ground cloves 1/8 teaspoon	
salt	½ teaspoon
black pepper to taste	
cilantro, optional	3-4 tablespoons

Directions:

1. Rinse the cauliflower, remove the stems, cut in half down the middle and cut once more along the stem. Cutting off the stem allows to spate the head of the cauliflower to the florets. Cut finely into 1-2-inch small pieces.
2. Put the chopped florets into the blender (or a food processor) and push the button. Wait until the florets will be of the rice size (less or more is also possible if you wish).
3. Put the cauliflower rice into the Crock Pot, add the species – like cumin, turmeric, ginger, cinnamon, cardamom, garlic, black pepper and salt and stir well everything.
4. Add butter and olive oil, cauliflower rice must be fully covered with oil and species.
5. Cover and cook on LOW 3 hours.
6. Wash the cilantro and chop finely. Set aside.
7. Once the cooking time is over, remove rice to a plate, serve with fresh cilantro.
8. Bon Appetite!

321.Cauliflower with mustard butter

Mustard-browned butter is not new to you, I guess. It is just a usual butter that is cooked until it gets the brown color. I usually do this in such a way – place the butter into a skillet over medium or low heat, cook a little bit and reduce heat at once. Water in my butter must be cooked off. Don't be surprised if you'll see that the butter will be of light brown or golden color. It doesn't mean something gets wrong. No. There are the milk solids one usually want to leave behind while drizzling over the veggies. In this recipe you don't need to get the cauliflower of rice consistency, it is better to leave the florets as they are or larger pieces. Still, if the florets fall apart, don't worry! Take more heads of cauliflower and make larger «steaks». I hope, once you or your family members try to cook cauliflower in such a way, there will be no other way of cooking it.

Ingredients (6 servings):

Cauliflower	1 large head
olive oil (or more if needed)	3-4 tablespoons
salt	
freshly ground black pepper	

mustard browned butter:

unsalted butter	1 stick
garlic	2 cloves
coarse-grain mustard	2 tablespoons
fresh parsley	2 tablespoons
salt	
freshly ground black pepper at will	

Directions:

1. Rinse the cauliflower, remove all stems, cut cauliflower in half down the middle and cut once more along the stem. Cutting off the stem allows to spate the head of the cauliflower to the medium florets.
2. Spread the bottom of the Crock Pot with olive oil or cooking spray, put the cauliflower florets there.
3. Drizzle the florets with olive oil, season finely with pepper and salt.
4. Cover and put the Crock Pot on LOW for 2-3 hours. Turn the florets from time to time.
5. While cooking prepare the browned butter – take a little saucepan, place it over low heat. Peel garlic and mince it finely. Wash the parsley and chop too.
6. Melt the butter in a little saucepan, add mustard, minced garlic, black pepper, parsley, and salt. Stir everything well. Be very careful not to burn the butter. It must get light golden color. Set aside.
7. Once the cooking time is over, remove the cauliflower into a plate and pour the mustard browned bitter over a hot cauliflower.
8. Add chopped fresh parsley and pepper if needed.
9. Bon Appetite!

322. Low Carb Spinach & Artichoke Dip Cauliflower Casserole

I'm a huge fan of a light combination of milk, shredded Parmesan (or Swiss) and mozzarella cheese. I think, any dish – it doesn't matter meat, fish, vegetables, couldn't be spoiled with cheese…. In no way! I use milk in a better part of my recipes, the same as butter or cheese. I don't only drink it or prepare boring cereals. Milk gets my recipe tenderness and silky. I'm happy that I can prepare such plain dishes using only milk, cheese, and vegetables in the Crock Pot.

Ingredients (13 servings):

raw cauliflower florets	4 cups
butter	1/4 cup
Silk Cashew Milk	1/2 cup
Full-fat cream cheese	8 oz
kosher salt	1/2 tsp
ground black pepper	1/8 Tsp
ground nutmeg	1/4 tsp
garlic powder	1/4 tsp
smoked paprika	1/4 Tsp
chopped spinach (frozen or fresh)	1 cup
canned or frozen artichoke hearts	3/4 cup
whole milk mozzarella cheese	1 1/2 cup
Parmesan cheese	1/4 cup

Directions:

1. Rinse the cauliflower, remove all stems, chop the florets into medium pieces.
2. Drain the liquid from the artichoke hearts, chop them finely.
3. If you use fresh spinach – wash and chop it finely.
4. Shred the Parmesan cheese into a plate and cut the mozzarella also.
5. Take a large bowl, combine the butter, milk, cream cheese, pepper, nutmeg, salt, garlic powder, paprika. Stir everything well. Place the cauliflower florets into this mixture, they must be fully covered with it.
6. Place the cauliflower-cheese mixture into the Crock Pot, cover and put on LOW for 2 hours.
7. Once two hours are over, open the Crock Pot, add chopped spinach, shredded Parmesan, and chopped mozzarella cheese. Add also chopped artichoke hearts. Cut this layer with remained Parmesan and mozzarella cheese.
8. Cover and put on LOW for 1 additional hour until the top will be golden.
9. Serve hot with keto bread or meat!
10. Bon Appetite!

323.Coconut lime cauliflower rice

Today I would like to present you amazing coconut lime rice – cauliflower rice! The coconut milk powder makes this dish luscious and tasty, you don't feel like you just eating cauliflower. It is something delicious and flavor! The lime is perfectly well here because it adds a really nice tang and freshness. All the time you taste this side dish you want to back again and try it. The pleasant texture of the cauliflower rice is amazing and appetizing, it is an Asian or Indian wonder! The best addition to this side dish is beef or pork curry prepared in the Crock Pot. Their combination is great and it satisfies your keto diet.

Ingredients (6 servings):

chopped cauliflower	2 cups
coconut milk powder	3 Tbsp
coconut oil	2 Tbsp
water	2 Tbsp
fresh cilantro	1 Tbsp
fresh lime zest	1 tsp

pepper and salt to taste

Directions:

1. Rinse the cauliflower, remove the stems, cut in half down the middle and cut once more along the stem. Cutting off the stem allows to spate the head of the cauliflower to the florets. Cut finely into 1-2-inch small pieces.
2. Wash the fresh cilantro and chop finely.
3. Wash the lime and peel the zest a little bit.
4. Place the cauliflower florets into a large bowl, add the coconut oil, milk powder, water, season with pepper and salt. Combine everything well.
5. Pour the mixture into the Crock Pot, cover and cook on LOW 2-3 hours until cauliflower rice will be tender.
6. Serve hot with pepper, salt, and fresh cilantro.
7. Bon Appetite!

324.Crock Pot cauliflower hummus recipe

This recipe is a real finding for those who can't stand without hummus. I have tried to change the real recipe of hummus preparation several times and found the cauliflower is the best veggie for this. When it is cold the cauliflower puree is like a hummus, that's why you need just to add the right species and ingredients and you'll get the dish you need. Of course, it is not a real hummus like you prefer to eat, but don't forget about the allowed foods in your keto diet and you'll find it is the best variation it could only exist!

Ingredients (10 servings):

raw cauliflower florets	3 cups
water	2 Tbsp
avocado or olive oil	2 Tbsp
salt	1/2 Tsp
garlic	3 cloves
Tahini paste	1.5 Tbsp
lemon juice	3 Tbsp

garlic   2 cloves (additionally to the quantity above)

extra virgin olive oil   3 Tbsp

kosher salt   3/4 tsp

smoked paprika and olive oil optional

Directions:
1. Rinse the cauliflower, remove the stems, cut in half down the middle and cut once more along the stem. Cutting off the stem allows to spate the head of the cauliflower to the florets. Cut finely into 1-2-inch small pieces.
2. Peel the garlic cloves and mince finely.
3. Take a medium-sized bowl, combine the cauliflower florets, olive or avocado oil, water, salt, a half of all cloves of minced garlic.
4. Put the mixture to the Crock Pot, cover and put on LOW for 2 hours. Stir well from time to time.
5. Once the cauliflower is done, place the mixture in the blender or food processor. Put additionally Tahini, juice of lemon, the rest of minced garlic cloves, salt if necessary and blend until tender smooth consistency.
6. Place the cauliflower hummus on a plate (or a bowl) drizzle it with oil and add the paprika.
7. Enjoy with veggies.
8. Bon Appetite!

325.Roasted Summer Squash with Lemon, Mint, and Feta

This recipe is for those who like mint or who eat it without hate) This side dish is a perfect idea for the sunny days. Firstly, as I found this recipe I was a little bit skeptical about it, but as I cooked this one in the Crock Pot I understood the real taste of lemon, mint and Feta combination. It is amazingly fresh! This combination of tastes is fully soaked up by squash (or zucchini if you will). This recipe is great for chicken, beef or pork. It gets the freshness, tenderness, and flavor. Enjoy it together with your family and friends!

Ingredients (6 servings):

yellow summer squash (zucchini   is also possible)   5-6 pcs

olive oil   1/4 cup

lemon juice   1/4 cup

mint leaves   1/2 cup

salt to taste   about 1/2 tsp

Feta cheese (more or less at will)   1 cup

black pepper at will, optional

Directions:
1. Wash the squash (or zucchini), cut into 8-inches long. Remove the stems, flower ends. Set aside.
2. Squeeze fresh lemon into a cup.

3. Wash and chop finely mint.
4. Crumble the Feta cheese.
5. Spray the bottom of the Crock Pot with cooking spray. Put the squash (zucchini) into the Crock Pot.
6. Take a medium-sized bowl, combine the juice of lemon, olive oil, salt, and mint. Pour over the squash. Toss the squash finely until all the pieces are covered with the mixture.
7. Cover and put on HIGH for 2 hours. Check until the squash (zucchini) are cooked until golden brown.
8. Once the cooking time is over, remove the ready squash (zucchini) to a plate, dress with crumbled Feta cheese.
9. Season with black pepper and salt at will.
10. Bon Appetite!

326.Keto Spicy Broccoli Stems

You may wonder, what I'm cooking today as a side dish. Yes, this dish is always on the list of non-appreciated veggies and don't get a huge respect for the majority of people. Usually, people don't save the broccoli stems – it is like a rubbish. But! Wait. It could be served as a side dish too! Why not!? I used to eat the broccoli stems in salads. As I have gathered a large package of broccoli stems I decided to cook them finally! You may use any variations of them – combine the stems with Feta or another kind of cheese, add the preferred sauce or topping, dress with black pepper, cilantro and lime! I realized that I could eat this spicy broccoli stems like a main dish. Here is my recipe!

Ingredients (8 servings):

broccoli stems	1 lb. (ca. 8 thick stems)
oil (avocado or olive)	1 Tbsp.
minced garlic	1 Tbsp.
green onion for garnish (optional)	1/4 cup
Sauce Ingredients:	
soy sauce (low sodium)	1 Tbsp.
Hoisin sauce	2 Tsp.
Chili Garlic Sauce	2 Tsp.
Splenda or Stevia	1 Tbsp.
Pepper and salt at will	

Directions:

Wash the broccoli stems, this time you have to trim away all discolored parts. Using a sharp knife, trim away the extra leaves, ribs from stems. Take a vegetable peeler and peel them. Cut the ready-prepared stems into slices (cut diagonal), ca. ½-inch thick.

1. Take a medium bowl and mix soy sauce, chili garlic sauce, Hoisin sauce, sweetener. Peel the garlic, mince it and add to the mixture.
2. Whisk everything well. Slice thinly green onions.

3. Spray the oil over the bottom of the Crock Pot, place the stems, pour the sauce over the stems. Stir well everything.
4. Cover and put on HIGH for 1 hours. Stir from time to time the stems.
5. Check the broccoli stems, don't let them burn. They must get a little crisp.
6. Serve hot, dress with the rest of green onions, black pepper and salt at will.
7. Bon Appetite!

DESSERTS

327.Keto Crock Pot quick cake

The ingredients for this quick cake are rather simple, moreover, you can use already prepared at the store chocolate chips. Remember only, they must be sugar-free. This recipe of the quick keto cake is great to prepare when the guests are coming and you still don't have something tasty.

Ingredients (8 servings):

Butter	1 tbsp
almond flour	3 tbsp
sweetener	1 tbsp
cinnamon	1 pinch
yolk	1 egg
vanilla extract	1/8 tsp
salt	1 pinch
sugar-free chocolate chips	2 tbsp

Directions:

1. Melt butter in a medium-sized pan, let it brown a little.
2. Mix the browned butter with the mentioned amount of almond flour in a bowl.
3. Add sweetener and cinnamon. Mix everything well.
4. Add the egg yolk, after this add vanilla extract, a pinch of salt.
5. Add the sugar-free chocolate chips. Stir to combine.
6. Open the Crock Pot and spray a surface and sides with cooking spray or oil and place your mixture.
7. Close the Crock Pot and put on high for an hour.
8. Once the time is over, let it cool some minutes and then dig in!
9. Enjoy with ice cream.
10. Bon Appetite!

328.Almond Butter Fudge Bars

Almond fudge bars is a great recipe to make with the whole members of your family. One can enjoy the bars as a quick snack, breakfast, lunch-time, or night dessert)) Homemade desserts are always better than bought at the storage. The Almond Butter Fudge Bars, I advise you to bake, have a crispy crust and are great with heavy-creamy or some toppings.

Ingredients (9 servings):

almond flour	1 cup
unsalted butter	1/2 cup
powdered erythritol (sweetener)	6 tablespoons

ground cinnamon	1/2 teaspoon
heavy cream	1/4 cup
almond butter	1/2 cup
vanilla extract	1/2 teaspoon
xanthan gum	1/8 teaspoon

80% dark chocolate or sugar-free chocolate chips 1 ounce

Directions:
1. Open the Crock Pot and spread the cooking spray over the sides and the bottom.
2. Melt the butter and divide into portions.
3. In a medium-sized bowl whisk together almond flour, melted butter, powdered erythritol, cinnamon. Combine everything well.
4. Spread the mixture on the bottom of the Crock-Pot, cover and set on HIGH for one hour. The mixture must get golden brown.
5. Take off the almond base and let it cool. Chop the dark chocolate finely.
6. Whisk together in a large bowl heavy cream with almond butter, remained butter and powdered erythritol.
7. Add the vanilla and xanthan gum and blend everything well.
8. Spread the mixture over the cooled almond base and sprinkle with chopped dark chocolate or if desired with chocolate chips.
9. Freeze overnight, slice the base into bars and serve.
10. Enjoy!

329.Chewy ginger cake Crock Pot

My Chewy Ginger Cake is made with erythritol that allows for our keto rules. I usually bake this cake for holidays and weekends. It is great making in the Crock Pot, simple and tasty. Why not trying to prepare?

Ingredients:

almond flour	1.5 cups
coconut flour	3/4 cup
ground ginger	1/2 tbsp
ground cinnamon	1 tsp
sea salt	1/4 tsp
unsalted butter	3/4 cup
powdered erythritol	3/4 cup
eggs	1 large

Directions:
1. Open the Crock Pot and spread the cooking spray over the sides and the bottom.
2. Whisk in a medium-sized bowl almond flour, coconut flour, cinnamon, ginger, and salt.

3. Take another medium bowl, combine together butter with erythritol until fluffy and light.
4. Crack the egg and slowly beat it in the dry mixture.
5. Turn out the dough ball knead until it comes everything together. Scoop into a ball.
6. Roll the dough ball in powdered erythritol, place it into the bottom of the Crock Pot.
7. Put on LOW for 2-3 hours and bake until golden brown.
8. Bon Appetite!

330.Halloween Mud Pie Keto Recipe

Trick or Treat… Or both? When the Halloween is around the corner you must bake this pie definitely! Yes, it takes you some time to prepare this tasty one. If you can find sugar-free gummy worms in the store, feel free to prepare them.

Ingredients (18 servings):

Sugar-Free Gummy Worms:

sugar-free Jell-O (8 grams each)	2 packets
gelatin (8 grams)	2 packets
water	1/2 cup

Cake Base:

almond flour	2 cups
coconut flour	2 tbsp
cocoa powder	1/2 cup
erythritol	1 cup
baking soda	1.5 tsp
salt	1/2 Tsp
butter (melted)	1 cup
eggs	3 large
vanilla extract	2 tsp
heavy cream	1/2 cup
almond milk	1/4 cup

Frosting:

Butter	1/4 cup
cocoa powder	1.5 tbsp
powdered erythritol	1/2 cup
almond milk	2 tbsp

Directions:

1. Begin to prepare the sugar-free gummy worms: put a small pot on low heat, whisk together sugar-free Jell-O, gelatin and a cup water.
2. Once all the clumps of gelatin are done, pour the ready-made liquid into the gummy molds. Refrigerate them overnight.

Baking the base:

1. Open the Crock Pot and spread the cooking spray over the sides and the bottom.
2. Whisk together all the dry ingredients in a medium-sized bowl - almond flour, coconut flour, baking soda, salt, erythritol.
3. Melt the butter.
4. Add also the wet ingredients - butter, cracked eggs, vanilla extract, heavy cream, almond milk.
5. Open the Crock Pot and spread the cooking spray over the sides and the bottom.
6. Pour the batter into the Crock Pot, cover and set on LOW for 4 hours.
7. Once the time is over, let it cool completely.
8. Prepare the frosting that will hold the end result together: take a saucepan and melt the butter.
9. Turn off the heat, stir in the cocoa powder, erythritol, almond milk. Whisk everything until smooth.
10. Once the cake is cooled, put it in a large mixing bowl and crumble it completely with your hands, pour the frosting, mix everything again.
11. Put (press) in the gummy worms you have made already. Make sure to press them firmly.
12. Once you get to the top layer, press everything good. Add the last part of the gummy worms to the top, being as creative as you like. Add some sugar-free chocolate chips to the cake top.
13. Enjoy and Happy Halloween!

331.Pumpkin Pie Keto Fat Bomb

Never heard about pumpkin pie keto fat bomb? Pure you! I decided to use the coconut butter in this recipe and I must tell you it is great and must get enough attention by preparing the desserts. It tastes like coconut, has a texture of peanut butter and is great for preparing cakes. It is ideal for keto diet and my family like it very much!

Ingredients (7 servings):

pumpkin puree	1/2 cup
coconut butter	2 oz.
coconut oil	1/2 cup
sweetener	1/4 cup
pumpkin pie spice	2 tsp
cup pecans	½
almond flour	1 cup

Directions:

1. Melt the coconut oil if it's not already liquid.
2. In a medium-sized saucepan melt the coconut butter until softened.
3. Combine in a mixing bowl the pumpkin puree, coconut butter, and coconut oil and stir everything well.
4. Add the sweetener.
5. Add the pumpkin pie spice as well. If you don't have it, just add cinnamon! Add flour.
6. Once your fat bomb is combined, pour this into the Crock Pot. Don't forget the spread the bottom and the sides of the Crock Pot with cooking spray!
7. Toast up chopped pecans a little in a dry pan until slightly browned and fragrant.
8. Add the pecans to the mixture.
9. Cover the Crock Pot and set on LOW for 2 -3 hours.
10. Enjoy warm!
11. Bon Appetite!

332. White Chocolate Green Tea Mug Keto Cake

Green tea mug keto cake is one of my lovely and unusual cakes ever. Firstly I tried it in the restaurant, its colored has surprised me at once! But what an amazing taste it has! I cooked it at home and found it was nothing difficult to prepare. The only necessary ingredient you have to put there is matcha powder. This ingredient makes the dessert flavorful, decadent, rich and funny!

Ingredients (11 servings):

powdered erythritol	1.5 tbsp
liquid stevia	5-10 drops
egg	1 large
coconut oil (or melted butter)	1 tbsp
vanilla extract	1/2 tsp
almond flour	1/4 cup
matcha powder	1/2 Tsp
baking powder	1 Tsp
xanthan gum	1/8 Tsp
sea salt	1 pinch
frozen sugar-free white chocolate chips	2 tbsp

Directions:

1. Freeze the sugar-free white chocolate chips beforehand to ensure they stay as chips while baking.
2. Open the Crock Pot and spread the cooking spray over the sides and the bottom.
3. Take a large bowl, whisk the erythritol and stevia into the egg.
4. Add the coconut oil (or if you use the butter - melted butter) and vanilla extract and whisk everything well to combine.

5. In another medium-sized bowl combine together almond flour, matcha powder, baking powder and xanthan gum.
6. Add this mix to the other wet ingredients. Add also a pinch salt, combine everything very well.
7. Fold in the white chocolate chips.
8. Pour in the Crock Pot, cover and set on LOW for 2 hours.
9. Once the baking time is over, let the cake cool and enjoy!
10. Bon Appetite!

333.Keto Peanut Butter Cake

Peanut butter cake has a special place among my keto desserts prepared in the Crock Pot. There are only three ingredients needed for the cake. They are the sweetener, peanut butter, and a fresh egg. It is simple enough, even kids can prepare this delicious cake.

Ingredients (3 servings):

peanut butter   1 cup

granular erythritol   1/2 cup

egg   1 large

Directions:

1. Open the Crock Pot and spread the cooking spray over the sides and the bottom.
2. Blend a half of an amount of granular erythritol into a food processor and blend for some seconds. You should get a finely powdered sweetener.
3. In a medium-sized bowl combine peanut butter with powdered erythritol and the fresh egg, mix everything well.
4. Roll the cake into a medium-sized ball and place on a bottom of the Crock Pot.
5. Cover the Crock Pot and set on LOW for 3 hours. Check the readiness from time to time, the cake edges must turn a darker brown.
6. Once the baking time is over, take off the cake and let it cool.
7. Enjoy with a glass of milk!

334.Black and white keto cake

An amazing keto cake that consists of chocolate and… chocolate! White and black! Always more chocolate for chocolate fans! Yes, I'm sure, you will not forget this texture! Don't forget to use sugar-free and keto-friendly ingredients in this recipe! It is a perfect alternative to sweets and chocolate!

Ingredients (16 servings):

For Cake

Almond flour   2 cups

coconut flour   2 tbsp

sweetener   1 cup

baking soda   1.5 tsp

salt	1/2 Tsp
butter	1 cup
cocoa powder	1/2 cup
water	1 cup
eggs	3 large
vanilla extract	2 tsp
sour cream	1/2 cup

White Chocolate Glaze:

Cocoa Butter Wafers	2 oz.
powdered erythritol	3 tbsp
vanilla extract	1 tsp
heavy cream	2 tbsp

Topping

| Cocoa Nibs | 20 grams |

Directions:

1. Open the Crock Pot and spread the cooking spray over the sides and the bottom.
2. In a medium-sized bowl whisk together almond flour with coconut flour, sweetener baking soda, and salt. Set aside.
3. Take a small pot, heat together butter, cocoa powder, water on a high heat. Whisk everything until combined and take it off from the heat.
4. Pour a half of chocolate mixture into dry ingredients (first bowl) and stir to combine. Once the mixture is thick and difficult to stir, pour the other half. Combine once more.
5. Add in 1 egg, after this add sour cream and vanilla extract, stir everything well.
6. Pour the batter into the Crock Pot and set on LOW for 5 hours, until the wooden toothpick comes out clean.
7. While the cake is baking, it is time to prepare white chocolate glaze.
8. In a little saucepan melt cocoa butter wafers.
9. Add powdered erythritol and mix to combine.
10. Add heavy cream and put the mixture in the fridge, stirring every 6-7 minutes.
11. Once the chocolate has chilled to the thick consistency, pulse it for some seconds in a blender until smooth.
12. Once the cake is ready, let it cool for about 10 minutes, then put it on a plate and let it cool completely.
13. After this glaze the cake. Let the glaze drape over the top of the cake.
14. Dress with the nibs.
15. Enjoy!

335.Keto pumpkin cake Crock Pot

Keto pumpkin cake prepared in the Crock Pot is great for everyday desserts. It is delicious creamy pumpkin base with a coffee cake crumble flavor topping. I'm sure, it will magically disappear from the kitchen once it is ready!

Ingredients (16 servings):

coconut flour	1/3 cup
pumpkin pie spice	2 tsp
cinnamon	1 tsp
salt	1/8 Tsp
eggs	2 pcs
organic pumpkin puree	1/3 cup
sweetener	1/3 cup
coconut milk	1/4 cup
coconut oil	2 tbsp
vanilla extract	1 tsp
baking soda	½ tsp
Crumble Topping:	
pecan meal	1/2 cup
coconut flakes	3 tbsp
coconut sugar	2 tbsp
cinnamon	1 tsp
coconut oil	3 tbsp

Directions:

1. Open the Crock Pot and spread the cooking spray over the sides and the bottom.
2. Take a medium-sized mixing bowl and combine coconut flour, pumpkin pie spice, cinnamon, and sea salt. Mix everything thoroughly. Set aside.
3. Take another large mixing bowl and combine eggs, coconut milk, pumpkin puree, melted coconut oil or butter, sweetener, and vanilla extract. Mix together until combined.
4. Add baking soda to the egg mixture. Mix together thoroughly.
5. Add coconut flour mix to the egg mix and stir until combined.
6. Pour into the Crock Pot and set aside.
7. In a little bowl combine pecan meal, coconut flakes, coconut sugar, oil, and cinnamon, use a fork to mix until paste forms.
8. Take the crumble topping all over the top of the pumpkin batter in the Crock Pot.
9. Cover the Crock Pot and set on LOW for 4 hours until top is browned, and a toothpick comes out clean.

10.   Cool the cake completely, then refrigerate for one hour or longer.

11.   Bon Appetite!

336.Keto Pumpkin Chocolate Chip

This dessert recipe is something special because of the mix sweet coconut flour, chocolate chips with cardamom, ginger powder and ground cloves. But be sure, it rather tasty, flavor and simple.

Ingredients (13 servings):

almond butter unsweetened	1/2 cup
pumpkin puree unsweetened	1/4 cup
erythritol granulated	1/4 cup
ginger powder	1/4 tsp
nutmeg	1/4 tsp
cardamon powder	1/4 Tsp
ground cloves	1/4 tsp
cinnamon	1 tsp
stevia powder	1/4 Tsp
baking soda	1/2 tsp
coconut flour	1 tbsp
chocolate chips	2 tbsp
egg	1pcs

Directions:

1. Open the Crock Pot and spread the cooking spray over the sides and the bottom.
2. Mix in a large bowl pumpkin puree, almond butter, sweetener, ginger powder, nutmeg, cardamom powder, freshly cracked egg, ground cloves, cinnamon, stevia powder, baking soda, coconut flour. Stir everything well.
3. Add chocolate chips.
4. Put the mixture into the Crock Pot, cover and set on HIGH for 2 hours.
5. Take out and let it cool.
6. Bon Appetite!

337.Keto Crock Pot Cheesecake

When I tried to cook this recipe for the first time I couldn't believe the cheesecake could be so easy!!!! It is amazing, flavor and tender cake! I think I don't need to tell you more about the cheesecake. You may serve it with low carb fruit sauce, berries. The best way – to let it cool in the refrigerator for a night, but I can't stand it!

Ingredients (4 servings):

cream cheese	3 8 oz. packages
eggs	3 pcs
Splenda	1 cup
Vanilla	½ Tbsp.

Directions:

1. Let the cheese (cream cheese) get the room temperature. Place it in a medium-sized bowl, add Splenda.
2. Using a blender mix everything well, until cheese and Splenda are blended thoroughly.
3. Add the cracked eggs, one after one blending all the time the mixture.
4. Spray the bottom and the sides of the Crock Pot with cooking spray, pour the egg-cheese mixture into the Crock Pot.
5. Cover and put the dish on HIGH for 2 hours.
6. Look after an hour from time to time. Check the readiness of the cheesecake – the knife must go out from the cake clean.
7. Let it cool.
8. Bon Appetite!

338. Keto Crock Pot pumpkin custard

This pumpkin custard is one of my favorite because it is baked in the Crock Pot. It is very flavorful and creamy. I just mix all the ingredients in a large bowl, blend well and after this pour to the Crock Pot. I usually use Stevia in my recipes (blended variation) or you may use another sweetener if you want. Instead of the vanilla extract, you may use the maple syrup if you like.

Ingredients (8 servings):

Eggs	4 large
granulated stevia	1/2 cup
pumpkin puree (canned)	1 cup
vanilla extract	1 teaspoon
superfine almond flour	1/2 cup
pumpkin pie spice	1 teaspoon
sea salt	1/8 teaspoon
butter, ghee	4 tablespoons

Directions:

1. Blend the granulated Stevia. Set aside.
2. Break the eggs into a bowl, compound them until smooth consistency (the mix must thicken slightly). Add a little bit the vanilla extract, put the pumpkin puree. Combine everything well once more.
3. Add slowly pie spice, salt, flour and stir thoroughly. Go on the blend.
4. Melt butter or ghee, pour slowly into the blended mixture. Stir everything well.

5. Spray the cooking spray over the bottom of the Crock Pot, pour the compound into the Crock Pot.
6. Put the paper towel over the top of the Crock Pot, a cap must be covered. So, it means the towel is arranged between the cap and the top. It must absorb the condensed damp.
7. Put the Crock Pot on LOW for ca. 3 hours. Check from time to time. When the dish is ready, the sides must put off from the Crock Pot.
8. Take off the custard from the Crock Pot, serve with Stevia whipped cream and nutmeg at will.
9. Bon Appetite!

339.Lemon Crock Pot Cake

This amazing lemon keto cake was prepared during 3 hours without any strong efforts. I must say, this keto cake tasted better the next day as it was kept all the night in the refrigerator. I think the cakes made of coconut or almond flour taste better when you keep them at least some hours in the refrigerator.

Ingredients:

Baking a cake:

almond flour	1 1/2 cup
coconut flour	1/2 cup
Puree all-purpose (or Swerve)	3 teaspoons
baking powder	2 teaspoons
xanthan gum optional	1/2 teaspoon
butter melted	1/2 cup
whipping cream	1/2 cup
Juice of lemon	2 tablespoons
Zest from two lemons	
Eggs	2 pcs

Cooking a topping:

Puree all-purpose (or Swerve)	3 teaspoons
baking powder	2 teaspoons
boiling water	1/2 cup
butter melted	2 tablespoons
lemon juice	2 tablespoons

Directions:

Baking a cake:

1. Take a medium-sized bowl, conjoin the coconut flour, sweetener, almond flour, baking powder, xanthan gum. Stir well everything
2. In another bowl whisk the butter, squeeze the lemon juice, xanthan gum, whipping cream, zest, crack the egg in a bowl.
3. Combine both mixtures dry and wet one.
4. Spray the cooking spray over the Crock Pot, pour the mixture into the Crock Pot. Cover and put on HIGH for 3 hours until the inserted in the center knife comes out clean.
5. While the cake is cooking, prepare the topping – conjoin the baking powder, water, melted butter and lemon juice.
6. Take off the cake once it is ready for a large plate. Pour the topping over it.
7. Add whipped cream or fresh fruits by serving, if desired.
8. Bon Appetite!

340.Keto chocolate cake Crock Pot

This should be definitely the best low carb cake recipe one has ever tried to cook and to eat! It is reach and flavor! I guess, it is no need to describe the chocolate cake prepared in the Crock Pot. It is delicious. Just cook it following the directions below.

Ingredients (10 servings):

almond flour	1 cup and additionally 2 tbsp
sweetener	1/2 cup
cocoa powder	1/2 cup
whey protein powder	3 tbsp
baking powder	1 1/2 Tsp
salt	1/4 Tsp
eggs	3 large pcs
butter melted	6 tbsp
unsweetened almond milk	2/3 cup
vanilla extract	3/4 tsp

Directions:

1. Spray the bottom and all the sides of the Crock Pot with cooking spray.
2. Take a bowl, mix well the almond flour, cocoa powder, sweetener, protein powder, baking powder, salt. Stir everything well.
3. Add butter (melted), cracked eggs, milk, vanilla. Combine everything.
4. Pour the ready-made mixture into the Crock Pot, cover and put on LOW for ca. 2 hours. It must look like a pudding.
5. Take off from the Crock Pot and let it cool.
6. Serve warm with whipping cream.
7. Bon Appetite!

341.Crock Pot raspberry-vanilla pudding cake

If you have a small container of fresh raspberries, don't hesitate to cook this amazing cake! It is a flavor, appetizing, tender pudding cake. The mixture is rather simple, it contains egg-free texture with an addition of boiling hot water at the end of cooking process. This dessert is amazing, keto-friendly, simple. Top this cake with vanilla, fresh raspberries and whipping cream.

Ingredients (10 servings):

Sweetener	2 cups
almond flour	2 cups
baking powder	4 Tsp
salt	1 Tsp
milk	1 cup
butter	4 Tbsp
vanilla	1 tsp
fresh raspberries	2 (6 oz) container
vanilla pudding mix	1 Tbsp
boiling water	1 3/4 cup

some fresh raspberries for dressing

Vanilla or whipped cream

Directions:

1. Take a medium bowl, combine flour, sweetener, baking powder, vanilla, salt, milk. Whisk everything. Melt the butter and add to the mixture.
2. Open the container with raspberries and pour them into the mixture.
3. Spread the cooking spray over the sides and bottom of the Crock Pot.
4. Put the mixture into the Crock Pot and spread it on the bottom.
5. Sprinkle the pudding mix over the top of the mixture but don't stir it.
6. Take a little bowl, let the water boil.
7. Pour the water carefully over the top of the pudding mix and the mixture.
8. Cover and put on HIGH for 2 hours.
9. The ready-made pudding will be on the bottom of the cake.
10. Serve with whipping cream or vanilla and fresh raspberries.
11. Bon Appetite!

342.Crock Pot Mocha Pudding Cake

This dessert cooked in the Crock Pot is something between a pudding and a chocolate cake. It has a tender, velvety texture, the chocolate and coffee notes give this dessert an amazing mocha taste! It doesn't need too much time, everything is rather simple. I would say, this cake could be cooked even by beginners!

Ingredients (10 servings):

Butter	¾ cup
unsweetened chocolate	2 ounces
heavy cream	½ cup
instant coffee crystals	2 tablespoons
vanilla extract	1 teaspoon
cocoa powder	4 tablespoons
almond flour	1/3 cup
salt	1/8 teaspoon
eggs	5 large pcs
Stevia	2/3 cup

coconut oil spray for the sides and bottom of the Crock Pot

Optional: whipped cream for serving

Directions:

1. Cut butter into large chunks.
2. Chop finely unsweetened chocolate.
3. Spray the bottom of the Crock Pot with cooking spray.
4. Take a little bowl, melt butter together with unsweetened chocolate. Whisk it all the time, don't let it burn. Set aside and let it cool.
5. Take another medium bowl, whisk coffee crystals, heavy cream, vanilla extract.
6. Take one more bowl and combine the cocoa, salt, almond flour. Stir well.
7. Using a mixer or a blender, whisk the eggs on a high speed until thickened slightly. Add sweetener.
8. Turn the speed of the mixer (or blender) on low, pour the butter with chocolate. Continue mixing.
9. Stir almond flour, salt and cocoa mixture too.
10. Add also to the blending mixture coffee, cream and vanilla mix.
11. Pour the compound into the Crock Pot. Put a paper (towel) over the Crock Pot and cover with cap.
12. Put on LOW for 3 hours.
13. Check the readiness of the cake – the edges must be like a cake, the center – must have a soft consistency.
14. Serve the cake with whipped cream if desired.
15. Bon Appetite!

343.Keto black raspberry cheesecake

Do you prefer raspberries? Do you like cheesecake? If yes – this amazing flavor combination is definitely for you! I have combined the best ingredients I had in my refrigerator. It is very simple, keto cake you must try! I promise you will not be upset!

Ingredients (8 servings):

black raspberries (fresh)	1 pint (frozen are also possible)
lemon juice	2 Tbsp
cream cheese softened	16 ounces
Greek-style yogurt	6 ounces
vanilla extract	2 tsp
liquid stevia	25 drops
eggs	2 pcs
black raspberries, for garnish	½ cup

Directions:

1. Tale a medium-sized skillet and put over medium heat, place the raspberries. Stir them frequently. They must reduce the jam. It takes about 15 minutes.
2. Use a potato masher, break the raspberries up. Any pieces must remain.
3. Add lemon juice and let the mixture cool.
4. Take a large bowl combine liquid stevia and cream cheese, Greek yogurt, vanilla. Using a blender mix everything well, until the ingredients are blended thoroughly.
5. Add the cracked eggs, one after one blending all the time the mixture.
6. Spray the bottom and the sides of the Crock Pot with cooking spray, pour the egg-cheese mixture into the Crock Pot.
7. Cover and put the dish on HIGH for 2 hours.
8. Check the readiness of the cheesecake – the knife must go out from the cake clean.
9. Take off the cake from the Crock Pot and pour the raspberry on top. Dress with fresh raspberries.
10. Place in the refrigerator for 2 hours.
11. Bon Appetite!

344.Crock Pot Blueberry Lemon Custard Cake

Today I recommend you to cook very tasty lemon-blueberries custard cake. It is a light amazing combination of berries and creamy lemon. I like the recipes especially desserts, prepared with coconut flour as it gets delicious and moist. Garnish this perfect dessert with light cream or fresh blueberries!

Ingredients (9 servings):

Eggs	6 pcs
Coconut Flour	1/2 cup
lemon zest	2 teaspoons
lemon juice	1/3 cup
lemon liquid Stevia	1 teaspoon
Swerve sweetener	1/2 cup

Salt	1/2 teaspoon
light cream	2 cups
fresh blueberries	1/2 cup

lemon slices and fresh blueberries for garnish

Directions:

1. Break the eggs into a bowl, compound them until smooth consistency (the mix must thicken slightly). Add Swerve sweetener and salt. Combine everything well once more.
2. Add flour and stir thoroughly. Go on the blend.
3. Mix the lemon zest, juice, and liquid Stevia, blueberries, stir well everything.
4. Spray the cooking spray over the bottom of the Crock Pot, pour the compound into the Crock Pot.
5. Put the paper towel over the top of the Crock Pot, cover with lid. The paper towel must absorb the condensed damp.
6. Put the Crock Pot on LOW for ca. 3 hours.
7. Take off the custard from the Crock Pot, serve with fresh blueberries, lemon slices, and light cream at will.
8. Bon Appetite!

345.Crock Pot keto crème Brulee

To prepare this amazing crème Brulee needs only 4 simple servings and 2-3 hours in the Crock Pot. The preparation process, I mean making some circles of foil, seems a little bit difficult than just to put the mixture to the Crock Pot at once. But in no way, it is not so difficult as you think. Just follow the directions and enjoy!

Ingredients (4 servings):

egg yolks	3 large
heavy whipping cream	1/2 cup
Sweetener	1/4 cup plus 2 teaspoons
vanilla bean	1/4 pcs

(or vanilla extract – 1 teaspoon)

Directions:

1. Take a medium saucepan, mix the egg yolks, 1/4 cup of Sweetener, whipping cream. Stir everything well.
2. With helping of a special dull knife, try to take off the seeds from the bean. Add them to the mixture. Once you couldn't scrape out the seeds, use the vanilla extract and add it also to the crème mixture.
3. Take medium-sized pieces (about 2 12") of foil, make a so-called «snake shape» rolling them up. Make it in a circle, pinch the ends together. Put this circle into the bottom of the Crock Pot, do the same with next piece.
4. Put each ramekin on a top of the circle of foil.
5. Let the water boil in a little bowl, pour it. Be careful! The water must reach about 1/3 of the way on ramekins.

6. Put the Crock Pot on LOW for 2,5 -max. 3 hours. Check the custard once the time is over.
7. Chill custard for 5 hours.
8. Before serving spread the remained sweetener over the custard.
9. Bon Appetite!

346.Crock Pot keto cinnamon almonds

The keto cinnamon almonds are super both as dessert and as an appetizing. It makes amazing smell all over your house! The cinnamon almonds are the favorite keto-dish of all my family.

Ingredients (7 servings):

Sweetener	1 cup
Cinnamon	3 Tbsp.
Salt	⅛ tsp.
Egg White	⅛ tsp.
Vanilla	2 tsp.
Almonds	3 Cups
Water	⅛ Cups

Directions:

1. Take a bowl, conjoin sweetener, salt, cinnamon.
2. Take another one bowl, whisk thoroughly the egg white, vanilla. Place almonds and toss thoroughly. The cooking procedure let the sweet mix stick to almonds.
3. Spread the spray over the Crock Pot, put the cinnamon mixture with almonds, put it to LOW. Toss until the mix cover well all the almonds.
4. Cook ca. 3 hours. Stir all the time every 15 minutes. Add a little bit water and stir well.
5. Remove the almonds from the Crock Pot to the baking sheet, spread them and let them cool. Separate them from one another.
6. Enjoy!

347.Keto lemon coconut cake with cream cheese icing

The base of this keto Crock Pot cake is flavor, tender and delicious! I can't describe it with words, this is amazing and appetizing! The icing on this cake cooked with cream cheese, lemon zest, and vanilla is a perfectly integral addition to the cake!

Ingredients (12 servings):
Coconut Cake:

Coconut Flour	1/2 Cup
Eggs	5 pcs
Erythritol	1/4 Cup
Butter Melted	1/2 Cup

Lemon Juiced	½ Tsp
Lemon Zest	1/2 Tsp
xanthan gum	1/2 Tsp
Salt	1/2 Tsp

Icing:

Cream Cheese	1 Cup
Natvia	3 Tablespoons
Vanilla Extract	1 tsp
Lemon Zest	½ Tsp

Directions:

1. Firstly, separate the yolks and whites of eggs. Whisk the whites until smooth in a large bowl.
2. Place the coconut flour, juice of lemon, zest, xanthan gum, salt in the same bowl. Melt the butter and pour also. Continue whisking.
3. Spread the cooking spray over the Crock Pot (bottom and sides), pour the mixture into it.
4. Cover and put on LOW for 3 hours.
5. While the cake is cooking, take a little bowl, whisk there Natvia, cream cheese, vanilla, zest together with a blender.
6. Once the cake is ready, remove it to a plate and top with the icing.
7. Bon Appetite!

348.Crock Pot keto coffee cake

This recipe is for those who like coffee most of all. I think you will definitely like this brown, tender cake. It is amazing, delicious, flavor cake. The syrup will be a great addition to the ready-made cake!

Ingredients (10 servings):

sour cream	1/2 cup
coffee	1/3 cup
softened butter	½ cup
eggs	3 pcs
sugar substitute (Swerve)	1/2 cup
almond flour	2 1/4 cup
baking powder	2 1/2 Tsp

Syrup:

Water	1/3 cup

| sweetener | 1/3 cup |
| instant coffee | 1/2 Tsp |

Directions:

1. Take a medium bowl, conjoin the sour cream, coffee, until smooth. Add softened butter, stir well. Mix everything until smooth. Add the eggs, whisk all the time.
2. Stir the sweetener.
3. Take another bowl, conjoin baking powder and almond flour. Put this mixture into the coffee mix.
4. After you have combined all the mixtures, pour this into the Crock Pot covered with cooking spray.
5. Cover and cook on LOW for 2-3 hours.
6. Check with a toothpick if the cake is ready.
7. Prepare the syrup – mix the water and Swerve on a medium heat. Whisk until all the ingredients are dissolved. Pour the instant coffee. Let it cool a little.
8. Once the cake is ready, remove it to the plate, pour the syrup over it.
9. Cut and enjoy!
10. Bon Appetite!

349.Crock Pot Angel food cake

The Angel food cake is light like a cloud or a fresh air! The cream of tartar that I have firstly used in this recipe stabilizes all the beaten egg whites that are of special importance in this recipe for the Crock Pot. I like to eat this cake with macerated berries and whipped cream because I think it is the best combination I could only imagine! You may also use the other berries of your keto diet you prefer more, but don't forget about forbidden and allowed products!

Ingredients (8 servings):

Sweetener	¾ cup
Almond flour	½ cup
Kosher salt	¼ teaspoon
Egg whites	5 large
Cream of tartar	½ teaspoon
Vanilla extract	1 teaspoon
Macerated Strawberries	
Whipped cream	
Strawberries for dressing	

Directions:

1. Firmly wring a 3-foot length of foil (aluminum foil), after this shape it into a zigzag form width-wise the oval or round Crock Pot. Just try to create a rack, adding 1 cup of water.
2. Place the top of the Crock Pot and set on LOW after this.
3. Take a medium bowl, whisk together flour, sweetener, salt and set aside everything.

4. Take another little bowl, crack the eggs (whites) and add slowly tartar. Using the blender or the food processor, mix everything on a medium speed. It takes usually 1-2 minutes. You may increase the speed slowly until the texture gets foamy. Add vanilla.
5. Pour the mixture with sweetener from the first bowl into the second one, whisk all together.
6. Transfer the batter to a loaf pan and smooth top.
7. Place the loaf pan into the Crock Pot, press into the aluminum foil rack just to ensure the level of the pan. Take a clean kitchen towel and drape over the Crock Pot. Put the lead over it.
8. Put the Crock Pot on LOW approximately 2-3 hours. Once 1,5 hours is over start to check the readiness of the cake in the Crock Pot.
9. Once the cake is ready, remove the pan from the Crock Pot and let it cool about 20 minutes.
10. Using a knife, run it around the edges separating the ready cake from the pan.
11. Remove it to the serving plate.
12. Dress with macerated strawberries at will and the whipped cream.
13. Bon Appetite!

350.Crock Pot milk cake low-carb

I hope this recipe will be the real beginning for those who have never used his/her Crock Pot. This recipe for the delicious cake is definitely for you! The main option here, I think, it is that you don't need to sit all the time waiting for your cake and controlling the Crock Pot. That is what I exactly like my Crock Pot for!

Ingredients (8 servings):

For Cake

eggs	3 pcs fresh
Condensed Milk 14 oz	2 cans
Evaporated Milk substitute	14 oz (1 can)
Almond Flour	2 1/2 cups
Butter softened	3 tablespoons
sweetener	1/4 cup

For Topping

Milk 14 oz	1 can
sweetener	2 tablespoons
vanilla extract	0,5 tablespoon

Directions:

For Cake

1. Take a large bowl and mix there cracked eggs whisked thoroughly, condensed milk, evaporated milk substitute, almond flour, butter softened, add sweetener. Stir everything well together.

2. Spray the cooking spray over the bottom and the sides of the Crock Pot, pour the mixture into the Crock Pot.
3. Put the paper towel on the top of the Crock Pot and put the Crock Pot on HIGH for 3 hours.

Prepare the topping:

1. Take a medium saucepan and mix sweetener, condensed milk, and vanilla let it boil until smooth texture.
2. Once the cake is ready, remove it from the Crock Pot on the plate and top with ready-made topping.
   Let the liquid absorb. You may serve it both warm or cool.
3. Bon Appetite!

351.Crock Pot giant chocolate pie recipe

A giant chocolate pie is a delicious, flavor recipe that is perfect for daily eating and for a party! You may also serve this pie with whipped cream. What is better – it is coking this pie in your Crock Pot that lets you mix all the ingredients and forget about cooking for some period of time. I'm sure, this chocolate pie recipe will be great adding for your supper or dinner!

Ingredients (8 servings):

butter at room temp	0,2 lb
sweetener	4 tablespoons
eggs	2 pcs fresh
vanilla extract	1 tablespoon
almond flour	0,4 lb
baking soda	1/2 teaspoon
salt	1/4 teaspoon
dark choc chips or dark chocolate low-carb	0,3 lb

Directions:

1. Take a middle bowl, mix together butter, sweetener, vanilla extract. Crack the fresh eggs. Whisk everything together.
2. Take another little bowl, conjoin flour, salt, and baking soda.
3. Stir the flour mixture into the mix of butter. You have to stir everything well until biscuit texture. The right consistency of the mixture means the sides of the bowl are clean.
4. Stir the choc chips and spread them thoroughly.
5. Spread the Crock Pot with the cooking spray, pour the mixture into the Crock Pot.
   Put the Crock Pot on LOW for 3 hours, it may also be needed to put the Crock Pot for 30 minutes on HIGH last 30 minutes.
6. Once the time is over, take off the pie from the Crock Pot and let it cool for 20 minutes.
7. Bon Appetite!

352.Keto brownies Crock Pot

If you prefer the delicious combinations of peanut butter and chocolate chips low-carb, this one will be definitely for you! So easy to cook, so great to eat! For this recipe, you need only simple ingredients that could be bought at any market.

Ingredients (8 servings):

unsalted butter (melted)	½ cup
cocoa powder low-carb	2/3 cup
sweetener	1 1/3 cup
salt	1/2 teaspoon
eggs	2 pcs fresh
almond flour	3/4 cups
chocolate chips low-carb	2/3 cups
creamy peanut butter (melted)	1/3 cup

Directions:

1. Take a mixing bowl medium-sized, conjoin together melted butter, sweetener, cocoa, mix until smooth.
2. Add salt crack the fresh eggs, stir everything until incorporated.
3. Add the chocolate chips, distribute them thoroughly.
4. Spray the cooking spray over the Crock Pot bottom and sides, pour the batter into your Crock Pot.
5. Melt the peanut butter in a little pan, drizzle it over the brownie batter, swirl with a toothpick.
6. Add the remained chocolate chips over the brownie.
7. Cover the Crock Pot and cook on LOW for 2-2,5 hours mostly.
8. Once the time is over, open the Crock Pot and remove the cake.
9. Let it cool and enjoy!

353.Crock Pot Pumpkin Pecan Bread Pudding

I'm excited to present you today the pumpkin pecan bread pudding! I think it is high time to bake this delicious one. I hope you have already got a little bit experience and have already tried to cook the keto bread that's why it will be easy for you to perform this recipe. Have a little patience!

Ingredients (13 servings):

Keto bread cubes	8 cups
toasted pecans	1/2 cup
cinnamon chips	1/2 cup
eggs	4 pcs
canned pumpkin	1 cup
half n half	1 cup

sweetener	1/2 cup
butter melted	1/2 cup
vanilla	1 tsp
cinnamon	1/2 tsp
nutmeg	1/2 tsp
ginger	1/4 tsp
ground cloves	1/8 tsp

Vanilla ice cream if desired

Caramel ice cream topping at will

Directions:

1. Cut the bread slices into cubes. I remember you how to cook the keto bread – You have to take a medium bowl, mix butter and cream cheese. Stir until the creamy consistency. Add rosemary, sage, parsley to the mix and proceed to stir. Add cracked eggs and blend up to the smooth consistency.
   Mix with baking powder, coconut and almond flour. Spray the Crock Pot with cooking spray. Pour the consistency to the Crock Pot. Cover and put on LOW 3-4 hours. Keto bread should be golden on top and come out clean. After the keto bread is done you may use the bread slices cut into cubes (use the old bread mostly).
2. Peel and shred the ginger. Peel the cloves. Chop the pecans.
3. Mix all together in a large bowl freshly cracked eggs, canned pumpkin, half-n-half, sweetener, melted butter, cinnamon, vanilla extract, nutmeg, ginger, and cloves.
4. Pour the mix on the top of the cubed bread. The mixture must coat the cubes gently.
5. Cover the Crock Pot and put it on LOW for 3,5 hours. Check until the toothpick inserts in the center and gently comes out clean.
6. Serve the bread pudding warm and top it with vanilla ice cream or if you prefer.
7. Bon Appetite!

354.Crock pot Cocoa Zucchini Bread

If you have some zucchinis at your refrigerator and you would like to cook something tasty, new and delicious – this unusual cocoa-zucchini bread is for you! After some hours (I mean actually two hours in the Crock Pot) you get a really new bread, flavorful and moist! I always put a little bit more cocoa chips than it is mentioned in the recipe because I like them very much, and I must say, it tastes even more wonderful! If you like to eat sweet bread, you may also put a little bit more sweetener. I hope you will try one day.

Ingredients (10 servings):

Eggs	3 pcs
Sweetener	1 1/2 cups
vegetable oil	1 cup
almond flour	3 cups

baking soda   1 tsp

cinnamon   2 tsp.

vanilla   3 tsp

salt   1/4 tsp.

cocoa chips low-carb   1 cup

zucchini   2 cups

Directions:
1.   Wash the zucchini, peel and grate them. Set aside.
2.   Take a medium-sized bowl, mix almond flour, baking soda, vanilla, cinnamon, salt. Combine everything well.
3.   Take another little bowl, mix the sweetener, vegetable oil and cracked fresh eggs. Whisk together.
4.   Join the shredded zucchini, cocoa chips and mix everything together from all the bowls. Stir well.
5.   Spray the bottom and the sides of the Crock Pot with the cooking spray.
6.   Pour the batter into the Crock Pot, cover and set on LOW for 3 hours.
7.   Once the time is over, remove the cake to a plate and serve warm!
8.   Bon Appetite!

355.Chocolate-Cinnamon Latte Cake Recipe

When we are speaking about the tasty and delicious cakes I always remember this recipe because I like coffee. This super easy Crock Pot recipe is based on a white cake mix that you have to prepare yourself following my instructions. It is easy and quick. Further, you add the ingredients listed below, pour the mixture into the Crock Pot (I recommend you to use the foil) and put on HIGH. Serve the ready-made cake with ice cream or whipped cream.

Ingredients (12 servings):
For cake mix (homemade):

Almond flour   2 3/4 cup

Sweetener   1 3/4 cups

baking soda   2 teaspoon

salt   3/4 Tsp

For cake:

unsweetened cocoa   1/3 cup

ground cinnamon   1/2 teaspoon

butter melted   1/2 cup

strong hot brewed coffee sugar-free 1 1/4 cups

eggs	3 large
evaporated milk unsweetened	1 (12-oz.) can
Vegetable cooking spray	
dark chocolate morsels	1 (10-oz.) package
whipped cream or coffee ice cream at will	

Directions:

1. Whisk together the ingredients for a cake mix in a medium-sized bowl (sweetener, almond flour, salt and baking soda).
2. Mix the previous ingredients with unsweetened cocoa, cinnamon, melted butter, coffee, cracked fresh eggs and unsweetened evaporated milk (substitute) in a large bowl. Stir everything well.
3. Spray with the cooking spray the bottom and the sides of the Crock Pot.
4. You may use the aluminum foil, allowing 2-3 inches to extend over the sides. Don't forget to grease the aluminum foil with cooking spray also. Pour the mixture into the Crock Pot and cover it. Cook on HIGH 1 ½ hours maximum.
5. Remove the lid and let it cool for 30 minutes.
6. Remove the cake from Crock Pot on a plate (use the foil sides as handles).
7. Serve warm or cool with whipped cream if desired or ice cream.
8. Bon Appetite!

356.Berry cobbler Crock Pot recipe

Summer is the time of easy and delicious cake recipes full of vitamins. Today I would like to bake the cobbler in my Crock Pot. I would like to use blueberries, raspberries, strawberries, and blackberries. What a rainbow I have! My berry cobbler is simply easy and ideal for any party, family dinner. It is a classic cobbler recipe that is used by me many years. Let enjoy it together!

Ingredients (13 servings):

baking soda	1 1/2 teaspoons
ground cinnamon	1/2 teaspoon
almond flour	1 1/4 cups
sweetener	3/4 cup
whole milk	1/4 cup
salted butter	2 tablespoons
fresh egg	1 large
fresh raspberries	1 cup
fresh blueberries	1 cup
fresh blackberries	1 cup
fresh strawberries	1 cup

| fresh lemon juice | 1 tablespoon |
| kosher salt | 1/4 teaspoon |

Directions:

1. Take a medium bowl and combine baking soda with cinnamon, almond flour, and ¼ cup sweetener, stir well everything. (Divide flour and sweetener into halves).
2. Whisk together in a small bowl whole milk, melted butter, freshly cracked egg.
3. Add dry ingredients to milk mixture; stir just until moistened and set aside.
4. Wash all the berries thoroughly. Toss the berries in a large bowl, add lemon juice and salt, the remaining amount of sugar and remained almond flour in a medium bowl.
5. Spray the cooking spray over the bottom and sides of the Crock Pot.
6. Transfer the berry mixture to the Crock Pot, cover and cook on LOW for 2-3 hours.
7. Bon Appetite!

357.Cranberry Upside-Down Cake Recipe

What could be easier to cook than the cranberry upside-down cake? Really, I don't know! Everything you need to do here – it is to mix all the ingredients listed below (follow my instructions) and pour the mixture into the Crock Pot. Turn on the mentioned position and wait with patience until the cake is done! Enjoy it right now!

Ingredients (12 servings):

Sweetener	1 cup
butter melted	1/2 cup
whole-berry cranberry sauce	1 (14-oz.) can
fresh cranberries	1 (12-oz.) package
milk	3/4 cup
eggs	2 large
almond extract	1/2 teaspoon
Vanilla ice cream (if desired)	

For cake mix (homemade):

Almond flour	2 3/4 cup
Sweetener	1 3/4 cups
baking soda	2 teaspoon
salt	3/4 Tsp

Directions:

1. Whisk together all the ingredients for the cake mix using a medium-sized bowl (sweetener, almond flour, salt, baking soda).
2. Take a small bowl and toss the sweetener, melted butter, and sauce. Mix until smooth texture.

3. Spray the Crock Pot with cooking spray and pour the mixture into the Crock Pot. Top with the cranberries.
4. Using the blender or the food processor, mix cake mix (homemade), milk, fresh eggs, almond extract, vanilla until smooth. It takes you usually 1 minute.
5. Pour the batter over cranberries in the Crock Pot. Cover it and cook on HIGH for 1,5-2 hours, check with a toothpick inserted in the center. It must come out clean.
6. Turn off the Crock Pot and let the cake cool for about 25 minutes.
7. Remove the cake to a serving plate.
8. Serve with the ice cream, at will.
9. Bon Appetite!

358.Cinnamon Bread Pudding Crock Pot

The cinnamon bread pudding is great for supper, dinner, and breakfast! You may eat it even at your lunchtime, it is perfectly well! All the ingredients are easy to find in the stores and they don't cost too much. Try to cook it for your family and friends.

Ingredients (10 servings):

eggs, beaten	3 large
sweetener	1/2 cup
ground cinnamon	1 teaspoon
ground nutmeg	1/4 teaspoon
milk	1 cup
whipping cream	1 cup
vanilla extract	1 teaspoon
butter melted	2 tablespoons
cinnamon keto bread loaf, cut into 1-inch cubes	1 (1-pound)
pecans toasted	1/2 cup

Whipped cream at will

Directions:
1. Take a middle-sized bowl and blend together fresh cracked eggs, sweetener, cinnamon and nutmeg. Chop the pecans.
2. Stir in milk, vanilla, cream and melted butter.
3. Add the cubes of bread, after conjoining the pecans. Stir thoroughly until bread is almost moistened. Cover and roast about an hour.
4. Spray the Crock Pot with the cooking spray, pour the mixture into the Crock Pot; cover with the aluminum foil.
5. Pour a cup of water into the Crock Pot (put a wire rack to fit cooker on the bottom).
6. Cover the lid and cook on LOW 5 hours or until a fork comes out clean.
7. Cool bread before serving.
8. Serve warm with whipped cream, at will.
9. Bon Appetite!

359.Matcha Crock Pot Souffle

This tasty dessert treats for those who like souflles! The Matcha Crock Pot Souffle is a sweetened whipped dessert with green matcha, fresh raspberries with chocolate and whipping cream.

Ingredients (9 servings):

Eggs	3 large pcs
Swerve confectioners	2 tablespoons
vanilla extract	1 teaspoon
matcha powder	1 tablespoon
butter	1 tablespoon
raspberries	7 whole
coconut oil	1 tablespoon
unsweetened cocoa powder	1 tablespoon
whipped cream	¼ cup

Directions:

1. Separate the eggs into whites and yolks.
2. Whip the egg whites in a bowl of a medium-size with the one tablespoon of Swerve confectioners. Add matcha powder. Continue to whip until smooth consistency.
3. Take another large bowl, using a fork break up the yolks. Mix in the vanilla, after this, add a small amount of the already whipped whites. Fold the rest of the egg whites into the yolk mix.
4. Open the Crock Pot, add the melted butter. Add the souffle mixture to the Crock Pot. Set on LOW for 2 hours and put the raspberries on top.
5. Once the cooking time is over or the top starts to brown, remove the soufflé from the Crock Pot.
6. Melt the coconut oil in a saucepan, whisk in the cocoa powder and the rest Swerve confectioners. Drizzle across the top.
7. Serve with whipped cream.
8. Bon Appetite!

360.Keto Brownies Crock Pot

Today I decided to cook our lovely brownies flourless in the Crock Pot. I think you love the brownies too… don't waste time and run to the kitchen!

Ingredients (7 servings):

low-carb milk chocolate	5 ounces
butter	4 tablespoons
eggs	3 large pcs
Sweetener	½ cup

mascarpone cheese   ¼ cup

unsweetened cocoa powder ¼ cup

salt   ½ teaspoon

Directions:

1. Melt the chocolate in a medium-sized saucepan over a medium heat for a little, stirring each time until smooth consistency.
2. Melt the butter and stir everything well. Continue until smooth. Set aside and let it cool.
3. Take a large bowl, beat the eggs and whisk with granulated sweetener on high until the mix becomes frothy and the eggs are pale. It should take about 4-5 minutes.
4. Add the mascarpone cheese to the bowl and beat until smooth.
5. Add the cocoa powder and salt and mix everything well.
6. Sift in the rest of the cocoa powder and stir.
7. Be sure the chocolate is still melted. Pour the melted chocolate into the batter and mix thoroughly until it is creamy.
8. Open the Crock Pot, pour batter and set on HIGH for 2 hours.
9. Remove from the Crock Pot and let it cool completely!
10. Bon Appetite!

Index

Conclusion

Trying something new, for example, new diet, we usually wonder – if the chosen method suitable for me? How can I avoid eating forbidden products? What must I cook today? Is it boring? How many times should I go shopping? It is a total misconception, I think if a person thinks the ketogenic diet is just eating boring food without some variety of recipes and tasty combinations. The recipes of this cookbook contain a huge number of recipes from single portions to full meals that could feed the whole your family and friends, reasoning how easy and tasty could be the keto diet. But what about if you are always in a hurry, busy, have a big family? Maybe you have no mood to cook at all? Is the cooking process boring for you? You don't like washing pile of dishes all the time, don't you? I have gathered all the keto-friendly recipes that you may cook in the Crock Pot! It solves all your problems. No need to spend a lot of time on the stove, no need to search on the Internet for hours trying to follow the keto-rules and keeping in the mind necessary information all the time. I have done all these jobs for you! I think the ketogenic diet is the easiest and simplest way one could choose to burn fat in the body for energy. This cookbook will definitely help you to say «Goodbye» to preferred bread, potatoes, rice and pasta, and to say warm greetings to oils and cheese. The ketogenic diet really works if you follow the rules posted on the food list (forbidden and allowed products) and the genius Crock Pot helps you in the achievement of the aim. Think about your health – Could you do something useful for it right now? Consuming of heart-healthy fats decrease the possible risk of heart diseases, the limitation of sweets and sugar lowers the risk of diabetes type 2. Of course, eating keto-friendly food doesn't mean to consume ice cream or any kind of fat all the time. There is a huge variety of products low in carbohydrates and full of fat that is advised you at the recipes of this keto Crock Pot cookbook.

Author's Afterthoughts

Thanks ever so much to each of my cherished readers for investing the time read this book!

I know you could have picked from many other books but you chose this one. So big thanks for downloading this book and reading all way to the end.

If you enjoyed this book or received value from it, I'd like to ask you for a favor. Please take a few minutes to post an honest and heartfelt review on Amazon.com Your support does make a difference and to benefit other people.

www.ingramcontent.com/pod-product-compliance
Lightning Source LLC
Chambersburg PA
CBHW072254260726
48658CB00001BA/18